D0209855

Differential Diagnosis
in Neuropsychiatry

Differential Diagnosis in Neuropsychiatry

by

JEREMY K. A. ROBERTS
M.B.Ch.B., L.M.C.C., M.R.C.P.(U.K.), M.Phil.,
M.R.C.Psych., D.P.M.(Lond), F.R.C.P.(C) Psychiatry

*Consultant in Neuropsychiatry, Neuropsychiatry Unit,
The Royal Ottawa Hospital; Assistant Professor of Psychiatry,
University of Ottawa, Canada.
Formerly Senior Registrar in Psychological Medicine,
The National Hospital for Nervous Diseases, Queen Square, London, England.*

A Wiley Medical Publication

JOHN WILEY & SONS
Chichester · New York · Brisbane · Toronto · Singapore

Copyright © 1984 by John Wiley & Sons Ltd.

All rights reserved.

No part of this book may be reproduced by any means, nor
transmitted, nor translated into a machine language
without the written permission of the publisher.

Library of Congress Cataloging in Publication Data:

Roberts, Jeremy K. A.
  Differential diagnosis in neuropsychiatry.

  (A Wiley medical publication)
  Includes bibliographical references and index.
  1. Neuropsychiatry.   2. Diagnosis, Differential.
I. Title.   II. Series.   [DNLM: 1. Nervous system disease—
Diagnosis.   2. Organic mental disorders—Diagnosis.
3. Diagnosis, Differential.   4. Neurologic examination—
Methods.   5. Psychological tests. WL 141 R645d]
RC343.R7   1984   616.89′075   83-23289
ISBN 0 471 90402 3

British Library Cataloguing in Publication Data:

Roberts, Jeremy K. A.
  Differential diagnosis in neuropsychiatry.
  1. Neuropsychiatry
  I. Title
  616.8   RC341

ISBN 0 471 90402 3

Phototypeset by Dobbie Typesetting Service, Plymouth, Devon.
Printed by St. Edmundsbury Press, Bury St. Edmunds, Suffolk.

*To my Father, Nasreen,
Clifford and Soraya*

"Science . . . admits no sharp
boundary between knowledge and use"

(Bronowski, 1956)

Acknowledgements

I would like to particularly thank Dr M. R. Trimble for the support and encouragement which started me on this book; the late Dr R. T. C. Pratt for his assistance with the cases; and Dr A. Hennessy for her helpful comments on the manuscript. Helpful comments were also provided by Drs J. Beitchman, R. Chandrasena, A. Guberman, E. Koranyi, Y. D. Lapierre, N. Nayar, D. Stuss and R. Trites. Thanks are also due to those physicians of the National Hospital for Nervous Diseases, Queen Square, London, England, and the Royal Ottawa Hospital, Ottawa, Canada, who gave permission for the use of those cases under their care. Appreciation is due to Mr J. Parker and the Medical Art Department of the Royal Ottawa Hospital, for their help in producing many high quality figures.

Special thanks are due to Mrs R. Sawdon whose contribution to this manuscript goes far beyond the enormous hours she has spent typing it. Her help has been invaluable.

Contents

Foreword

It is with pleasure that I have accepted the offer to write a foreword to this book, and there are two fundamental reasons why I am delighted to be associated with it. First, the author has chosen to use the term 'Neuropsychiatry' in the title. Although thought by many to represent an old-fashioned branch of medicine with its practitioners being neither neurologists or psychiatrists and thus failing to do either adequately, there are others who recognize its growing potential. Thus it is a subject in a field where the clear dichotomy between the two independent disciplines has led to many conceptual problems and some disservice to patients. The disorders covered in this book represent a clinical specialty that is truly independent, in the sense of being intermediate between traditional neurology and psychiatry, requiring specialist information from both fields, but possessing in addition its own special knowledge or expertise in clinical evaluation and treatment. Although some may feel that other terms are more appropriate, for example, the popular designation of Behavioural Neurology, used widely in America, the appellation Neuropsychiatry rightly emphasizes the psychiatric component of the specialty, so often lacking from a strictly neurological approach to behaviour disorders.

Secondly, this work is essentially clinical. So often textbooks are full of elaborate descriptions of diseases, with their signs and symptoms, and fail to emphasize the essence of the clinical evaluation and differential diagnosis. Dr Roberts has dissected out for us the important elements of evaluation of patients and decision-making in these difficult conditions, providing a text that is not only informative but practical. The inclusion of case histories at the end of the main material further emphasizes some important issues, and also shows the rich and diverse nature of presentations in Neuropsychiatry.

Neuropsychiatry has a healthy future. This book, I hope, will provide further inspiration to the interested to seek further.

MICHAEL R. TRIMBLE
December, 1983

Introduction

Eight years ago the eminent British neurologist Macdonald Critchley wrote "I do not believe that neurology should be orientated too closely towards psychiatry . . . A neuropsychologist is far less of an anomaly than a neuropsychiatrist" (Critchley, 1975). Since then many have ceased to hold this view and this is substantially due to the development of new techniques for investigating brain structure and function, including Computerised Axial Tomography and, more recently, Positron Emission Tomography and Nuclear Magnetic Resonance. Such advances have helped to blur the dividing line between neurology and psychiatry, and prompted Janice R. Stevens to write recently "neuropsychiatry . . . is a specialty whose time has come, and for which appropriate training programmes are urgently needed by both psychiatrists and neurologists" (Stevens, 1982).

This book is intended as a contribution towards this field for those training in psychiatry and neurology, and other medical and non-medical health workers who are involved in the large area of medicine where neurology, neurosurgery, neuropsychology and psychiatry overlap. The first six chapters are concerned with the examination and investigation of the neuropsychiatric patient. Chapters 7 and 16 deal with certain diagnostic problem areas that are commonly encountered in neuropsychiatry. Much of the material covered in this book deals with those questions raised by interested undergraduate and postgraduate students, during teaching sessions. An attempt is made to maintain a practical orientation as far as possible. With this intention in mind Chapter 17 consists of a series of brief case histories that are selected in order to emphasise or illuminate certain points from the previous chapters.

In addition to the references cited in the text, certain 'source" books have been used, which can be used for further elaboration on a particular topic. The books used are Filskov and Boll (1981) and Walsh (1978), for neuropsychology; Lishman (1978) and Trimble (1981a) for neuropsychiatry; Beeson and McDermott (1971) and Hart (1979), for medicine; Merritt (1979) and the Handbook of Clinical Neurology series (edited by P. J. Vinken and G. W. Bruyn), for neurology; and Nicholi (1978) and Sim (1974), for psychiatry.

CHAPTER 1

The Neuropsychiatric History

1.1 INTRODUCTION

As the physician's time is limited it is necessary for him to direct his questions in such a way as to get the maximum relevant information from the patient and any other informants available within this limited period. Though flexibility is needed during the interview, the following outline is suggested as a general guide to the kind of information that is most relevant in the assessment of a neuropsychiatric problem.

The importance, provided the patient does not object, of consulting a reliable second source, cannot be over-emphasised. This "secondary" informant may be able to provide a more objective view of the development of the patient's illness, identify any errors or omissions in the patient's history, and provide an assessment of the patient's premorbid personality. Though there may have been a change in the patient's personality since his illness began, this may not be evident from his history for reasons such as a lack of motivation, a defective memory, or an impairment in his ability to compare his current and premorbid levels of functioning. Such difficulties are commonly encountered in patients with organic brain disease. If available the patient's mother should be interviewed as she is usually the best source of information about the patient's early life, e.g. prenatal factors, birth details and developmental milestones.

The steps involved and the areas that should be enquired about in the evaluation of the neuropsychiatric patient are listed in Table 1.1. The rest of this chapter is concerned with that information which is most likely to be relevant to such cases. Though it is not possible to be totally comprehensive in the space allowed, an attempt will be made to clarify the significance of some of this data.

While evaluating the patient it is helpful to bear in mind the different disorders that can cause, or be associated with, neuropsychiatric illness. As this involves an extensive differential diagnosis, many of these disorders have been classified, as shown in Table 1.2, in such a manner as to facilitate their recall.

Table 1.1 The neuropsychiatric history

Basic data	Name, age, country of origin
	Presenting complaints
History of current illness	
Family history	Neurological and psychiatric disorders (including deaths at an early age, epilepsy, mental retardation, metabolic disorders)
Antenatal events	Foetal exposure to alcohol, drugs, toxins, infections or physical agents
	Complications during pregnancy
Birth	Gestational age and weight, complications of delivery
Early development	Developmental milestones, febrile convulsions, other neurological events
Personal development	Neurotic traits, e.g. school phobia
	Interpersonal relationships, academic performance at school, antisocial behaviour
Occupational history	
Psychosexual history	Females (menarche, menstrual cycle, abortions)
	Males (onset of shaving, masturbation, voice breaking)
Past medical history	Childhood illness(es)
	Head injury, encephalitis, meningitis, migraine, epilepsy
	Previous surgery (especially neurosurgery)
Previous psychiatric history	Alcohol, drug abuse, suicide attempts
Premorbid personality	
Forensic history	Litigation pending
Current home situation	

1.2 BASIC DATA

Valuable information may be provided by the patient's behaviour and the presenting complaints he makes during his initial contact with the physician. How did he come to the hospital? What is his attitude to the doctor? Why does he think he is here? Even at this early stage in the interview it is possible to surmise certain things about the patient, e.g. if he can find his own way to the hospital and keep his appointment at the correct time and place, this tells us something about his memory, motivation and topographical orientation. A patient with early dementia is often brought to the hospital by an exasperated spouse and is frequently vague about his problems. Errors may occur if he is unaccompanied, as in the early stages of cognitive decline the patient's deficits may not be obvious to anyone meeting him for the first time.

The common causes of any particular neuropsychiatric disorder will vary with the patient's age. In the young adult an acute onset of a psychotic illness will often be due to illicit drug ingestion or acute schizophrenia. In the elderly such behaviour, appearing for the first time, is more likely to be due to an affective disorder or delirium. Though common disorders should be considered initially

Table 1.2   The differential diagnosis of neuropsychiatric disorders

Alcohol and other toxins	Lead, manganese, thallium, carbon disulphide
Blood vessel disease	Intracranial (aneurysm, infarction), extracranial (cardiac disease, hypertension, carotid stenosis)
Collagen disorders	Systemic lupus erythematosus, temporal arteritis
Congenital and inherited	Huntington's chorea, dystrophia myotonica, porphyria, Marfan's syndrome, tuberose sclerosis, Wilson's disease, XYY, XXY
Degenerative	Dementia of Alzheimer's type, Pick's dementia, normal pressure hydrocephalus, Parkinson's disease, multiple sclerosis, Creutzfeldt–Jacob's disease
Drugs	Hallucinogen, stimulant, neuroleptic, anti-depressant, anti-convulsant, sedative
Endocrine, metabolic, vitamin disorder	Disorder of thyroid, parathyroid, adrenal, pituitary; hypoglycaemia, liver disease; deficiency of B_{12}, thiamine, folate, or nicotine acid
Epilepsy	Ictal, inter-ictal, post-ictal, peri-ictal
Functional	Neurosis, psychosis, personality disorder
Growth	Carcinoma (primary, secondary, remote effect), subdural haematoma
Hypoxia	Cardiac or respiratory failure
Idiopathic	
Injury or post-operative	Head injury (open or closed), psychosurgery
Infection	Abscess, encephalitis (encephalitis lethargica, herpes simplex, rabies)

when assessing a patient, certain uncommon neurological disorders, e.g. Wilson's disease, can present with prominent psychiatric symptoms, and may also show a predilection for certain age groups. It is important to bear them in mind because they are often potentially treatable and, if they are genetically determined, their diagnosis may have implications for other family members who are at risk. Sternleib and Scheinberg (1968) studied patients with *Wilson's disease*, an inherited abnormality of copper metabolism resulting in damage due to the deposition of excess copper mainly in the central nervous system and liver. They found that 7 out of 8 of the patients' asymptomatic siblings who had a low serum caeruloplasmin (the globulin necessary for binding copper) and an elevated level of hepatic copper, subsequently developed the clinical features of the disorder on follow-up. This contrasted with the progress of another 40 siblings who had the same biochemical abnormalities and who were treated with penicillamine and a low-copper diet. The latter all remained asymptomatic during the same follow-up period.

In certain cases the patient's racial background or his country of origin may indicate that he is at an increased risk of developing a particular disorder. In such cases the predisposing factors may be genetic or environmental. *Genetic predisposition* is important in relation to Huntington's chorea (particularly common in the Moray Firth area of Scotland, and Tasmania), porphyria variegata (South Africa), and dystonia musculorum deformans (Ashkenazi

Jews). In certain mountainous areas there is a low iodine content in the water and this can cause goitre and hypothyroidism. Such areas include the peak district of Derbyshire (England), the central region of North America, and the European Alps. Inhabitants of temperate areas, notably Scandinavia and Canada, are prone to infestation with the tapeworm, diphyllobothrium latum, which can cause vitamin B_{12} deficiency. Multiple sclerosis, an important neuropsychiatric disorder of uncertain aetiology, is particularly associated with temperate climates and is rare in people who have spent the first years of their life in tropical or subtropical regions (Fischman, 1982).

Certain *culturally based practices* may be prejudicial to health and may result in the development of neurodegenerative disorders. This has been seen in strict vegetarians (vegans) who are at risk of developing a dietary deficiency of vitamin B_{12} deficiency (Hughes-Jones, 1973). In another study Ali *et al.* (1978) reported on a series of Asian children who were found to have elevated blood levels of lead. This was the result of their being exposed to Surma, a lead containing powder that is used by certain people of Asian extraction. It is applied to the conjunctiva for cosmetic (cosmetic plumbism) or therapeutic reasons. People from the underdeveloped countries who subsist mainly on a diet of polished maize are prone to develop pellagra, due to nicotinic acid deficiency, a syndrome that includes depression, dementia, dermatitis and diarrhoea. However, the belief that the Marchiafava–Bignami disease (extensive cerebral demyelination) was confined to male italians who drank wine, is now known to be erroneous (Lishman, 1978).

Kuru is a condition of considerable theoretical importance. It is a degenerative disorder of the CNS that is clinically and pathologically very similar to *Creutzfeldt–Jacob (CJ) disease*, and is found to have a high prevalence in the natives of New Guinea. It was the demonstration that Kuru could be transmitted to primates (Gajdusek *et al.*, 1966), that led to the investigation of CJ disease and the demonstration that both disorders were due to a transmissible replicating agent (Gibbs and Gajdusek, 1969). These findings contributed to the development of the concept of the "slow virus" as a cause of neurological illness (Johnson, 1982).

Also of theoretical importance is the high prevalence of *Amyotrophic Lateral Sclerosis* (ALS), and the *Parkinsonism–Dementia complex*, found in the Western Pacific, on the island of Guam. These disorders clinically overlap with each other and there appears to be a genetic predisposition to develop them. Excessive levels of manganese have been found in the spinal cord of some Japanese patients with ALS, which raises the possibility of an interaction between genetic and toxic factors (Yase, 1972).

1.3 FAMILY HISTORY

Genes may play a role in relation to neuropsychiatric disorders, in several ways. They can have a direct effect in causing a disorder (Huntington's chorea); it may be as a result of their interaction with the environment (febrile convulsions);

or they may indirectly influence the environment in which the patient lives. The term "cultural inheritance" has been used to describe the transmission of behaviour from one generation to another by a process of learning (Partridge, 1979). An example of this phenomenon might be the development of aggressive behaviour in a person who is exposed to an aggressive paternal model. Similarly, a parent with Huntington's chorea will often create a disturbed home situation which can adversely affect the development of his children and may cause mental disturbance in them, even if they have not inherited the gene for the choreiform disorder.

When there is a genetic contribution to the development of a disease it may result from the inheritance of a single dominant gene (tuberose sclerosis); two recessive genes, one from each parent (Wilson's disease); more than two genes (polygenetic inheritance); sex-linked genes (Hunter's type of mucopoly-saccharidosis); or as a result of an interaction between the environment and certain genes. In some cases the cause may be even more complicated, e.g. the inheritance of a disorder being understandable as the result of an interaction between the environment, a dominant gene and polygenes (Shields, 1977). Currier *et al.* (1982) suggested that modifying genes may vary in their effects on autosomal dominant disorders. They may function in a compensatory way and cause the disorder to present with a later onset and a slower course, or they may be additive in their effects, producing an earlier onset and a more rapid course. These variations may be reflected in clinical and neuropathological differences, and they may explain some of the differences found between certain disorders that are essentially similar, e.g. Alzheimer's dementia and senile dementia.

In *autosomal dominant conditions* it is usual for one of the patient's parents to be affected. If penetrance of the gene is complete then 50% of the affected parent's offspring will be at risk of inheriting the gene. *Huntington's chorea, febrile convulsions and the cerebral dysrhythmia of petit mal epilepsy, are the commonest autosomal dominant neuropsychiatric disorders in which the responsible gene has almost total penetrance.* However, even in such disorders, a family history may be absent. This was the case in 20% of patients with Huntington's chorea, in one study (Heathfield, 1967). The lack of a positive family history in a patient with a dominantly inherited disorder may be due to one of the following:

1. The disorder has developed as a result of a gene mutation.
2. The gene has only partial penetrance.
3. The age of onset of the disorder is late and the affected parent died before it became apparent.
4. Relatives may be unaware of or reluctant to admit to a family history of a particular disorder, for certain reasons, e.g. ignorance, denial or guilt.
5. There may be wide variation in the clinical manifestations of the gene which may be influenced by the presence of other genes or certain environmental

conditions. This can result in a failure to recognise certain of these incomplete forms (formes frustes) of the disorder.

6. The patient may be unaware (due to adoption) or incorrect (due to illegitimacy) about the real identity of his biological parents.

Autosomal dominantly inherited conditions of neuropsychiatric significance include tuberose sclerosis, Huntington's chorea, certain forms of epilepsy (petit mal and febrile convulsions), dystrophia myotonica, dystonia musculorum deformans, neurofibromatosis, phaeochromocytoma, porphyria, Marfan's syndrome, pseudohypoparathyroidism, and possibly Pick's dementia and dementia of the Alzheimer's type (DAT) (see Table 1.2). Some of the physical features of these inherited disorders are shown in Figure 1.1. Not all cases of Pick's or DAT show this pattern of inheritance and sporadic cases often occur (Lishman, 1978). Heston *et al.* (1981) found evidence of a subgroup of patients with DAT who were characterised by a relatively early onset of the dementia with a rapid course. Among the blood relatives of these patients there was an increased incidence of dementia, lymphoma, Down's syndrome, and disorders related to the abnormal functioning of the immune system, especially diabetes mellitus.

Those disorders listed in Table 1.3 may present to the psychiatrist because of movement disorder (1,4), mental subnormality (2,6,10,12), dementia (4,8,11), epilepsy (3,9,10,12), suspected hysterical conversion (1,9,10), or acute episodes of anxiety/ autonomic overactivity (5,7,9,10). Intracranial tumours may develop (6,12) and cause neuropsychiatric consequences in their own right. Some of the physical signs of these disorders are shown in Figure 1.1.

The genes predisposing to petit mal and febrile convulsions are unusual in that their expression is strongly age-dependent. In *petit mal epilepsy* the EEG characteristically shows bilateral generalised 3 cycles/second spike and wave discharges that are sometimes, but not always, accompanied by a brief loss of awareness (absence). Each attack lasts a matter of seconds only. The EEG abnormality is inherited as an autosomal dominant disorder with full penetrance only between the ages 4 and 8 years. Only about 25% of those carrying the gene actually develop clinical absences (Metrakos and Metrakos, 1961).

A febrile convulsion is a major seizure occurring between 6 months and 5 years of age, when the body temperature is over 38°C. About 5% of the population in this age range are genetically at risk of developing convulsions when febrile. The gene that is responsible is dominant and almost fully penetrant between the age of 6 months and 2½ years in girls, and 6 months and 3½ years in boys (Taylor and Ounsted, 1971). This difference in the duration of the vulnerability periods reflects a sex-related difference in the process of neurological maturation.

Marfan's syndrome is an autosomal dominantly inherited connective tissue disorder in which the patient characteristically has long thin extremities, with the arm span measuring greater than the height, and the lower segment (pubis to ground) measuring greater than the upper segment (pubis to vertex). He is also predisposed to dislocation of the lens of the eye (ectopia lentis) and chest deformities, notably pectus excavatum ("funnel" chest) and pectus carinatum ("pigeon" chest). The gene has a variable expression and it is particularly important not to confuse this disorder with *homocystinuria*, which also shows these features. The latter is also a connective tissue disorder, and it results from a recessively inherited deficiency of the enzyme cystathionine synthetase. Unlike Marfan's, mental retardation, epilepsy and intravascular thromboses, which may involve the cerebral vasculature, are not uncommon. Aortic incompetence, mitral valve prolapse and dissecting aneurysm of the aorta, are found in Marfan's only. The diagnosis of homocystinuria can be confirmed by looking for excess homocystine in the urine, and the complications can be avoided by treatment with large doses of pyridoxine or using a low-methionine diet with supplemental L-cystine (Perry, 1981).

Other autosomal recessively inherited conditions of neuropsychiatric importance include Wilson's disease, dystonia musculorum deformans, Friedreich's ataxia, and Hallevorden–Spatz disease. Such inherited neurological disorders commonly present in children, but occasionally they can be seen in adults, when they are prone to create problems of diagnosis. For a discussion of the genetic and biochemical bases of such disorders the reader is referred to Rosenberg (1981).

A genetic aetiology should always be considered in any patient who is exhibiting one or more of the following—mental subnormality; epilepsy; a dermatogical abnormality, e.g. a disorder of pigmentation or an unusual rash; and an unusual facial configuration, or some other congenital abnormality of physical appearance.

Genetic factors may have more subtle neurobehavioural effects. In general, dominant cerebral hemisphere (i.e. verbal) functions are superior in women, when compared to those in men, and the reverse is true (non-verbal functions are superior) in males when compared to females. It is clear that a variety of factors, including genotype, can influence the development of cerebral function. Females normally have an XX sex chromosome complement, but women with Turner's syndrome are deficient in one X chromosome (XO) and have been found to have superior verbal skills when compared with normal XX females. It has also been found that, in general, in patients who have extra X-chromosomes, *the greater the number of additional X chromosomes the less efficient are their psychological functions based on verbal ability*. Not only does the genotype appear to be important in cognitive development, but hormonal factors appear to be as well. Exposure to androgens during intrauterine life has been associated with more efficient non-verbal skills in later life (Flor-Henry, 1978).

On balance the evidence suggests that *there is less lateralisation of higher cortical functions in females, than in males*, and this is reflected in studies of the clinical consequences of damage to the dominant hemisphere. Aphasia, as a result of damage to this side of the brain, has been found to be three times more common in males than in females. Even in the absence of aphasia, verbal skills remain more sensitive to such damage in males (Springer and Deutsch, 1981).

8

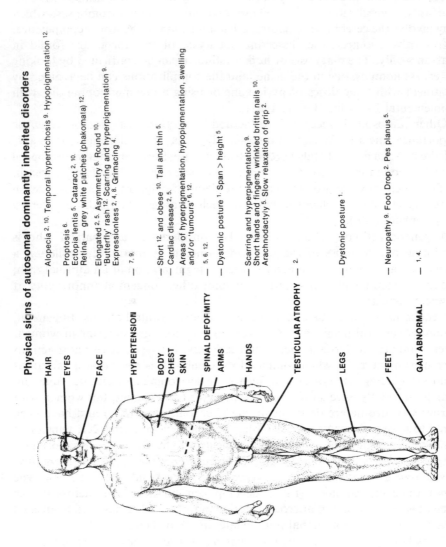

Physical signs of autosomal dominantly inherited disorders

HAIR — Alopecia 2, 10. Temporal hypertrichosis 9. Hypopigmentation 12.

EYES — Proptosis 6.
Ectopia lentis 5. Cataract 2, 10.
Retina — grey white patches (phakomata) 12.

FACE — Elongated 2, 5. Asymmetry 6. Round 10.
'Butterfly rash 12. Scarring and hyperpigmentation 9.
Expressionless 2, 4, 8. Grimacing 4.

HYPERTENSION — 7, 9.

BODY — Short 12. and obese 10. Tall and thin 5.

CHEST — Cardiac disease 2, 5.

SKIN — Areas of hyperpigmentation, hypopigmentation, swelling and/or 'tumours' 6, 12.

SPINAL DEFORMITY — 5, 6, 12.

ARMS — Dystonic posture 1. Span > height 5

HANDS — Scarring and hyperpigmentation 9.
Short hands and fingers, wrinkled brittle nails 10.
Arachnodactyly 5. Slow relaxation of grip 2.

TESTICULAR ATROPHY — 2.

LEGS — Dystonic posture 1.

FEET — Neuropathy 9. Foot Drop 2. Pes planus 5.

GAIT ABNORMAL — 1, 4.

Figure 1.1   Physical signs of autosomal dominantly inherited disorders. Refer to Table 1.3 for key

Table 1.3	Autosomal dominantly inherited disorders

1. DYSTONIA MUSCULORUM DEFORMANS
2. DYSTROPHIA MYOTONICA
3. EPILEPSY — PETIT MAL
      — FEBRILE CONVULSIONS
4. HUNTINGTON'S CHOREA
5. MARFAN'S SYNDROME
6. NEUROFIBROMATOSIS
7. PHAEOCHROMOCYTOMA
8. PICK'S DEMENTIA
9. PORPHYRIA
10. PSEUDOHYPOPARATHYROIDISM
11. ? DEMENTIA OF THE ALZHEIMER'S TYPE
12. TUBEROSE SCLEROSIS

1.4 ANTENATAL, BIRTH AND EARLY INFANTILE EVENTS

Teratogens and other antenatal factors

A *teratogen* has been described as *any environmental agent which acts during pregnancy to cause birth defects* (Hanson, 1979). Teratogens can be drugs, including alcohol, chemical agents (methylmercury), physical agents (uterine abnormalities), or maternal metabolic factors (diabetes mellitus).

The first trimester of pregnancy is generally accepted as that stage in foetal development when it is most important to avoid exposure of the foetus to potentially teratogenic agents. However, the central nervous system (CNS) appears to be particularly vulnerable to noxious agents at a different stage of pregnancy. During the first trimester the gross morphology of the CNS is determined and the differentiation of the primitive cells that are destined to become neurones, occurs between the tenth and the eighteenth week. The main brain growth spurt is when the glial cells begin to multiply rapidly (Dobbing and Smart, 1974). This stage begins in mid-pregnancy and extends at least into the first two postnatal years. Rapid myelination overlaps with and follows this stage, continuing into the fourth post-natal year. Developing organs appear to be particularly vulnerable to damage during their periods of rapid growth and this is in keeping with the clinical evidence that the prognosis for head injury (Rutter, 1981), and febrile convulsions (Annegers *et al.*, 1979), is particularly bad when they are sustained in the first two years of life. Development of the CNS does not cease at this stage, of course, and it is not clear for how long dendritic arborisation and synaptic connectivity continue to develop.

Teratogens and other factors may have subtle effects on the child which are not clinically obvious in the period following birth. Pasamanick and Knobloch (1966) coined the term "continuum of reproductive casualty" to describe the concept of foetal damage as a spectrum of disorders of varying severity. At the extreme end of the spectrum is stillbirth, and at the other end, it is suggested, the effects on the developing child are more subtle and may influence behaviour.

The study of the behavioural consequences that result from exposing a child to adverse factors in utero has been called "behavioural teratology" (Werboff and Gottlieb, 1963). These concepts raise the question of how frequently do insults to the developing CNS cause later effects which arc masked as a result of the functional plasticity of the CNS during this period. One example of behavioural teratology is *Foetal Minamata disease*. In this disorder methylmercury, used in the manufacture of chloralkali and paper, contaminated the seawater in Minamata Bay (Japan). This caused delayed cancer, cerebral palsy and behavioural changes in children who had been exposed to the toxin in utero (Matsumoto *et al.*, 1965).

Alcohol is a low molecular weight substance and so can easily cross the placenta by diffusion. It is also a potent teratogen, and foetal exposure to alcohol is now recognised as causing the *Foetal Alcohol syndrome*. There is evidence that this condition may be quite common in the children of alcoholic mothers and it has been suggested that it can be seen to some degree in up to 6 out of every 1000 live births (Hanson *et al.*, 1978). The full syndrome is less common (less than 1/1000 live births) and consists of a characteristic facial appearance, with a small head, short palpebral fissures, an underdeveloped philtrum, a thin upper vermilion and retrognathia. All these features, together with mental retardation and pre- and postnatal growth retardation, have been described by Smithells (1979) as being present in about 80% of reported cases. He recommends that the presence of failure to thrive with impaired development and growth in infancy, should prompt a careful examination of the child for the characteristic facial appearance and abnormalities of the palmar creases. The latter involves either a single transverse crease or an abnormal crease which runs from the ulnar side of the palm to the gap between the index and middle fingers. A wide number of other features have been described less frequently, involving skin haemangiomas, abnormalities of the eyes, skeleton, heart, joints and kidneys. Many of these children eventually develop hyperactivity. The practical importance of being aware of the Foetal Alcohol syndrome is in making pregnant women conscious of the risks to their foetus if they abuse alcohol and in suspecting alcoholism in mothers who produce children with the features of the syndrome. As this condition has only been fully recognised in the last decade (Jones *et al.*, 1973) there may be many adults with disorders of behaviour and mental retardation who will be found to exhibit some of these stigmata on examination. By identifying the cause of their behavioural disorder the clinician will then be alerted to the possibility of other congenital physical disorders being present, e.g. cardiac or renal disease.

In the past, intrauterine exposure to treponema pallidum was not uncommon and could result in *congenital syphilis*, which can cause mental retardation in childhood or dementia in adolescence. Now this infection is uncommon and it is usual for pregnant women to be screened for antibodies to treponema pallidum. Adequate treatment of serology positive women almost eliminates the risk of foetal infection, though there is now evidence that what in the past was thought to be adequate drug treatment may, in some cases, have not been sufficient to eradicate the infection (Tramont, 1979). Intramuscular penicillin may not produce effective blood levels and the intravenous route may be necessary (Budell, 1976; Ducas and Robson, 1981). Clinically the adult with congenital syphilis characteristically exhibits the "Bulldog" face, consisting of a flattened saddle nose, maxillary under-development and frontal bossing. Scarring of the cornea, nasal septum, mouth, palate and retina, and dental abnormalities, e.g. Moon's molars and Hutchison's teeth, may be seen. Interstitial keratitis and eighth nerve deafness may progress despite adequate treatment and do not appear to be the result of active infection. The neurological and laboratory findings in congenital syphilis are similar to those found in adult acquired syphilis.

Other intrauterine infections are more common now. *Cytomegalovirus* is responsible for up to 10% of cases of infantile microcephaly. It may also cause hydrocephalus, choroidoretinitis, blindness, jaundice and a characteristic radiological finding of intracranial paraventricular calcification. *Rubella* may cause the characteristic features of infantile cataracts, deafness, micropthalmia and congenital heart defects. However, there may not be a history of maternal infection as it may be subclinical and not apparent in the obstetric history, and the congenital consequences may be non-specific, e.g. premature delivery, low birth weight and mental retardation. Other infections that are potentially able to cause congenital neurological damage include herpes simplex, mumps and measles (Caplan, 1982).

Though schizophrenia is relatively unaffected by pregnancy, other psychiatric disorders tend to be less severe and occur less frequently during this period (Brockington, 1979). When it is necessary to use drugs it is best to restrict the dose, use several small doses rather than a single large dose, and keep the duration of treatment to the minimum period necessary. Of the drugs used in psychiatry, meprobamate and diazepam have been particularly suspected of being teratogenic. The official position of the US Food and Drug Administration is that tranquillisers of the benzodiazepine type are teratogenic. However, the British Committee on the Safety of Medicines does not support this view (Hollingsworth, 1977). Lithium has been suspected of being teratogenic and causing cardiac abnormalities, but there is no evidence of it causing an increased incidence of significant congenital malformations, above the 2.5% incidence found in the general population, in children born to mothers taking this drug (Weinstein, 1976). *There is no convincing evidence that the minor or major tranquillisers, antidepressants of the monoamine oxidase inhibitor (MAOI) or non-MAOI type, are teratogenic* (Ellis and Fidler, 1982).

It is particularly difficult to evaluate the teratogenic effects of specific drugs of abuse, e.g. lysergic acid diethylamide (LSD), because polydrug use, often in association with alcohol, is common in drug abusers. In addition, in such a population there are other factors which put the health of the foetus and developing child at risk, such as a genetic predisposition to psychiatric disorder, maternal infection and nutritional deficiencies (Hawkins, 1976). There are unconfirmed reports of chromosomal damage resulting from LSD use (Robinson *et al.*, 1974).

In contrast, patients receiving anticonvulsants have an increased risk of foetal abnormalities, especially cleft lip and palate. However, it is not clear if this increase in foetal abnormalities is related to genetic or environmental factors other than the drug itself (Friis *et al.*, 1981).

About 50% of epileptic patients have an increase in their seizures during pregnancy, particularly between the eighth and sixteenth week. The majority of the remaining patients will have no change in seizure frequency. Unfortunately which group the patient will fall into is difficult to predict (Ramsay, 1979). For optimal control of epilepsy during pregnancy, it is necessary to carefully control the dose of the anticonvulsant drugs. Regular blood anticonvulsant level monitoring is necessary as the blood levels tend to fluctuate during pregnancy.

Maternal use of the anticonvulsant phenytoin has been found to be associated with a characteristic clinical picture in the neonate. This is called the *Foetal Hydantoin syndrome* and involves a characteristic facial appearance consisting of an underdeveloped maxilla, microcephaly, wide separation of the eyes (hypertelorism), a low nasal bridge and an exaggerated Cupid's bow of the upper lip. Neurological disorders and mental deficiency also occur, as well as cardiovascular, skeletal and limb abnormalities (Hanson, 1979; Hanson and Smith, 1975).

Birth and postnatal factors

Other disorders can damage the developing CNS of the foetus, especially toxaemia of pregnancy or intra-uterine bleeding. Major risk factors at birth are a caesarian section, a high forceps delivery, prematurity (weight under 2.5 kg) and a short gestational age. The latter has been shown to be very important in predicting survival, especially if the gestational age of the child is under 38 weeks at delivery and he weighs under 2.5 kg (Alberman, 1978). Other risk factors are being the first, fourth or later born, hypoglycaemia, hyper-bilirubinaemia, a low Apgar score, a prolonged delay before respiration starts, and being the second born of twins (Berg and Kirman, 1960). However, even the first born of twins are at an increased risk of neurological damage (Howard and Brown, 1970).

An interaction between birth factors and subsequent events in the environment may occur, a good example of which is provided by the *Battered Child syndrome*. There is an increased incidence of battering found amongst low birth weight children or those who are otherwise "handicapped". Developmental disability predisposes to such abuse but, alternatively, such disability may also be a consequence of neurological damage caused by battering. The infant's brain is particularly vulnerable to such trauma which can cause a subdural haematoma, intellectual impairment or some other type of neurological damage (Solomons, 1979). In contrast, though children who are hyperkinetic and have poor impulse control are at an increased risk of sustaining head injuries, it is usually the behaviour disturbance that causes the head injury, more often than the reverse (Rutter, 1981).

Parents may have difficulty in remembering accurately the dates of their child's developmental stages. The accuracy appears to be influenced by how long ago the event was and the particular behaviour inquired about. In one study it was the date that the child started walking that was remembered most easily by the parents (Hart *et al.*, 1978). It is best to commit to memory the normal age range for a few basic developmental stages. For an English population the stages shown in Table 1.4 could be used (Illingworth, 1979; Meadow and Smithells, 1978). If milestone dates are unavailable or unreliable it may be helpful to ask the parent to compare the child's development to that of his siblings. Over-activity, attentional difficulties and temper tantrums should be enquired about.

Table 1.4 Some developmental stages

Age (yrs)	Gross motor	Fine motor	Language	Social behaviour	Copying ability	
					Blocks	Drawing
1	Walks holding on to furniture	Picks up objects using index finger and thumb	1–2 words	Repetitive play		
1½	Runs	Scribbles spontaneously		Mimics domestic work	Can build tower of 3 cubes	
2	Up and down stairs on feet	Opens doors. Turns single pages	Uses "I", "me", etc. Joins words	Plays *near* other children	"Tower" of 6 to 8 cubes	| or —
3	Rides tricycle Dresses self		Counts up to 10. Knows nursery rhymes	Plays *with* other children	"Bridge" of 3 cubes	

1.5 PERSONAL DEVELOPMENT

There are certain periods in a child's life which are particularly likely to cause stress and may reveal an underlying neurotic predisposition. Such a time is when the child first starts attending school, when the anxious/dependent child may exhibit school refusal. This involves his developing physical or psychological symptoms each morning before the start of school, the symptoms disappearing quickly when the parents, who are often overprotective, allow the child to remain at home. In contrast, though the child with a conduct disorder may avoid attending school, he does not stay at home, and his parents may be unaware he is playing truant.

A long-standing neurotic tendency may be indicated by a history of certain symptoms persisting since childhood or developing for the first time in adult life, e.g. night terrors (pavor nocturnus), and sleep walking (somnambulism). Kales *et al.* (1980b) found that underlying psychopathology was most likely in patients who developed *sleep-walking* for the first time after the age of 10 years, particularly when there was a high frequency of episodes occurring in response to stressful events. In a further study Kales *et al.* (1980a) found that *night terrors* were particularly associated with psychopathology when their onset was after the age of 12 years, they were preceded by a major life-stress event, and they occurred frequently. They further suggested that the onset of night terrors in middle or old age may indicate the presence of organic brain disease. In both types of disorder the absence of a family history of the behaviour is also evidence in support of there being underlying psychopathology, which was usually a neurosis or a personality disorder.

The quality of the interpersonal relationships between the child and his peers is important. A failure to establish satisfactory interpersonal relationships with peers may be due to rejection by them and this occurs in children with attentional deficit disorders (with or without hyperactivity), aggressive tendencies or other antisocial behaviour that brings them into conflict with their peers. Alternatively the anxious child may be sociophobic, having experienced frustration at his unsuccessful attempts to socialise. This may result in his deliberately avoiding contact with his peers. If the child was not bothered by his lack of social interaction with his peers or adults, and did not actively seek such relationships, this suggests a schizoid tendency. Such children may subsequently progress into an adult schizoid personality, and are at risk of developing schizophrenia later (DSM III, 1980). Information which indicates long-standing behavioural problems may not be volunteered spontaneously, or even in response to vague questions such as "did you have a normal happy childhood?" So, where appropriate, more specific inquiry should be made.

Academic performance at school may have been impaired due to a specific developmental disorder of reading, arithmetic or language. Special education may have been required or school years repeated, due to academic failure. For people of borderline intellect school often forms the most difficult barrier to overcome in their life. A person of such intellect may make a good, though sometimes precarious, adjustment to the responsibilities of adult life, after leaving school. Intellectual retardation, and reading disability, have been particularly associated with psychiatric disorders in the young (Rutter, 1981).

Other information of importance includes the highest grade attained at school, whether any more advanced training was undergone, the types of occupations obtained on leaving school, the number of positions held and the duration of the longest, the reasons for leaving, if the patient was ever fired and the reasons why.

1.6 OCCUPATIONAL HISTORY

The patient's occupational history can suggest certain things about him, such as his type of personality and his intellectual abilities. It may also indicate that he has been at an increased risk of exposure to a toxic agent, e.g. alcohol. Occupations requiring extensive social interaction, such as bar-tending, carry a high risk of alcoholism. Other occupations may result in exposure to industrial toxins, e.g. lead, mercury or manganese. The clinical effects of some of these toxins are listed in Table 1.5. Table 1.6 shows some of the occupations that have, at some time or another, been associated with a risk of exposure to these agents (LeQuesne, 1982; Lishman, 1978; Mena *et al.*, 1967). Such exposure may be relatively indirect, e.g. Foetal Minamata disease.

Extensive travelling is involved in some jobs and exposes the patient to the risk of contracting certain diseases, such as cysticercosis (Mexico), cerebral malaria (Africa), schistosomiasis (Far East), or one of the meningoencephalitides which may be caused by infections endemic to the area visited, e.g. trypano-somiasis in tropical Africa.

A cumulative effect may result from repeated exposure to neurological insults. An example of this is the recurrent head trauma sustained during a career in boxing. A rough idea of the degree of brain damage resulting from such a career may be obtained from the number of fights and head blows (especially "knockouts"), sustained. This may result in the *"Punch-Drunk" syndrome* or *"Dementia Pugilistica"*, and involves dementia with cerebellar and extrapyramidal signs (Mawdsley and Ferguson, 1963). In some cases cognitive deterioration may develop following a latent period after the damage has been sustained. The possibility of a comparable disorder developing in other occupations involving similar risks, should be borne in mind. Foster *et al.* (1976) described five National Hunt jockeys who had all had recurrent head injuries during the course of their careers. One died of a mesencephalic haemorrhage, three developed temporal lobe epilepsy, and the fifth underwent a personality change with disinhibition, memory impairment and other cognitive changes. Other sports where recurrent head trauma has been suspected of causing brain damage include rugby football, association football (soccer), and wrestling (Lancet, 1976).

1.7 PSYCHOSEXUAL HISTORY

If the patient is married or cohabiting, a reasonable assessment of sexual interest can be obtained by the frequency of sexual intercourse after the first year or two of marriage. This can then be compared to the patient's current rate of intercourse and his level of sexual interest, to identify whether or not there has been any change in sexual drive. The reliability of such questions depends on the marriage being satisfactory. If this is not the case the level of extramarital sexual activity, and/or masturbation, may give a better indication of the level of libido. In women the age of menarche and subsequent regularity of periods

Table 1.5 Clinical features of industrial toxin poisoning

Toxin	Neuropsychiatric manifestations	Neurological symptoms and signs	Other features	Diagnosis
1. Inorganic lead	Delirium Neurasthenia Fits	Motor neuropathy ("wrist drop") Transient focal signs (raised intracranial pressure in children)	Gastrointestional disturbance and pain Hypertension Gum "lead line" Gingivitis Anaemia and basophilic stippling of red cells	Elevated lead levels in blood and urine Elevated urinary coproporphyrin III
2. Organic (tetra-ethyl) lead	Delirium Fits Mania and other psychoses Sleep disturbances	Coarse tremors of face and limbs	Gastrointestinal disturbance Weight loss Metallic taste	Elevated lead levels in blood and urine
3. Inorganic mercury	"Erythism" (anxiety, sociophobia, dysphoria) Episodic sweating and blushing	Coarse tremors of the face and limbs	Salivation Gingivitis	Excessive mercury in blood, urine and hair Slit lamp examination of the eyes for mercurialentis
4. Organic (methyl) mercury	Mental slowing Restlessness	Sensory disturbances including paraesthesia, deafness, visual field constriction Cerebellar signs	Salivation Gingivitis	Excess mercury in blood, urine and hair

	Psychiatric symptoms	Neurological symptoms	Physical signs	Investigations
5. Manganese	Hypersomnia, insomnia Bizarre impulsive behaviour including pathological laughing, crying, running and aggression) Mental deterioration Psychotic symptoms	Nocturnal leg cramps "Cock Step" gait Parkinsonism and other movement disorders	Impotence Liver damage	Manganese levels in urine, serum and hair shaft
6. Arsenic	Mental deterioration Delirium Neurotic symptoms Memory impairment	Sensory neuropathy Headache Vertigo	Dermatitis Conjunctivitis Lachrymation Rhinorrhoea "Raindrop" skin pigmentation, and keratosis Weight loss Mees' lines (white bands) on nails	Arsenic level in urine, nail and hair Increased urinary coproporphyrins
7. Thallium	Delirium Depression Paranoia	Rapidly progressing peripheral neuropathy Ataxia Movement disorder Retrobulbar neuritis	Abdominal pain, vomiting, stomatitis, salivation Nail dystrophy Renal damage Hypertension Alopecia and loss of outer $\frac{1}{3}$ eyebrows	Proteinuria and amino-acidemia
8. Carbon disulphide	Personality change Mania and other psychotic symptoms Mood swings Memory impairment	Motor and sensory polyneuritis Auditory and visual symptoms and signs Headache	Anorexia Insomnia Loss of Libido	Blood level of carbon disulphide

Table 1.6   Occupations associated with industrial toxin poisoning

Battery manufacturing[1,]
Bleaching[5]
Brass founding[1]
Chemical worker[3]
Enamelling (vitreous)[1]
Felt hat industry[3]
Finger printing[3]
Fur industry[6]
Glass manufacturing[1,6]
Lead smelting and refining[1]
Meter (direct current) repairing[3]
Ore working[3,5,6]
Painting[1,8]
Paper manufacturing[4]
Petrol manufacturing and petrol tank storage cleaning[2]
Photoengraving[3]
Pigment manufacturing[1]
Plumber[1]
Poison handling and absorption
    — Disinfectant[6]
    — Fungicide[4]
    — Insecticide[6]
    — Pesticide[6,7]
    — Weed killer[6]
Pottery glazing[1]
Rayon manufacturing[8]
Rubber and rubber solvent manufacturing[1,8]
Ship building[1]
Thermometer making[3]
Type metal handling (Compositor)[1]
Welding (electric)[5]

1 — Inorganic lead.
2 — Organic (tetra-ethyl) lead.
3 — Inorganic mercury.
4 — Organic (methyl) mercury.
5 — Manganese.
6 — Arsenic.
7 — Thallium.
8 — Carbon disulphide.

should be enquired for. Sexual experience should be tactfully enquired about, particularly with a view to assessing any deviancy or hyposexuality. The presence and health of any offspring, any deaths among the patient's children, and (in the case of female patients), any previous miscarriages or still births should be enquired for.

Blumer and Walker (1975) reviewed the higher cortical centres concerned with sexual activity in man and pointed out the importance of the hypothalamus, paracentral cortex and the temporal lobe. When epileptic seizures originate in the paracentral lobule, lateralised sensations in the genitals can be experienced, but this does not involve sexual arousal at the cerebral cortical level. The latter is occasionally associated with temporal lobe seizures (TLE); post-operatively, following successful temporal lobectomy for a seizure disorder (Blumer, 1970); and as a symptom of tumours (usually deep fronto-temporal), and infections involving the limbic system (rabies, encephalitis lethargica).

Disease of the posterior hypothalamus can cause precocious puberty, whereas antero-inferior hypothalamic lesions may cause delayed puberty (Bauer, 1959). Roberts *et al.* (1983) described a patient with subclinical obstructive hydrocephalus secondary to aqueduct stenosis, who had delayed menarche, presumably due to the effect of the enlarged third ventricle pressing on, and interfering with the function of, the hypothalamus.

Both sexual deviance and hyposexuality have been associated with TLE. *Inter-ictal hyposexuality is most common and is found in the majority of patients with TLE.* It involves impotence (in males) and/or a low level of sexual drive (Blumer and Walker, 1975). This hyposexuality may be reversible if the seizures are controlled, and a transient rebound hypersexuality may then be seen. Sexual deviation is much less commonly seen in TLE.

Both the sexual drive and the performance (arousal and orgasm) can also be affected by drugs of abuse, e.g. stimulants, opiates, hypnotics, and alcohol; by other drugs, e.g. neuroleptics; and in most psychiatric disorders. The performance alone may be affected as a result of damage in the pelvic region, e.g. post-operative; and certain drugs, e.g. the monoamine oxidase inhibitors (MAOI), the non-MAOI anti-depressants, and anticholinergic agents (Bebbington, 1979).

Though promiscuity may be seen occasionally, *frigidity appears to be particularly associated with the histrionic and passive-immature-dependent personality types* (Merskey, 1979). Sexual maladjustment was found in 59% (10 cases) of the former, and 47% (8 cases) of patients with the latter personality type, in one series (Merskey and Trimble, 1979). These patients were selected because they were suffering from hysterical conversion disorders, and only 17% (3 cases) of a control group of psychiatric patients, had comparable sexual problems. When a population of patients with oganic brain disease (including epilepsy in many of them) were looked at, only 26% had sexual problems.

A history of sexual promiscuity in young patients increases the risk of syphilis and other venereal diseases being contracted. *Syphilis* tends to be acquired by sexually active people in the 15–30 year age group, and more often if they are non-white, though this racial bias may be due to social factors. Though the prevalence of syphilis is declining, its incidence has remained relatively steady at 20,000 new cases/year in the United States, since 1960 (Tramont, 1979). A history of urethral discharge or some other indication of venereal infection, should be enquired for. Gonorrhoea may occur together with syphilis, and treatment of the former may disguise the presence of syphilis. Now that penicillinase-producing gonococci are being found there is the possiblity that gonorrhoea may be treated with an antibiotic, such as spectinomycin, that is not fully effective against a concurrent infection with treponema pallidum. Over

33% of patients with syphilis are homosexual (Tramont, 1979), and "clustering" of cases is particularly likely to occur in this population, with some of the patient's infected contacts being asymptomatic.

1.8 PAST MEDICAL AND PSYCHIATRIC HISTORY

This section will deal briefly with the development of the central nervous system (CNS) and its vulnerability to trauma, infection, anoxia and certain toxins. The neuropsychiatric significance of headache, and certain other previous medical events, will be mentioned.

The immature nervous system

Enquiry should be made for a history of febrile convulsions, and whether there have been any other seizures, head injuries, neurological infections (encephalitis or meningitis), middle ear or sinus infections, or any previous neurosurgery. It is important to know the age at which such events occurred. When the immature CNS is damaged the long-term effects differ in several ways from what would be expected if the adult CNS sustained comparable damage. The sequelae can be affected by factors such as the patient's age, his premorbid personality, whether the cerebral damage is unilateral or bilateral, whether epilepsy develops later, and psychosocial factors. Though there is substantial localisation of function in the child's CNS (Rutter, 1981), specific psychological syndromes, e.g. the frontal lobe syndrome, do not usually result from focal damage, unlike in adults. The cognitive functions of the immature nervous system are relatively resistant to the effects of lateralised brain damage (Annett, 1973), and usually require widespread bilateral damage, before significant cognitive impairment results (Rutter, 1981). In one study, persisting intellectual and psychiatric sequelae were usual when a child had sustained a head injury with a post-traumatic amnesia (PTA) of over 3 weeks (Brown et al., 1981; Chadwick et al., 1981a). They were, however, unusual when the PTA was less than 2 weeks. But at the 2 year follow-up period in this study, it was the PTA, more than persisting neurological or intellectual deficits, that correlated most closely with the presence of psychiatric disorder. This is partly due to the fact that neurological signs that develop in childhood will often show considerable resolution over the ensuing years (Solomons et al., 1963).

Brown et al. (1981) found that the two major determining factors for post-traumatic psychiatric morbidity in their study, were the premorbid adjustment of the child and psychosocial factors; and I have already mentioned that the CNS is most vulnerable to damage during the first 2 years of life. Psychiatric morbidity is also more likely to occur if epilepsy develops. In a random survey of the young on the Isle of Wight psychological disorders were most common when epilepsy was found in combination with structural brain damage. However, the presence of either of these alone was associated with an increased (to a lesser degree) rate of psychopathology (Rutter et al., 1970).

The psychiatric disorders that follow damage to the immature CNS have no specific features that differentiate them from other childhood psychiatric disorders that are unrelated to organic brain disease (OBD). The one exception is found in certain children who show a "frontal lobe" pattern of behavioural disinhibition (Brown *et al.*, 1981). The latter group were "out-spoken (with) a general lack of regard for social convention. Frequently they made very personal remarks or asked embarrassing questions . . . (were overtalkative) . . . careless in personal hygiene and dress" and impulsive (Rutter, 1981).

The immature medial limbic brain structures are especially sensitive to anoxia, and febrile convulsions in infancy may damage the medial temporal structures and cause *mesial temporal sclerosis*, as they are particularly vulnerable at this age. This is a common cause of TLE. The chances of recurrent seizures following childhood febrile convulsions is probably about 4.4%, though estimates vary in different studies. About a fifth of these epileptic cases develop their seizures after the age of 10 years. A particularly high risk of later epilepsy appears to be associated with the presence of mental retardation or cerebral palsy, or if the febrile convulsions lasted longer than 10 minutes, or if they were associated with focal neurological signs (Annegers *et al.*, 1979; Nelson and Ellenburg, 1976).

Head injury

Temporal lobe epilepsy is one of the commonest types of epilepsy that develop after a closed head injury (Marsden, 1976b). Penetrating head injuries increase the risk of focal seizures occurring without impaired consciousness (simple partial seizures), in contrast to TLE where consciousness is impaired during the seizure. The development of epilepsy brings with it the attendant risk of psychiatric complications such as "epileptic" personality change, neurosis and psychosis (Trimble, 1981a). Such changes appear to be less commonly found in association with simple partial seizures (Stevens, 1975), but secondary problems can develop as a result of other factors, e.g. brain damage, anticonvulsant treatment.

Recurrent seizures (epilepsy) occur in 5% of patients following a closed head injury. The incidence of seizures increases if there is a depressed skull fracture, dural penetration, an amnesia that follows the trauma (anterograde) and lasts over 24 hours, and a seizure within the first week following the accident. It all these features are present there is an 80% risk of epilepsy developing subsequently. If an uncomplicated closed head injury is associated with an anterograde amnesia of less than 1 hour, the subsequent risk of epilepsy developing is about 1%. The risk of developing post-traumatic epilepsy is particularly high in children under the age of 5 years. The risk of sustaining brain injury is also increased in those over 50 years of age, and in patients with a history of alcoholism (Levin *et al.*, 1982).

The period of anterograde amnesia following the head injury is a good indication of its severity, in contrast to the lack of predictive value of the duration of amnesia preceding the injury (retrograde). However, any question of prognosis must take into account all the relevant factors involved, including premorbid personality and psychosocial environment, and a balanced opinion given in the light of them.

Neurological infections

Encephalitis will be suggested by a past history of an illness involving impaired consciousness, seizures or focal neurological signs. It is not uncommon for such an illness, occurring in the first two decades of life, to cause a disturbance in personality development (Andrulonis *et al.*, 1980; Greenbaum and Lurie, 1948). A good example of this would be the consequences of the 1918 epidemic of encephalitis lethargica. Many of those afflicted with *encephalitis lethargica* subsequently showed a disturbance of behaviour characterised by aggressive, impulsive and sexually deviant tendencies. In some of these cases the behaviour improved spontaneously at puberty or as a result of post-encephalitic parkinsonism developing, in others there was a tendency for the disorder to worsen with time. This contrasts with the gradual "maturing" of behaviour that tends to be seen in "non-organic" personality disorders. Recently cases have been described which suggest that sporadic or atypical cases of encephalitis lethargica still occur (Greenough and Davis, 1983; Hunter and Jones, 1966) and may not be recognised. Herpes simplex is a common cause of sporadic encephalitis and those patients who survive may exhibit features of the Kluver–Bucy syndrome (Greenwood *et al.*, 1983).

Meningitis is characterised by headache, pyrexia and neck stiffness. The diagnosis is usually made more easily than in encephalitis and enduring sequelae are less common, though there is a slight risk of developing normal pressure hydrocephalus or epilepsy, subsequently. Even when there are pronounced neurological signs during the acute illness in children, a good recovery is possible. In one follow-up study of 100 children who had had tuberculous meningitis, 23% had enduring neurological deficits, but only 2% showed disturbance of personality without any associated neurological deficit (Lorber, 1961).

Cerebral anoxia

A history of attempted suicide may have significance other than indicating a previous psychiatric disturbance. Smith and Brandon (1973) followed up 63 survivors of *carbon monoxide poisoning* (the majority being attempts at suicide) 3 years later and found 8% of the patients had developed a severe dementia as a result; 43% had subjective complaints of memory deficits which were generally confirmed by neuropsychological testing and correlated with the severity of personality deterioration (33%). The latter included episodes of impulsive aggressive behaviour and dysphoric moods.

About 20% of people develop neuro-behavioural sequelae after a latent period of up to 3 weeks following excessive exposure to carbon monoxide. As the symptoms on relapse may fluctuate and involve a pronounced depressive or hysterical colouring, it is necessary to be aware of this complication (McEvoy and Campbell, 1977; Norris *et al.*, 1982).

A *delayed encephalopathy* can follow any episode in which there is a significant reduction in the cerebral blood flow or oxygen supply (Plum *et al.*, 1962). This has been seen after anaesthesia, seizures, drug overdoses, surgery and after attempted suicide by hanging. Dooling and Richardson (1976) described an 11-year-old boy who, 1 week after being attacked and almost strangled, developed "muteness, emotional lability, regression and flailing of the arms". This behaviour was thought to be a psychological reaction to the attack and he was discharged home. However he continued to deteriorate and began to show neurological signs. In the early stages of his deterioration his EEG was unremarkable and was even normal on one occasion, and he performed well on tests of higher cortical function, though he was amnesic for the events surrounding the assault. He died of broncho-pneumonia 14 weeks later. Abnormalities of movement are often prominent in such delayed encephalopathies, but are not always present (Plum *et al.*, 1962). The cause of the disorder is unknown and an accumulation of lactic acid has been implicated, possibly interacting with other factors (Dooling and Richardson, 1976).

Drug and alcohol abuse

The signs of *chronic alcoholism* should be enquired for, e.g. withdrawal phenomena after a period of abstinence (insomnia, nausea, vomiting, tremulousness, hallucinations, delirium, seizures), memory impairment, and early morning drinking, social and occupational disruption, and alcohol related driving offences. The absence of such a history, though, does not rule out alcoholic brain damage secondary to alcohol abuse. There is a marked variability in an individual's neurological susceptibility to alcohol, and there is evidence which suggests that it can produce cerebral impairment after a relatively short period of abuse (Lishman, 1981) and in the absence of overt signs of neurological damage secondary to alcohol abuse (Brewer and Perret, 1971). Such cognitive impairment may be partially reversible with abstinence and a similar reversible cognitive impairment may be seen in association with drug abuse. Judd and Grant (1978) found that EEG and neuropsychological abnormalities (52% and 40% respectively) were common findings in young adults who had a history of *sedative/hypnotic drug abuse*. The aetiological role of these drugs in causing the cerebral impairment was supported by the improvement in the test results found in many of these patients who had remained abstinent until they were re-examined at follow up, several months later. This improvement was not seen in those who continued to abuse drugs.

Drug abuse may occasionally cause lasting neurological damage and this is particularly well documented in relation to the intravenous use of *amphetamines* (Rumbaugh *et al.*, 1971a) and has been confirmed in animal experiments using cerebral angiography (Rumbaugh *et al.*, 1971b). Neurological infections, seizures and cerebrovascular accidents due to vasculitis, embolism or haemorrhage, may occur. Other drugs that have been associated with such complications include pentazocine, tripelennamine, and diamorphine (heroin). It has been suggested that chronic intravenous use of such drugs impairs the "filtering" function of the lungs, allowing the injected material to reach the cerebral circulation more easily and so facilitating the development of cerebral damage (Caplan *et al.*, 1982).

Prolonged heavy use of *cannabis* has been associated with mental dulling, apathy and loss of affect — the so-called *Amotivational syndrome* or *"burnout"* (Cohen, 1981). However, Grant and Mohns (1976) reviewed the pertinent literature and demonstrated that there was no hard evidence for cannabis causing such neurological damage.

The patient's current drug intake must be assessed and, if possible, any tablets at the patient's home should be brought into hospital, especially if he is cognitively impaired and his history is unreliable. In such cases a drug screen of the patient's blood and urine should also be undertaken. It is also preferable for there to be as few tablets as possible available to the patient when he returns home, in order to avoid the errors in medication intake that are particularly likely to occur in patients with organic brain disease.

It is important in some cases to note when certain drugs were used and the temporal relationship between these dates and other symptoms of disease. Huntington's chorea and Wilson's disease are two progressive neurological illnesses characterised by movement disorders. As behavioural disorder may antedate the development of these motor phenomena, there is a risk that the movements may be erroneously ascribed to a drug effect, especially if neuroleptic drugs have been used. In other cases the underlying organic disorder predisposes the patient to adverse drug reactions, e.g. in hypoparathyroidism, where the deposition of calcium in the basal ganglia occurs, the patient is prone to develop severe extrapyramidal reactions when treated with neuroleptic drugs (Schaaf and Payne, 1966). Acute exacerbations of porphyria can be precipitated by certain drugs, notably the barbiturates and phenytoin (Lishman, 1978).

Migraine and headache

Adult patients with *migraine* often give a history of recurrent abdominal pain in childhood, associated with symptoms such as nausea and vomiting (Bickerstaff, 1974). This has been called the *Periodic syndrome* and may be due to a short-lived disturbance of abdominal vascular perfusion similar to the transient cerebrovascular disturbance found in migraine. The presence of such a history may have a bearing on certain adult disorders and should be distinguished from other undiagnosed childhood physical disorders which are often neurotic in aetiology. It will indicate a predisposition to migraine, especially if a family history of migraine is present. Such a history is important since migraine can be protean in its manifestations and occasionally adult patients can develop transient neurobehavioural disorders as a manifestation of migraine. Such disorders may initially present as *"migraine equivalents"*, in which the headache is not a prominent feature (Lishman, 1978).

When a previous history of headache is obtained, the type of headache should be evaluated as to whether it is a manifestation of serious intracranial disease or not. Terms such as "like a band around the head" are said to characterise head pain due to psychological causes but there are usually other features in the history suggestive of common migraine. It is probably best to remember certain details that suggest intracranial disease is present. These features are a recent onset of headache in a middle-aged or old-aged patient; pain that remains confined to one particular side of the head; an acute onset; a progression in severity (Wolf, 1980); and pain that wakes the patient from his sleep. Both migraine and psychogenic headaches may occur in the same patient. Also, patients who suffer from attacks of recurrent anxiety, often give a past history of migraine headaches (Harper and Roth, 1962).

Other past medical events

Merskey (1979) has said "a pain in the stomach is quickly copied from another child if it promotes absence from school". Children tend to be suggestible and prone to develop physical symptoms in response to anxiety provoking situations. The ease with which *conversion symptoms* develop seems to be related to socio-economic background and emotional adjustment, being particularly frequent in the child who is anxious, poorly educated and from a poor rural background. Though the literature on this subject is limited there appears to be a particular predisposition to develop such symptoms around puberty and in females, visual impairment being a particularly frequent symptom (Merskey, 1979). Other common symptoms of hysteria are pain, dizziness, and motor phenomena, e.g. weakness, convulsions, etc. (Trimble, 1981a). A history of undiagnosed physical illness on one or more occasions, in any young person, may indicate a predisposition to conversion phenomena, and the features characteristic of such phenomena, such as a close temporal relationship to stress, should be looked for. *The prognosis of hysterical disorders depends on the underlying psychopathology and cannot always be assumed to be good.*

Epidemic hysteria is particularly prone to develop in the young. Moss and McEvedy (1966) provided evidence in one study that an outbreak of dyspnoea, in association with other symptoms, was a manifestation of hysterical hyperventilation. They demonstrated that the affected had neurotic traits in their personalities and a previous history of psychiatric disturbance, more frequently than the unaffected. Such a disorder should be borne in mind when there is an outbreak, in a young population, of an illness that is in some way atypical.

Previous surgery may predispose to delayed neuropsychiatric complications such as hypothyroidism and hypoparathyroidism (following thyroidectomy), vitamin B_{12} deficiency and reactive hypoglycaemia (gastrectomy), and normal pressure hydrocephalus (neurosurgery).

1.9   PREMORBID PERSONALITY

"The presentation of symptomatology in medicine can be markedly influenced by personality factors, and failure to assess these adequately is one step towards

26

Table 1.7 Probe questions to assess certain personality traits

HISTRIONIC TRAITS	Are you an emotional type of person?
	Do you think you would make a good actress (actor)?
	Are you drawn to activity and excitement?
	Do you form excessively intense emotional relationships?
PARANOID TRAITS	Do you tend to be suspicious of other people's intentions?
	Do you feel that other people take advantage of you?
	Are you excessively sensitive to what other people say about you?
	Do you feel other people tend to dislike you?
ANTISOCIAL TRAITS	Have you had difficulty maintaining long-standing relationships with other people?
	Have you been in trouble with the police?
	Do you resent being given orders?
	Did you play truant, steal, set fires or lie persistently when younger?
SCHIZOID TRAITS	Do you prefer your own company?
	Do you find it difficult to feel warmth for others?
	Do you have only one or two close friends?
	Are you unconcerned about what others say about you?
OBSESSIONAL–COMPULSIVE TRAITS	Are you always particular about being on time for appointments?
	Do you like everything to be just so?
	Do you have to follow one particular task to completion, while ignoring all other tasks?
	Do you have to repeatedly check certain things, e.g. is the door locked?

diagnostic confusion'' (Trimble and Grant, 1982). *Personality can be defined as those "deeply ingrained patterns of behaviour, which include the way one relates to, perceives and thinks about the environment and oneself''* (DSM III, 1980). A personality trait refers to one particular aspect of behaviour that is characteristic of the personality.

An example of this "diagnostic confusion" is seen in a patient who, unable to communicate a profound disturbance of mood because of the nature of his premorbid personality, e.g. a patient with a histrionic personality type may be only able to communicate emotion at a superficial level, and an "over-controlled" obsessional personality type, may avoid any outward expression of his emotions.

A reliable description of the premorbid personality of the patient from a "secondary" source is invaluable. This may not be available and it may be necessary to rely entirely on information from the patient. In such cases it is useful to have a stock of "probe" questions that can be used to assess premorbid traits of behaviour (See Table 1.7). Often these traits will be most obvious when the patient is under stress. Other questions can be devised by the clinician to pursue and clarify the answers to these questions, and to look for other personality traits salient to the clinical problem involved.

The patient's occupation and interests may give some indication of his personality traits, the hysterical personality type frequently favouring the dramatic arts, the schizoid personality type preferring to work with machines and in others areas which do not require a high level of personal interaction. The inadequate personality type and those of limited intellect may give a history of working in unskilled jobs, possibly with a tendency to drift from job to job. As already discussed, certain occupations are associated with an increased risk of neuropsychiatric morbidity.

As well as using probing questions, an evaluation of the patient's current attitudes can be enhanced by the use of a questionnaire such as the Minnesota Multiphasic Personality Inventory, bearing in mind that the patient's current behaviour need not be typical of his life-long style of personality functioning, even though he may claim it is.

1.10   FORENSIC HISTORY

A history of previous trouble with the police may only be elicited if the patient is asked directly. This may provide evidence of alcohol abuse or drug abuse, or an underlying predisposition to aggressive behaviour. An apparently stable patient may, under the appropriate stress, be prone to outbursts of violence, with a history of fights and other conflicts resulting in arrest by the police. Similarly, depressive or hypomanic swings in mood may be accompanied by antisocial actions that are not typical of the patient's normal behaviour. The patient who is cognitively impaired may manifest changes in behaviour involving sexual indiscretion, shoplifting or other impulsive actions, resulting from disinhibition and/or poor impulse control, that may lead to conflict with the law.

Where antisocial behaviour has occurred in early life it is not only important to know its nature and frequency, but also the age at which it began, and whether it was carried out as an individual or group activity. Antisocial behaviour in the first decade is frequently associated with a lack of guilt and peer group rejection. Such unsocialised disorders of conduct have a poor prognosis and the child often becomes an antisocial adult. In contrast, the post-pubertal adolescent whose antisocial behaviour is part of a group activity and who shows an ability to establish satisfactory relationships with his peers, has a better prognosis.

The presence of ongoing litigation or any other legal action involving the patient should always be enquired for, as it may have some influence on prognosis. This is particularly true when litigation involves an industrial accident or a motor vehicle accident. The importance of litigation in maintaining or producing a patient's neuropsychiatric disability varies, and all factors pertaining to the traumatic event and its sequelae must be evaluated. In head injury cases, information of prognostic importance includes the cerebral damage sustained; the degree to which the patient feels responsible for the accident; the extent he feels it was caused by the negligence of others; the occurrence of injury to other people, especially those personally close to the patient; and his premorbid personality.

1.11   CURRENT HOME SITUATION

Some basic knowledge in this area is essential to understand the salient features of the patient's home environment and its implications for the support the patient is receiving, as well as the stresses he may be under. Such information is important, not only because of its relevance to the evaluation of a particular case, but also because it will indicate what help the patient will receive following discharge. The cognitively impaired patient often requires help in coping with everyday life, in taking medications, and in attending follow-up appointments with the physician.

CHAPTER 2

Mental State Evaluation
and Other Diagnostic Procedures

2.1 INTRODUCTION

When a patient is admitted to the ward for neuropsychiatric evaluation the nurses' reports are a valuable source of information about his condition. Such observations are particularly helpful when the patient is unable or unwilling to cooperate in a formal mental state examination. The nursing staff invariably spend more time in contact with the patient than the doctor does and they have the advantage of contact with the patient throughout the day, including periods when he is unaware of being observed and so may be more spontaneous and natural in his behaviour. In addition, information obtained during the formal assessment by the doctor may provide some indication of those aspects of the patient's behaviour which the nursing staff should pay particular attention to.

Observations of importance would include the patient's behaviour on waking. Can he dress himself unaided? Does he pay attention to his personal appearance and hygiene? During meals — does he eat appropriately? Is his appetite normal? During the day — what is his level of activity? Is there any pronounced disturbance of mood? Is he withdrawn or does he interact with other patients, and if so, is this done in a socially appropriate manner? Can he find his way around the ward? Can he find the toilet or is he incontinent? If so, does he react appropriately to this or is he indifferent? At night-time any cognitive impairment will usually become more obvious. Is he disoriented? How does he sleep? If there is insomnia does he lie in bed or get up and about? If active at night is his activity appropriate and goal-directed?

2.2 MENTAL STATE EXAMINATION

Table 2.1 lists the aspects of the mental state which should be evaluated by the psychiatrist. It may be necessary to assess a patient in an out-patient emergency setting, with little objective information available from the nursing staff or other

29

informants, and in such cases the mental state findings assume particular importance.

Appearance and motor activity

The patient's appearance should be noted. He may appear dishevelled, unkempt and dirty, suggesting a degree of social deterioration. This change may be found early in the course of a depressive illness but occurs later in chronic schizophrenia or dementia. Excessive make-up, jewellery and flamboyant clothes are found as a transient phenomenon in association with hypomania, or as a more persistent characteristic of behaviour in the histrionic personality type. Facial asymmetry and abnormal movements should be noted and are discussed further in the next chapter.

It may have been necessary to medicate a patient before his initial mental state assessment and *a careful note must be taken of any drugs the patient has been given prior to his assessment*. Many drugs used in psychiatric practice are capable of decreasing motor activity and slowing the process of thinking. Their use may result in the patient performing in a manner suggestive of developmental or depressive psychomotor retardation. Such drugs can also induce or exacerbate an organic confusional state. Neuroleptics can cause misleading physical effects, particularly if the doctor is unaware that the patient has received such drugs. Depot neuroleptics can affect behaviour, even when the last intramuscular dose of the medication was received weeks or months beforehand. Drug-induced *akinesia, a paucity of automatic or voluntary motor activity*, may mimic depressive psychomotor retardation, and the associated lack of spontaneous facial expression may be mistaken for flattening of affect. *Akathisia is a motor restlessness accompanied by an unpleasant subjective feeling of restlessness*, and it should not be mistaken for agitation secondary to an anxiety state. Unlike akathisia, restlessness and over-activity due to other causes tend not to be complained of spontaneously, and they lack the same dysphoric quality. *Dystonic movements are involuntary, slow, sustained, contorting movements*, which usually affect the jaw, neck or trunk. They may appear to be psychogenic in origin, particularly when seen outside a psychiatric setting, e.g. dystonia may develop after one dose of prochlorperazine has been taken as an anti-emetic.

Restlessness or fidgeting may be a manifestation of an extrapyramidal disorder, which may or may not be drug induced. Patients with chronic movements disorders may become adept at disguising the involuntary nature of their movements. *Any tendency to sudden movements should be noted*, even if they appear to culminate in purposeful behaviour, such as the patient smoothing down his hair or making some other adjustment to his appearance. This is seen in Gilles de la Tourette's syndrome, where tics may involve coughing, grunting or even words or phrases, which may be obscene in nature (coprolalia). Involuntary obscene gestures (copropraxia) may also occur.

Communication

The manner in which the patient gives his history will provide information about his language functions (fluency of speech and use of correct words), his affective state (emotionally oriented content of speech), the coherence of his thought processes (the degree to which the words used and ideas expressed, follow a logical sequence), his motor activity (rate of word production), his memory (recall of events and dates), and attention (the ability to maintain the theme of the conversation and avoid distraction).

Table 2.1   Neuropsychiatric mental state examination

		Examples
Nursing observations		(Variability of cognitive impairment)
Appearance and motor activity	Voluntary	(Listening to auditory hallucinations)
	Involuntary	(Movement disorders)
Communication	Speech	(Dysarthria, aprosody)
	Language	(Aphasia, alexia, agraphia)
	Thought	(Delusions)
Emotion		(Pathological laughing or crying)
Orientation		(Disorientation for time, age disorientation)
Attention		(Distractable)
Memory		(Verbal, non-verbal or global dysmnesia)
Problem solving/proverbs		(Concrete thinking)
Biological functions		(Anorexia, insomnia, amenorrhoea, impotence)

Communication between the doctor and patient may be verbal or non-verbal. Benson (1979) divides verbal expression into that involving thinking, language, and speech. *A disorder of language (dysphasia) is a disruption of the semantic (meaning) and syntactic (grammatical) aspects of verbal expression, resulting from organic brain disease.* It usually results from damage to the left (language dominant) cerebral hemisphere and its nature is determined by whether the anterior (hesitant and non-fluent verbal expression) or the posterior (fluent verbal expression, involving circumlocution) part of the hemisphere is involved. In contrast these features are intact in a *disorder of speech*, which results from *an impairment of the neuromuscular mechanisms underlying speech and causes disorders of phonation and articulation*, e.g. dysarthria. *Thought* is a difficult term to define and has been described as *"a complex system of cognitive processes (e.g. pattern recognition, concept formation. . . .), probably involving both linguistic and non-linguistic mechanisms . . . (it) cannot be observed directly and can only be inferred from introspection, self report, or experimental approaches"* (Andreasen, 1982). Though Andreasen correctly regards the term as vague and unscientific it remains very much in use in psychiatric terminology. According to Benson's classification *both speech and language mechanisms are intact in disorders of thinking*, which can involve the stream (flight of ideas or perseveration), the possession (obsessional ideas or alien thoughts), the form (lack of logical connection between words or ideas, or concrete thinking), or the content (delusions) of thinking (Hamilton, 1974). Clinical separation of these disorders of verbal expression can be difficult and more than one of them may be present in a particular patient, e.g. cerebrovascular disease can cause damage to both cerebral hemispheres and result in dysphasia (due to involvement of the left hemisphere) and dysarthria (due to a pseudobulbar palsy).

It is not only what the patient says but how he says it, that is important. The patient's affect can be evaluated objectively (what is observed) or subjectively (what he complains of). The former involves the doctor's observations. Does the patient appear elated or miserable, does he laugh or cry easily and appropriately? Is he anxious, aggressive, suspicious, apathetic or inappropriately bland? Is there an emotional "coldness" of the type found in the chronic schizophrenic or the emotionally deprived psychopath, which effectively prevents the doctor from being able to establish an empathic rapport with him? Are the ideas expressed by the patient consistent with the mood state suggested by his non-verbal behaviour, e.g. the patient appears miserable and tearful and complains of a preoccupation with thoughts of suicide.

Prosody refers to the emphasis, intonation and melody of the voice, which may communicate affect, irrespective of the ideas expressed. The type of affect may or may not be consonant with that indicated by the content of the patient's speech, e.g. the words "I feel sad" may be said in a happy tone of voice that communicates an entirely different message with different clinical implications. When this non-verbal aspect of language is impaired as a result of brain damage, the term dysprosody is used. In contrast to the association between dysphasia and damage to the cerebral hemisphere dominant for language, there is evidence that dysprosody is more likely to result from damage to the non-dominant hemisphere (Ross, 1981; Ross and Rush, 1981; Tucker *et al.*, 1977). The patient's ability to perceive and express affect communicated non-verbally by body movements, such as facial expression, may also be impaired in association with the dysprosody. In extrapyramidal disorders, e.g. Parkinson's disease, spontaneous body movements can be reduced while prosody may be preserved, though speech may be dysprosodic in such disorders.

Any discrepancy between the subjective and objective findings will create diagnostic difficulties and allowance must be made for those variables that are liable to interfere with the reliability of these findings. In such cases it may be helpful to enquire about the biological functions of the patient, particularly his pattern of sleeping, eating (any changes in weight), and his sexual drive. Any recent change in these functions might be clinically significant. The relationship between depression and brain damage is discussed in Chapter 11.

Emotion

Apathy is one of the commoner emotional changes seen in dementia, but anxiety and depression are often found in the early stages. They are understandable developments in patients who are aware of their failing cognitive skills, and will disappear with time as the dementia progresses. Emotional lability is seen in diffuse organic brain disease and involves laughing or crying that the patient is unable to control. Poeck (1974) discriminates between this lability and pathological emotional outbursts (laughing or crying), on the basis that the former occurs in appropriate situations, it is always accompanied by an alteration of mood, it is not associated with a stereotyped sequence of facial expressions, and it can be interrupted by extraneous distracting events. However, in the next paragraph the author makes no distinction between the two types of emotional disorder.

Pathological laughter or crying involve laughter or crying that is unrelated, or disproportionate, to the provoking stimulus (Black, 1982). There appear to be three neurological levels involved in mediating this behaviour. The cortical level, which controls or modulates; the effector level, involving the brain stem nuclei; and the diencephalic region, where the two other levels are integrated. Lesions of these pathways can produce pathological emotional expression and this is most commonly seen in pseudobulbar palsy, where there is bilateral interruption of the corticobulbar pathways, usually as a result of diffuse cerebral disease.

An inappropriate stimulus, such as hearing sad news, may provoke laughter, and any accompanying facial expression may or may not be appropriate. The accompanying subjective affect experienced by the patient may or may not be one of pleasure. These variations from normality may cause some difficulty in the differentiation between organic disorders and the pathological emotion found in psychiatric disorders. Inappropriate affect is well recognised in schizophrenia (Bleuler, 1950), and has been described in other psychiatric disorders, including mass hysteria (Bean, 1967).

Another disorder causing this behaviour is gelastic (laughing) epilepsy. This is an uncommon form of epilepsy and the ictal focus can be found at the cortical or subcortical level. The quality of the laughter varies, and crying may occur. The accompanying emotion may or may not be appropriate. The attacks are usually associated with temporal lobe epilepsy (Poeck, 1974).

When a patient with organic brain disease becomes unable to respond in the manner required by the examiner, he may, if he is aware of his failure, exhibit a catastrophe reaction. This involves extreme distress and anxiety, the patient becoming unable to continue the examination.

Orientation and attention

Orientation is used in this text to refer to an awareness of time (the hour, day, month), place (town, country, hospital, ward) and person (recognising familiar people and their roles). *"Orientation in time requires that an individual should maintain a continuous awareness of what goes on around him and be able to recognise the significance of those events which mark the passage of time"* (Hamilton, 1974). From this description it is easy to see how the cognitively impaired patient, unable to efficiently and appropriately process and retain information pertaining to the events occurring around him, will rapidly become disorientated in a strang environment where there are no familiar cues to help him. *Disorientation for time is an early sign of delirium*, preceding disorientation for place and person, which develop later (Lipowski, 1980). Disorientation itself is not diagnostic of organic brain disease as it can be found in any disorder where a patient is distracted, withdrawn or otherwise preoccupied. However, *a tendency to misidentify the unfamiliar for the familiar is particularly characteristic of delirium*, e.g. misidentifying a doctor for a relative (Levin, 1956).

Temporal orientation should be specifically enquired about as Benton *et al.* (1964) found that marked temporal disorientation can be missed otherwise, and it shows a significant correlation with the severity of general mental impairment, being particularly associated with bilateral cerebral disease. It was not related to age, education or intellectual level. Their patients had been in hospital for only a short period, whereas Stevens *et al.* (1978) found *age disorientation* in 25% of their institutionalised schizophrenics. They defined age disorientation as a 5-year discrepancy between the patient's true age and the age he claims. When other features of disorientation for time are present as well, it appears to indicate a more progressive form of schizophrenia (Crow and Stevens, 1978).

Attention can be defined as "selectivity in that aspect of the environment the subject responds to, or as an activity of central mediating processes that enhance the effects of a sensory stimulus while other such stimuli are inhibited or ignored" (Hebb, 1972). A disturbance of the attentional system can be manifest behaviourally in different ways and Geschwind (1982) emphasised five aspects of this system — selectivity, coherence, distractability, universality, and sensitivity. Selectivity refers to attention to certain specific stimuli in the environment, and this selective attention must be maintained for a certain period to allow organised thinking and behaviour to occur (coherence). In order to switch attention under the appropriate circumstances (sensitivity) it is necessary to maintain some awareness of other unselected stimuli in the environment (universality) whilst avoiding being distracted by irrelevant stimuli.

Cognitive processes are all dependent on intact attentional mechanisms. *Cognition* is a broad term that *is used here to refer to those higher cortical functions of perceiving, conceiving, remembering, reasoning, imagining and judging* (Drever, 1964).

Observation of the patient during the examination will indicate if he is able to respond briskly and appropriately to his surroundings, without being distracted by events irrelevant to the task he is engaged in. Formal testing can be carried out using digit span and serial 7's tests. In the serial 7's test he is asked to subtract 7 from 100 and then continue taking 7 from the product until instructed to stop. If he is unable to perform the subtractions this will be due to either a lack of cooperation, a lack of education, impersistence, inattention or dyscalculia. If the latter is present there may be other evidence of impaired function of the left temporo-parietal (angular gyrus) region, notably the other features of Gerstman's Syndrome (left–right disorientation, finger agnosia, agraphia), sensory aphasia, or alexia (reading disability acquired as a result of brain damage). A simpler sequence of subtractions, such as serial 5's, can then be used to clarify the importance of factors such as persistence and attention. *Motor impersistence is the inability to maintain a particular pattern of motor behaviour despite frequent requests to do so.* It is seen in organic brain disease (OBD) and has been particularly associated with lesions in the right frontal region (Joynt *et al.*, 1962). It may also be seen as a manifestation of minimal brain dysfunction (Kaufman, 1981).

Memory

Clinically memory can be crudely classified as immediate, short-term and long-term. If a patient fails to recall some event it should be remembered that this may be a result of factors other than an inability to remember (amnesia). For example, in patients with frontal lobe damage a failure of recall may be present (Hecaen and Albert, 1975). In these and other patients, a deficit in motivation may also play a role.

Normally the adult can remember and repeat back a sequence of about seven digits forwards, and five digits in reverse order. The patient's immediate memory span is the duration of his digit span forwards. This normally has a duration of about 25 seconds and involves a limited capacity. It has been suggested that when it is impaired by a focal brain lesion the lesion is usually in the left parietal area (Warrington and Gautier-Smith, 1977), but it is more often impaired by factors interfering with attention and perception.

The reversal of digits involves holding them in the short-term memory store and then mentally manipulating them into the reverse sequence. The reverse digit span has a greater tendency to be reduced in OBD, than the digit forward span, and so OBD will tend to cause an excessive discrepancy between the length of the two spans.

Testing memory correctly and knowing how to interpret the patient's responses is particularly important as memory impairment is a prominent and early feature in many disorders, e.g. dementia of the Alzheimer's type. Sometimes it is the only obvious clinical sign of brain damage, e.g. Korsakoff's psychosis. In the latter the patient may attempt to hide his deficit or may be unaware of it. Such "denial" is common in memory impairment due to alcohol and can result in the amnesia being missed on superficial memory testing.

Short-term memory (STM) can be tested by asking the patient to remember certain information and, after repeating it back immediately, he is then asked to recall it again, after an interval of about 5 minutes. The author has found it a more effective test of STM if the patient is not specifically informed that he will be asked to repeat the words back 5 minutes later, thus avoiding the problem of his attempting to rehearse the words during the intervening period. The mechanisms underlying STM differ from those involved in immediate memory, and it is the former that is affected in certain important memory disorders secondary to OBD. The material to be remembered can be a name and address, or a sequence of paired words, e.g. colour/red, library/book, table/chair, camera/film, and so on. If this sequence is within the patient's immediate memory span then failure to recall it after a 5 minute delay indicates an impairment in his ability to either learn or to recall new material. Such a memory deficit is typically seen in alcoholic patients with mamillothalamic damage (Korsakoff's psychosis) or as a result of bilateral hippocampal disease (often post-encephalitic). Some task can be given to the patient in the period intervening between learning and recall, and this will introduce inappropriate memory traces which may interfere with the recall of the material learned previously. Such interference effects have been found in association with frontal lobe disorders. The use of an intervening task will also help to minimise the effects of "rehearsal".

If both of a pair of words are forgotten after 5 minutes then the first of the pair can be given as a cue to the patient, to see if he can then remember the second word. A good response to cueing is seen in patients with "mamillo-thalamic" amnesia, whereas it tends to be absent in "hippocampal" amnesia (Walsh, 1978). If the patient then recalls the second word of the pair this suggests that the deficit is more one of recall, than an inability to learn. In addition, recall can be tested by asking the patient to select the correct words from a suggested list, and incorrect words can be used to test for suggestibility. The characteristic features of these two forms of amnesia may not always be present and other data, e.g. a previous history of encephalitis or alcoholism, must also be taken into account.

An alternative test of verbal memory is the repetition of a Babcock sentence such as "the one thing a nation needs in order to be rich and great is a large secure supply of wood" (Institute of Psychiatry, 1973). Such a sentence will usually require several attempts before it is repeated correctly, and it requires the use of short-term memory rather than just immediate memory.

Some amnesic patients perform well when set specific memory tasks and a better indication of memory functions may be the patient's ability to recall what he ate for breakfast or the details of some other incidental event occurring a few hours beforehand. Long-term memory can be tested by the ability to recall important dates and events in the past. Such dates should be noted during the early stages of history taking and then re-checked for any inconsistencies, later in the interview. A knowledge of current events in the world should be enquired for but minor errors are often of uncertain significance and may just reflect the patient's self absorption and preoccupation with other matters.

Visual memory can be evaluated by using the immediate and delayed recall of various diagrams (e.g. a Greek cross) of different degrees of complexity. This can be combined with testing for constructional apraxia.

Confabulation may be present and *is the "falsification of memory occurring in a clear consciousness in association with an organically derived amnesia"* (Berlyne, 1972). Such falsification of memory may vary from just an incorrect date, to a detailed account of a major nonexistent event. In some cases fantastic confabulations, that are obviously false, may be produced ("I visited Mars in a spaceship''). Such phenomena should be differentiated from delusions or deliberate lying (where the patient will hope to gain some advantage from his fabrication). Differentiation between a delusion and confabulation can be very difficult at times. When lying becomes greatly exaggerated it is called *"pseudologia fantastica"* and this is particularly associated with Munchausen's syndrome.

The patient with OBD will usually attempt to overcome his inability to answer questions by producing confabulatory answers (Q. Who is the prime Minister? A. Lloyd George), or *"near miss" answers* (Q. What year is it? A. 1983). Near miss answers should not be confused with *answering past the point* (vorbeireden). *In vorbeireden the patient answers in such a way as to indicate he understands the question but is deliberately making an incorrect answer* (Q. What colour is an orange? A. Blue). This type of answer has been particularly associated with the Ganser syndrome but clinically it is more commonly seen in other disorders. The excessive use of *"don't know" responses* suggests a negativistic attitude that is particularly seen in depression. It is also seen in other disorders where the patient is uncooperative, in frontal lobe disease, and in subcortical dementia.

Suggestibility is often seen with confabulation, the patient claiming an incorrect response, that has been suggested by the doctor, as being the forgotten memory. The patient's response to increasingly inappropriate suggestions, e.g. "we went out for a meal together yesterday, didn't we?" can be used to test the degree of suggestibility.

Perseveration is the "continuation or recurrence of a purposeful response which is more appropriate to a preceding stimulus than to the succeeding one which has just been given, and which is essential to provoke it" (Allison, 1966). It is frequently found in association with confabulation (Shapiro *et al.*, 1981). It is commonly found with frontal lobe lesions, but it has little localising value in organic brain disease. It may involve speech, e.g. Q. What day is it? A. Tuesday. Q. What year is it? A. Tuesday. It may also be seen in non-verbal motor responses.

Other symptoms and signs

Concrete thinking is the inability to think abstractly and it is found in mental retardation, organic brain disease and chronic schizophrenia. This *"loss of the abstract attitude" can result in a failure to form concepts, to focus attention on the fundamentals of a particular problem, to plan ahead, and to adjust to changing circumstances* (Lezak, 1976). The latter may result in "stimulus-bound" behaviour, where the patient is unable to switch attention from a matter of previous concern, to one that has now become more important.

Problem solving and proverb interpretation involve abstract thinking. In assessing the patient's response to such tests due allowance must be made for variables such as education, intellect, cultural background, and experience. Proverbs can be varied from the simple "a rolling stone gathers no moss" to the more difficult "people in glass houses shouldn't throw stones". Problem solving should be tested but the difficulty of the problem should be adjusted to the patient's expected level of ability, assessed on the basis of his educational and occupational history. The problem can be varied in degree of difficulty from digit reversal to a mathematical problem involving several sequences.

The *positive symptoms of psychosis*—hallucinations, bizarre or disorganised behaviour, delusions, and disorder in the form of thinking, e.g. incoherence, lack of logic, tangentiality (Andreasen and Olsen, 1982), should be enquired for, and any behaviour on the part of the patient that suggests they are present, looked for. These symptoms are easier to recognise and more responsive to neuroleptic treatment, than the negative symptoms of psychosis (Crow, 1980). The latter include asociality, flattening of affect, poverty of speech and apathy, features typical of chronic schizophrenia, but also found in frontal lobe disorders and subcortical dementia (Roberts, 1983).

A delusion is a false unshakeable belief that is out of keeping with the patient's social, educational or cultural background. If there are several delusions present that are persistent and based on one particular theme, then they are said to be "systematized". Such delusions are particularly found in older patients, in those with chronic organic brain disease, paranoid personality disorders or chronic paranoid schizophrenia. In contrast the unsystematized delusions are evanescent, changing in response to differing environmental cues. They are usually associated with acute confusion, whether it is organic in origin (e.g. delirium), or not (e.g. hypomania, acute schizophrenia). The affected tend to be young and there is considerable impairment of social functioning (Detre and Jarecki, 1971).

The important signs of aphasia, apraxia and agnosia will be discussed in Chapter 3.

2.3 HYPNOSIS

Hypnosis "is an unusual (or altered) state of consciousness in which distortions of perception (possibly including those of place and time) occur as uncritical responses of the subject to notions from an objective source (usually the hypnotist) or a subjective source (his own memory) or both" (Mellett, 1980).

Merskey has suggested that hypnosis can be regarded as a procedure involving collusion between the patient and the hypnotist to attain a goal that is mutually agreed upon. This view implies that the hypnotised patient maintains a significant degree of awareness of his surroundings, despite being in a "trance". Investigations have supported his view insofar as patients in a hypnotic state of relaxation exhibit EEG changes that are not significantly different from what would be expected in the non-hypnotised alert patient (Merskey, 1979). Also, though patients undergo surgery under the influence of hypnosis, they usually experience some pain during the procedure (Hilgard and Hilgard, 1975). Furthermore, Halliday and Mason (1964) found normal cerebral evoked potentials in patients after stimulating body areas rendered anaesthetic by hypnotic suggestion. This indicates that whatever the patient might say, his central nervous system is responding normally to the stimulation applied to the "anaesthetised" area. This discrepancy between the subjective and objective findings is consistent with the patient being in a state which might be described as one of dissociation.

If such a state of altered consciousness can be induced by suggestion, it is reasonable to expect to be able to remove it by the use of suggestion. Hypnosis can be used to remove hysterical conversion phenomena in suitable patients. It has the advantage of being easier and safer to carry out than the use of intravenous barbiturates (amytal), it does not cause significant EEG changes, and it is a simple technique to learn (for further details see Waxman, 1980).

Though other underlying psychopathology may become evident, it is a safe procedure provided appropriate evaluation is carried out beforehand, and other forms of treatment are used when indicated (Merskey, 1979). After the conversion phenomena have been removed then some form of psychotherapy is usually indicated to maintain the improvement and avoid a recurrence of symptoms.

Requirements for its effective use include a cooperative patient and his susceptibility to induction. The latter is reduced by severe psychopathology and so the usefulness of hypnosis is restricted mainly to less severe cases (Frischholz, 1982). For a discussion of the possible psychophysiological basis of the process, the reader is referred to Mellett (1980).

2.4 THE AMYTAL INTERVIEW

The use of intravenous amylobarbitone (amytal) can be a useful adjunct in the diagnosis and treatment of certain neuropsychiatric conditions. The drug acts to reduce anxiety, producing sedation and disinhibition. It is particularly useful in the diagnosis and treatment of conditions resulting from dissociation (such as hysterical conversion states), and in stupor. It has also been recommended as a quick and effective treatment for emotional disorders induced by specific stressful events, e.g. post-traumatic neurosis (post-traumatic stress disorder). In such cases the patient may, under the influence of the drug, become able to relate the details of the traumatic event. This will not only be helpful in clarifying the diagnosis, but may also be therapeutic by bringing about an abreaction. *Abreaction is the bringing into consciousness of forgotten affect-laden experiences, with an associated discharge of the accumulated emotion* (Perry and Jacobs, 1982).

In some cases a single dose of the drug can result in a dramatic response, e.g. producing speech in a catatonic patient who had been mute for several years (Bleckwenn, 1931). In such patients negativistic behaviour, such as refusing to eat, may be life-threatening and require urgent treatment. In the malingering patient the procedure may be refused, or the patient may be difficult and defensive during it. In these cases it may be of help by disinhibiting the patient, leading to more obvious lying.

Clinical improvement resulting from this procedure is usually only temporary. In severely depressed patients retardation can be reduced, depressive ideation revealed, and there may be an improvement in mood. In schizophrenic patients psychotic symptoms may be revealed (Woodruff, 1966). Patients with organic brain disease tend to be sensitive to the cerebral effects of amytal and impairment of cognition may appear for the first time or, if already present, become more pronounced. Sedation, usually indicated by slurring of speech and rapid lateral nystagmus, is usually found after a dose of between 150 to 350 mgm of amytal has been given, in adult patients without organic brain disease (OBD). However, it may occur with a dose of under 150 mgm in those patients with OBD (Perry and Jacobs, 1982). This "organic sensitivity" to barbiturates was confirmed in another study comparing a group of elderly demented patients, to another age-matched group with depression in remission (Hemsi *et al.*, 1968).

Weinstein *et al.* (1954) found disorientation for place and time, anosognosia (denial of illness), and misidentification of people in the patient's environment, were the most frequent results of this procedure in patients with OBD. Plum and Posner (1980) found that neurological signs may be revealed in the patient who is in an organic stupor. If such signs develop or the conscious level of the patient deteriorates, the procedure should be stopped. This is to limit the effects of the drug interfering with the monitoring of the patient's vital signs, and to allow a full neurological evaluation to be carried out looking for new neurological signs.

As a general rule, in the absence of contra-indications, *the judicious use of intravenous barbiturates tends to clarify a diagnosis*, rather than confuse it. If an EEG is considered appropriate then the amytal is best withheld until later, to avoid confusing the interpretation of the EEG.

Perry and Jacobs (1982) recommended giving intravenous sodium amytal at a rate not exceeding 50 mgm/minute and not exceeding a total of 1000 mgm on any single occasion. Once sedation is achieved it can be maintained by giving about 25 to 50 mgm every 5 minutes. Contra-indications to its use are renal or hepatic disease, barbiturate addiction, porphyria, hypotension or any airway obstruction. Cardiopulmonary resuscitation equipment should be at hand at all times in case of respiratory arrest or other complications, and the procedure should not be used if the patient resists. For further information on the practical aspects of the technique the reader is referred to Perry and Jacobs (1982).

2.5   THE DEXAMETHASONE SUPPRESSION TEST (DST)

There is a syndrome of depression involving an unpleasant mood with an inability to enjoy any activity and not even a temporary improvement in mood in response to some pleasurable event. If, in addition, there are at least three of the following—a worsening of the depression in the morning, a tendency to wake from sleep in the early hours of the morning, increased or decreased motor activity, anorexia, weight loss, and ideas of guilt, the DSM III describes this syndrome as depression with melancholia. In about 50% of patients with this condition, the pituitary gland will not be suppressed by dexamethasone. Non-suppression specifically means that there is a failure to suppress the activity of the pituitary–adrenal axis in the 24 hours that follow giving 1 mgm of dexamethasone. The drug is usually given by mouth at 11 pm. Failure to suppress is indicated by the level of at least one serum cortisol (usually at least two samples are taken at 4 pm and at 11 pm the next day) being greater than 5 mgm/100 ml.

The preliminary results of studies on this test suggest that it may be helpful in the diagnosis, management, and assessment of prognosis of affective disorders. As organic brain disease may disguise or distort the manifestations of depression, this test may well prove to be of particular usefulness in neuropsychiatry, as a means of identifying patients with masked depression or depressive pseudodementia. However, about 4% of patients with other psychiatric disorders without significant depression, have been found to be non-suppressors (Carroll, 1982). So the clinical state of the patients must be taken into account, before embarking on treatment for depression, as such treatment may be poorly tolerated by those with organic brain disease.

Patients who do not suppress, more often respond to treatment with electro-convulsive therapy (ECT) or antidepressants, than those who suppress normally. There is also evidence that those patients whose DST undergoes a change to suppression following treatment, tend to have a good prognosis. Alternatively those who appear to clinically respond to treatment, but continue to be non-suppressors, tend to relapse within a month or two of leaving hospital (Brown, 1981).

There is evidence that certain factors may cause a raised incidence (greater than the 4% of the healthy population) of false positive DST results. They are listed in Table 2.2 (Brown, 1981; Carroll et al., 1981; Dewan et al., 1982; Raskind

Table 2.2   Factors influencing the dexamethasone suppression test

FAILURE TO SUPPRESS

Depression with melancholia — 40 to 56%

Cushing's disease
Anticonvulsants and other
  liver enzyme inducers
Physostigmine
Pregnancy
Acute physical illness
Primary degenerative dementia
Chronic schizophrenia
Catatonic disorders
Schizoaffective–depressed

FALSE POSITIVE SUPPRESSION

Hypopituitarism
Hypoadrenalism
Steroids
High dose benzodiazepines

et al., 1982). Drug-induced "false non-suppression" is of particular importance in neuropsychiatry, and is seen in patients taking drugs which induce liver enzymes, such as the anticonvulsants. In another study elderly patients with primary degenerative dementia were found to be non-suppressors in 7 out of 15 cases (Raskind *et al.*, 1982), though none of these demented patients showed any significant evidence of depression. If this finding in demented patients is confirmed, and cognitively intact elderly patients suppress normally, as was found in one study (Tourigny-Rivard *et al.*, 1982), this raises the question at what level of cognitive impairment does the DST cease to be reliable? Questions of this type require clarification, before the full value of the DST in neuropsychiatry is recognised.

CHAPTER 3

Aspects of the Neurological Examination

3.1 INTRODUCTION

The physical and neurological examination of the neuropsychiatric patient will not be discussed in detail here as there are many excellent accounts covering this area in standard texts on neurology, such as De Jong (1970). However, the following topics will be mentioned in an attempt to clarify their causes, characteristics, and their clinical significance in neuropsychiatric diagnosis. The topics include physical asymmetry and abnormal movements, particularly with reference to the head and face (as it is abnormalities in this area of the body that arc, in many ways, most important to the psychiatrist), certain primitive reflexes, left handedness, minimal brain dysfunction and soft neurological signs, and aphasia, apraxia, and agnosia. Finally the differential diagnosis of hysteria and malingering will be considered.

3.2 FACIAL ASYMMETRY

Even before formal physical examination of the patient is started, certain physical signs may be noticed which may be of relevance to the understanding of the case. Facial asymmetry may be seen either as a localised phenomenon or as part of a more widespread physical asymmetry. Facial asymmetry can be associated with a number of conditions that are listed in Table 3.1.

Certain causes are of particular importance in neuropsychiatry. If the facial asymmetry is caused by a neurological disorder it is usually due to an upper (UMN) or a lower motor neurone (LMN) lesion of the 7th (facial) cranial nerve. UMN facial weakness spares the muscles of the upper part of the face so that the patient can raise his eyebrows to command, but has difficulty with voluntary movements involving the lower part of his face, e.g. smiling or puffing out his cheeks, on command. This is because both cerebral hemispheres control the upper facial muscles on the left (or the right) side. Acquired facial weakness in the elderly is usually UMN in type and due to cerebrovascular disease. If the right side of the face is involved, associated signs of left frontal lobe damage, usually motor aphasia and weakness of the right arm, will be present.

43

Table 3.1 Causes of facial asymmetry

Blood vessel disease	Cerebrovascular accident
Congenital and inherited	Sturge–Weber syndrome
	Meckerson Rosenthal syndrome
	Perinatal brain damage
	Neurofibromatosis
Degenerative	Romberg's disease (progressive hemifacial atrophy)
Metabolic	Syringobulbia, demyelination, motor neurone disease
Epilepsy	Diabetes mellitus
Growth	Temporal lobe epilepsy
	Sarcoidosis
	Frontal lobe tumour
	Tumour in the cerebellopontine angle
Injury and post-operative	Fracture of skull base
Inflammation	Mumps
	Bell's palsy
	Herpes Zoster of the geniculate ganglion
	(Ramsay–Hunt syndrome)

Such facial weakness is most noticeable on voluntary movement (performed to command) in contrast to spontaneous (reflex) emotional movements, which are often spared and involve different neurological pathways. Loss of such spontaneous facial movements can be seen with right frontal lesions (Ross, 1981) and may be an early sign of a frontal lobe tumour (Lishman, 1978). This is of importance because clinical signs and symptoms tend to be less pronounced with slow growing tumours in the frontal region of the brain, and they may progress insidiously and present to the psychiatrist clinically, as a dementia or a change in personality.

Difficulty arises in assessing the significance of minor degrees of facial asymmetry in the absence of hard neurological signs. Such a finding is not uncommon in patients without any neurological disorder and was present in 32% of 25 healthy controls in Remillard et al.'s study (1977). However, 80% of the 50 patients with TLE in this study had definite facial asymmetry and when there was a unilateral epileptic temporal lobe focus (present in 37 patients), 73% had a contralateral facial weakness and 13% an ipsilateral weakness. This weakness was of the UMN type, but was most evident on spontaneous emotional expression. The study excluded patients with any evidence of physical asymmetry in other areas of the body, or a cerebral tumour. Such findings require confirmation but provide support for the impression that minor degrees of facial asymmetry, even as an isolated physical finding, may have clinical significance.

Other evidence of asymmetry in body development should be looked for and may indicate perinatal brain trauma. Lesions of the parietal lobe or postcentral gyrus are particularly prone to produce this effect, and it is most marked if the damage occurs around the time of birth or in early childhood. The resulting asymmetry is more of a failure to develop, than a true atrophy (De Jong, 1970). This failure to develop may involve the face or even the entire half of the body, contralateral to the side of the lesion. The skin, subcutaneous tissues, muscles and bones, may fail to develop also. Such effects emphasise the importance of the nervous system as a trophic factor in normal bodily development (Poskanzer, 1975). UMN lesions do not cause marked muscle wasting though some degree of disuse wasting may occur in the affected limbs.

3.3 ABNORMAL MOVEMENTS OF THE FACE AND BODY

Abnormal involuntary movements of the face and head are a common finding in psychiatry and often represent a drug-induced *tardive dyskinesia*. This disorder is also called the *buccolinguomasticatory syndrome* because it typically involves rhythmic activity of these three muscle groups causing chewing, lip smacking, and similar movements. Tardive dyskinesia is probably usually a result of dopaminergic hypersensitivity caused by prolonged use of dopamine receptor blocking drugs (Marsden *et al.*, 1975). Early in the course of treatment, these drugs can cause Parkinson's syndrome and, less often, other types of abnormal movements. These movements include the sustained, contorting movements of dystonia, *chorea (variable dance-like, fidgety movements), tics (involuntary noises, words or movements in functionally related groups of skeletal muscles, usually being abrupt and unexpected), athetosis (irregular, slow, writhing movements)* and even *hemiballismus (wild flinging movements of the limbs)*. The differential diagnosis of such abnormal movements must take into account

Table 3.2   Causes of involuntary movements

Toxins	Manganese, carbon disulphide, thallium
Blood vessel disease, tumours or other insults	Thalamus, basal ganglia, subthalamic nucleus (corpus luysi)
Collagen disorders	Systemic lupus erythematosus
Congenital and inherited	Huntington's chorea, Wilson's disease, dystonia musculorum deformans, perinatal brain damage (especially kernicterus)
Degenerative	Senile orofacial dyskinesia, dental disorders, idiopathic parkinsonism, secondary dystonia
Drugs	Major tranquillisers, methylphenidate, amphetamines, cocaine, phencyclidine and structurally related drugs, L-dopa, methyl dopa, oral contraceptives, tricyclic antidepressants, anti-malarial drugs, anticholinergic agents, phenytoin
Endocrine and metabolic	Hyperthyroidism, pregnancy, Hallevorden–Spatz disease, hypernatraemia, inborn errors of metabolism (e.g. phenylketonuria, acanthocytosis, infantile gout, hypoparathyroidism)
Epilepsy	Temporal lobe epilepsy
Functional	Catatonic phenomena, tic disorders* (Gilles de la Tourette's syndrome)
Hypoxia	Carbon monoxide
Infection	Encephalitis, post-encephalitic, Creutzfelt–Jacob disease, Chagas disease, Sydenham's chorea

*There is evidence of a disorder of brain function contributing to the development of certain of these (Bruun and Shapiro, 1972).

other disorders listed in Table 3.2 and this subject is discussed further by Granacher (1981).

Certain conditions involving movement disorders are reversible provided the correct diagnosis is made, but if they are misdiagnosed serious consequences can result. Any of the parkinsonian signs of "cog-wheel" rigidity, akinesia, postural instability, and the "pill-rolling" tremor of the hands, can be produced by neuroleptic treatment. Such extrapyramidal signs can also be found in Wilson's disease, Huntington's chorea, manganese and carbon disulphide poisoning, idiopathic and post-encephalitic parkinsonism, and parkinsonism induced by drugs that are not particularly associated with psychiatric practice, such as the anti-hypertensive drug methyl dopa. *There is no easy way to separate idiopathic from drug-induced parkinsonism when the patient has had prolonged exposure to neuroleptics.* Idiopathic Parkinson's disease is suggested by the presence of asymmetrical extrapyramidal signs (akinesia, rigidity and tremor), which persist despite drug withdrawal, and the early onset of a "pill-rolling" tremor. Akathisia is uncommon in Parkinson's disease and would make a drug-induced aetiology more likely (Marsden *et al.*, 1975). When oculogyric crises occur, post-encephalitic parkinsonism should be suspected, particularly when it is associated with compulsive antisocial behaviour and a past history of encephalitis. Toxins can induce extrapyramidal disorders, and choreathetotic movements may be caused by manganese or thallium.

Wilson's disease and Huntington's chorea are two disorders of particular importance to the neuropsychiatrist. *Huntington's chorea* is an autosomal dominantly inherited disorder usually starting in the middle aged and characterised by the triad of progressive dementia, almost any type of psychiatric disorder, and choreiform movements. The disorder can present with any of these features initially, but commonly presents with the abnormal movements which usually involves the head, neck or upper limbs.

Wilson's disease is also called *hepatolenticular degeneration* because the abnormal deposition of copper, that characterises this disorder, occurs mainly in the liver (producing cirrhosis) and the basal ganglia (producing the rigidity, tremor, dystonic and athetoid movements). Copper deposition in Descemet's membrane produces a brown or green ring at the edge of the cornea. This is called the Kayser–Fleischer ring and though it may require slit lamp microscopy to be seen, it will confirm the diagnosis when the patient is over 10 years of age. Onset of the disorder is usually in the first two decades of life and it is caused by the inheritance of an autosomal recessive gene.

Both Wilson's disease and Huntington's chorea can occur at almost any age and the neurological features can be antedated by virtually any type of psychiatric disturbance. If the patient has received prior treatment with neuroleptic drugs, when the movement disorder starts it may be regarded as being drug-induced. Table 3.3 compares the features of the three types of disorders. Their separation is of more than academic interest and has implications for treatment, prognosis, genetic counselling, and awareness of the possible risk to the patient's relatives.

Table 3.3   Comparison of Wilson's disease, Huntington's chorea and tardive dyskinesia

	Tardive dyskinesia	Huntington's chorea	Wilson's disease
Prolonged use of neuroleptics	+	−	−
Family history	−	+	−
Age of onset	Commonest in older patients	30–50 yrs	0–20 yrs
Site of onset of movements	Orofacial	Head, neck and upper limbs	Upper limbs
Early dysarthria	−	+	+
Rapid intellectual decline	−	+	−
Abnormal EEG	−	+	+
Cerebral atrophy on CAT brain scan	−	+ *Low FH/CC ratio	+ **Atrophy of the lentiform nuclei
Pathognomonic features	−	−	Kayser–Fleischer ring, low serum caeruloplasmin
Treatment	Withdraw drugs	Palliative	Penicillamine
Prognosis	Good	Death usually in 10 to 15 yrs	Good (if treated)

+ = Usually present.
− = Usually absent.
FH = Frontal horn span.
CC = Intercaudate distance.
*Neophytides *et al.* (1979).
**Selekler *et al.* (1981).

The clinical presentation tends to vary with the age of onset and in younger patients it is more parkinsonian in Huntington's chorea, and liver involvement is the dominant feature in Wilson's disease. The prognosis is worse in both conditions in younger patients. Young adults and children with extrapyramidal disorders, no matter what the aetiology, tend to have their abnormal movements more pronounced in the trunk and limbs, the oro-facial region being preferentially involved in older patients (Marsden *et al.*, 1975).

The *dystonias* can be caused by most disorders that affect the basal ganglia (or the thalamus), particularly carbon monoxide, head injuries, tumours, infections, and cerebrovascular disease. Dystonias which have no apparent cause can arise spontaneously. Idiopathic localised dystonias such as spasmodic torticollis (episodic spasm of the sternocleidomastoid muscle) and blepharospasm, may occur (Marsden, 1976a). The secondary dystonias tend to be unilateral and focal, and the associated features and prognosis depend on the underlying cause. Such focal dystonias are often regarded as entirely psychological in origin. This is because of certain features that are often found in association with them: their unusual nature; their sensitivity to psychosocial stress; the ability to relieve them by means of unusual "tricks"; the absence of an "organic" cause; and their association with psychiatric disorders (Marsden, 1976a).

Dystonia musculorum deformans (DMD) or *torsion dystonia*, is an uncommon disorder that can be inherited in an autosomal recessive or dominant manner. Onset is usually in the first four decades of life. The alteration in muscle tone results in the body being distorted into abnormal postures. It tends to affect the axial and proximal musculature initially. The recessive form has an earlier age of onset, but a more rapid progression, and can result in crippling deformity. The dominant gene may clinically manifest itself in a partial way, and an abnormality of gait or a foot deformity, may be all that is seen. Such a partial presentation may mask the presence of a family history. Patients with DMD have no particular predisposition to any psychiatric disorder, but because their body can be distorted into bizarre postures, which may occur only with certain activities, e.g. the patient can walk backwards normally but has difficulty walking forwards, and because the course of the disorder often fluctuates over time, a diagnosis of hysteria may be considered (Lishman, 1978).

Tics are common findings in childhood, when they are usually temporary phenomena. The face is usually involved and blinking is particularly common. In *Gilles de la Tourette's syndrome* multiple tics, usually including coprolalia and other vocal tics, develop before the age of 15 years. The tics spread gradually to other parts of the upper body, and though the condition may fluctuate and the movements change and increase in complexity, it remains life-long. Mental coprolalia, obsessive doubting, a compulsion to touch objects and perform ritualistic movements, e.g. squatting or twirling when walking, may be present. Both a history and physical signs suggestive of minimal brain dysfunction, are common. The treatment of choice, when treatment is required, is usually haloperidol or pimozide (Trimble, 1981a). Patients may become adept at disguising their movements and utterances, but in one of the author's cases the patient drew attention to his problem by persistently requesting major tranquillisers to "relax his nerves". A similar disorder with multiple tics, including verbal tics, may be more benign and remit in adolescence (Transient Tic disorder). More localised tic disorders may be seen, which remain lifelong and may even start after the age of 40 years (Chronic Motor Tic disorder).

Tremor is a rhythmical movement about a joint, resulting from recurrent, rapid and alternating contractions of antagonistic groups of muscles (Bruun and Shapiro, 1972). It may be induced by a vast number of drugs, but it can also be inherited as an autosomal dominant disorder *(familial tremor)* with onset before the age of 30 years. Like most tremors this primarily involves the extremities, but it can progress to the head and neck, and may be accompanied by dysarthria. It is important not to misdiagnose this condition as parkinsonism or to mistakenly attribute the dysarthria to drug or alcohol use (Sutherland *et al.*, 1975).

Senile tremor can also occur, usually in the sixth decade (Wolf, 1980), and it is not a sign of organic brain disease. Initially it often involves shaking of the head and it may spread to involve the hands, but is not particularly incapacitating.

Myoclonus is a shock-like contraction of part of a muscle, the whole muscle, or a group of muscles. It can be found in, or caused by, many of the disorders listed in Table 3.2, but it is particularly important as an indication of a metabolic disorder (when it is usually found in association with tremor) and in Creutzfeldt–Jacob disease, when it accompanies the characteristic periodic EEG discharges found in the later stages of this condition. It can also be a normal phenomenon, e.g. a hiccough, and may be found during the initial stages of sleep.

Transient orofacial movements in psychiatric patients are not always indicative of tardive dyskinesia but may be caused by amphetamines, cocaine or other stimulant drugs. If consciousness is impaired in association with brief episodes of facial movements, temporal lobe epilepsy should be suspected. There is evidence that facial movements may occur in patients with schizophrenia who have not been exposed to neuroleptics (Owens *et al.*, 1982). Such movements may be mannerisms or stereotypies and can be seen in any disorder producing catatonic phenomena.

3.4 LEFT-HANDEDNESS

The clinical significance of a preference for the left hand (sinistrality) in performing motor activities, is not at all clear. *About 90% of the general population are right-handed*, but the other 10% are difficult to evaluate because they vary in their degree of left-handedness and the hand preference they claim for various activities, e.g. writing, throwing a ball or threading a needle, often differs from what is seen by an independent observer (Springer and Deutsch, 1981). It is helpful in considering the significance of sinistrality, to divide these people into those with a positive family history (FH +) and those with a negative family history (FH −) of left handedness.

The FH + group tend not to show an absolute preference for their left hand, nor a clear left hemisphere dominance for language or a right hemisphere dominance for spatial functions. They develop dysphasia with equal frequency whichever side of the brain is damaged, though they have a better prognosis for recovery than dextrals (Hardyck and Petrinovitch, 1977).

Support for the importance of genetic factors in relation to sinistrality is provided by studies of family incidence. About 2% of the offspring of dextral parents will be left-handed and this figure rises to 17% if one parent is sinistral, and 46% if both are (Chamberlain, 1928). 20% of twins are left-handed, but this figure is the same whether the twins are monozygotic or dizygotic, and discordance for handedness is present in 25% of twin pairs. These findings are difficult to explain but may be due, in part, to the increased risk of neurological damage that twins are exposed to at birth, compared with single births (Howard and Brown, 1970). A relationship between brain damage in early life and sinistrality has been claimed by many authors (discussed by Hardyck and Petrinovitch, 1977) and it is most pertinent to mention this in relation to the FH − group. The FH − group contrasts with the FH + group, in showing a more marked preference for the left hand. Dysphasia in the FH − group is almost always associated with lesions of the left hemisphere, and they show the same pattern of dominance for language and spatial functions, as the dextral population. Evidence linking left-handedness to brain damage includes an increased incidence of sinistrality among those with mental retardation, epilepsy, learning disability, twins (Springer and Deutsch, 1981), and fourth — and later — born children (Bakan, 1977; Bishop, 1980), but the evidence does not support the assumption that brain damage is responsible for many FH — sinistrals.

Sinistrality cannot be assumed to be of any clinical significance as an isolated finding (Bax, 1980), but taken in the context of a selected neuropsychiatric population it should not be discounted as being of no importance, without all other relevant factors, e.g. any history of perinatal complications, being taken into consideration. A brain insult to the left cerebral hemisphere in childhood can lead to a shift of cerebral dominance to the other side of the brain, with the development of left-handedness, but these so-called *"symptomatic" left-handers are probably very uncommon.*

3.5 APHASIA, APRAXIA AND AGNOSIA

The 3 A's, aphasia, apraxia, and agnosia, refer to those disorders of behaviour that are typically seen as a result of impaired function of the cerebral association cortex. The presence of these clinical signs is strong evidence for organic brain disease involving the cerebral cortex. Some disorders, e.g. dementia of the Alzheimer's type, typically involve the association cortex of the brain, initially sparing the primary motor and sensory cortices. The presence of constructional apraxia is an important early sign of this disorder. In contrast the posterior association cortex is relatively spared in Pick's disease and the subcortical dementias.

Aphasia is a disorder of communication that affects the semantic (meaning) and syntactic (grammatical structure) aspects of language, and usually results from cortical dysfunction in the language dominant (LD), usually the left, cerebral hemisphere. It may be difficult to clearly differentiate it from disorders of speech and thought, especially as the process of thinking is not an observable phenomenon, but certain observations and simple procedures will clarify the presence or absence of dysphasia in most cases.

The three most important aphasia syndromes are the motor, sensory and anomic aphasias. These three types of aphasia are compared and contrasted in Table 3.4. The reader is referred to Diagram 4.1 (see page 67) for the areas of the brain that will now be referred to with regard to the mechanisms underlying the aphasias. The clinical characteristics of these and other disorders of language can be more clearly understood by considering a model for language mechanisms, proposed by Geschwind (1979). According to this model a verbal instruction to the patient will be received at the cortical level, initially in the primary auditory cortex. Comprehension of these auditory impulses then occurs in Wernicke's area. The response is initiated in this region and passes via the arcuate fasciculus to Broca's area, where it "evokes a detailed and coordinated program for vocalization". In contrast, written information passes to the primary visual cortex initially, and then to the angular gyrus, before reaching

Wernicke's area. The angular gyrus integrates auditory and written language, and this gyrus appears to be necessary to evoke the auditory form of a written word in Wernicke's area. This process seems to be necessary before the writing can be understood and the response initiated.

Motor or non-fluent aphasia is also called *Broca's aphasia* because the responsible lesion involves Broca's area, which is antero-inferior to the premotor cortex of the LD cerebral hemisphere. The left frontal lobe is the part of the brain that plays the major role in controlling all aspects of motor behaviour, including propositional language. Hence it is characteristic of motor aphasia that speech is slow, hesitant and non-fluent. The patient says little and tends to leave out "connecting" words, e.g. "if", "from", "but". Despite this the information content of the speech is high and comprehension is relatively intact. This results in a "telegrammatic" style of speech. Evidence of muscle weakness of the UMN type, usually involving the face and arm on the right side of the body, is usually present.

Table 3.4   Essential features of motor, sensory and anomic aphasia

	Type of dysphasia		
	Motor	Sensory	Anomic
Obvious effort	+	−	−
Fluent speech flow	−	+	+
Right-sided UMN facial or limb weakness	+	−	−
Articulation	−	+	+
Meaningful information in speech	+	−	−
Comprehension	+	−	+
Circumlocutions/paraphasias	−	+	+
Repetition	−	−	+

+ = Usually present or intact.
− = Usually absent or impaired.

Sensory or fluent aphasia is also called *Wernicke's aphasia* because the lesion responsible involves Wernicke's area, which is in the posterior part of the superior temporal gyrus. Speech is usually fluent but the patient has difficulty finding certain words and so his speech wanders as he tries to talk around the missing word (circumlocution). In the case of the word "pen" he might say "well it's a . . . something you use to write with . . . you put ink in it". He will use substitutions for words or parts of words (paraphasias). Though speech output tends to be profuse, it conveys relatively little information. Comprehension is also impaired and this should be taken into account when the patient is given a command. In this type of aphasia the patients are often not aware of their impaired comprehension and as neurological deficits may be absent, this can cause diagnostic problems (vide infra).

Both these aphasias involve lesions in the region of the sylvian fissure and difficulty in repetition of spoken words is characteristic of these *perisylvian aphasias.* As mentioned it is the small "connecting" words such as "if" and "or", that are most difficult to repeat. This can be tested by asking the patient to repeat a phrase such as "No ifs, ands or buts".

There is frequently a degree of overlap between the two types of aphasia and this is seen in an extreme form in global aphasia, where the speech is characteristically non-fluent *and* comprehension is impaired. In such cases it is difficult to test comprehension as the patient has minimal speech output, but it may be possible to get around this difficulty by naming objects in his visual field and asking him to point at them.

Anomia is a pathological difficulty in finding correct words, either spontaneously or on specific testing. Though always present in aphasia it can also be found in a number of diffuse cerebral disorders. It is usually present in established dementia of the Alzheimer's type, where it tends to form part of a language disorder called *anomic aphasia*. Here speech is fluent but rambling with numerous circumlocutions and a poverty of meaningful content. Repetition and comprehension are relatively intact, and writing may also be normal. This language disorder has little localising significance, other than indicating diffuse cortical brain disease.

Many other types of aphasia can be found and those that result from lesions distant from the sylvian fissure, and do not involve repetition difficulties, are called the *transcortical aphasias*. In some cases subcortical lesions may cause language disturbance (Mohr *et al.*, 1975). However, for practical purposes, it is the motor, sensory, and anomic aphasias, that are mainly of importance in neuropsychiatry. They are important because they indicate the presence of disease of the cerebral cortex and can have a diagnostic value, e.g. the presence of motor or sensory aphasia early in the course of a dementing illness makes a diagnosis of Alzheimer's dementia unlikely and should lead to a search for other disorders, especially cerebrovascular disease or a tumour.

The ability to write is a very fragile skill and easily disrupted by organic brain disease (*dysgraphia*). Aphasic patients will usually be dysgraphic and the presence of an intact ability to write fluently to dictation, producing a neat product without misspellings, incorrect words or missed words, is incompatible with the presence of any significant aphasia or delirium (Benson, 1979; Chedru and Geschwind, 1972b). This skill should be assessed and will be helpful in differentiating organic from non-organic disorders.

Disorders of mood commonly accompany the focal aphasias. Depression is a common and understandable finding in motor aphasia. It may also occur, but is less common, in sensory aphasia. In the latter a denial of disability, and even euphoria, is often seen (Benson, 1979). There is evidence that depression is more likely to be seen with large lesions in Wernicke's area (Robinson and Benson, 1981). For further discussion of the aphasias the reader is referred to Benson (1979).

Apraxia is "a disorder of skilled movement that is not caused by weakness, sensory loss, abnormality of tone or posture, abnormal movements, intellectual deterioration, or poor comprehension" (Geschwind, 1965). Though the patient may be unable to produce the movement to command he may be able to perform it as a reflex activity. Lesions of the left hemisphere can produce disorders of skilled motor movement of varying degrees of severity. "Limb-kinetic" apraxia (usually due to a lesion of the premotor cortex) can be regarded as representing the mild end of this spectrum of severity, but as it also involves some degree of muscle weakness as well as clumsiness of the dominant hand, it does not conform fully to the above definition of an apraxia (Lishman, 1978). At the other end of the spectrum is the inability to perform complex motor sequences, e.g. miming the sequence of motor actions involved in opening a locked door using a key (ideational apraxia). An inability to perform less complex movements to command (ideomotor apraxia), e.g. waving goodbye, can be regarded as occupying the middle area of this hypothetical spectrum. Ideational and ideomotor apraxias tend to involve both sides of the body and are usually associated with left sided parieto-temporal disorders.

The apraxia may only be evident when the appropriate command is given, but in some cases it may also be found when the patient is asked to imitate movements demonstrated by the examiner (see Table 3.5). A patient with apraxia may be able to perform an activity requiring some object, only if he is given the necessary object (e.g. a door key, in the above example of testing for ideational apraxia).

Agnosia is "the impaired recognition of an object which is sensorially presented while at the same time the impairment cannot be reduced to sensory defects, mental deterioration, disorders of consciousness and attention, or to a non-familiarity with the object" (Frederiks, 1969). This term is used, with varying degrees of appropriateness, to describe a variety of disorders. It usually constitutes one part of a syndrome of cognitive deficits that are particularly associated with right hemisphere lesions.

Constructional apraxia and dressing apraxia, are most commonly associated with lesions of the right hemisphere and are probably more appropriately classified with the agnosic disorders. Constructional apraxia (visuospatial agnosia) is a "disturbance which appears in formative activities in which the spatial part of the task is missed, although there is no apraxia of single movements . . . (and it usually affects) tasks involving drawing or constructing and arranging blocks and objects" (Warrington, 1969). It is occasionally seen with left hemisphere lesions. The errors of construction tend to be qualitatively different depending on whether the lesion is left or right sided. Table 3.5 shows two diagrams (a greek cross and a cube) that the patient can be asked to draw. The value of his drawing a cross will be enhanced by telling him not to lift his pen off the paper while executing the drawing.

Dressing apraxia is basically an inability to dress oneself correctly. It is more specific for right-sided lesions and tends to be closely associated with constructional difficulties, though the latter is much more common. The patient cannot orientate himself correctly in relation to his clothes and may put his foot in his shirtsleeve, put his shirt on back to front, or put his clothes on in the wrong order, e.g. underpants over trousers.

Astereognosis is an agnosia in which there is a failure to recognise a familiar object by touch alone, though this is a simplified view of a complex phenomenon. It usually involves one hand and the lesion is usually in the contralateral parietal lobe. Less common forms of agnosia may be found and lesions of the left occipital lobe have been mainly implicated as the cause of colour agnosia and visual object agnosia. In the latter the patient is unable to name a familiar object, and also fails to recognise its significance, e.g. the colour red on a traffic light. Finger agnosia involves an inability to name and recognise fingers on both hands and it forms part of the Gerstmann syndrome. *Prosopagnosia is a relatively specific defect of the ability to recognise familiar faces* and it has tended to be associated with lesions of the posterior part of the right hemisphere (Lishman, 1978), but post mortem evidence indicates that there is usually bilateral inferomedial occipital lobe damage (Damasio *et al.*, 1982).

Table 3.5   Testing for apraxia and agnosia

TYPE OF DISORDER		COMMAND
IDEOMOTOR APRAXIA	Buccofacial	"Protrude tongue" "Blow out a match"
	Hand	"Wave good-bye" "Wind watch"
	Foot	"Tap on floor" "Kick a ball"

CONSTRUCTIONAL APRAXIA
(Visuospatial agnosia)

Examiner shows the patient a diagram   "Draw while looking
  e.g. Greek cross   at the diagram"

  e.g. Cube

ASTEREOGNOSIS

Examiner instructs the patient to close his eyes and then
  gives him an object, e.g. paper clip, coin, ring.   "Identify by touch"

3.6 PRIMITIVE REFLEXES

Primitive reflexes are believed to be those muscle reflexes that are found when there is a failure of the cerebral cortex to inhibit the subcortical centres controlling motor activity. They "are normally present during the early maturation of the central nervous system and they may reappear when the central nervous system has been altered by age and disease", according to Paulson and Gottlieb (1968). They are particularly found in the neurologically immature, in the elderly, and in patients with organic brain disease (OBD). However, some adults show reflexes of this type in the apparent absence of OBD (Jacobs and Gossman, 1980). I will mention three primitive reflexes that have been the subject of studies in different patient populations, and would suggest that it is useful for the clinician to attain some degree of experience and proficiency in eliciting a certain number of primitive reflexes. This will increase his awareness of the range of their variability and clinical significance.

The *grasp reflex* is produced by stroking the palm firmly in an outward direction and involves reflex grasping of the stimulating object. This reflex has been particularly associated with disease of the contralateral frontal lobe. Some patients may grasp the stimulating object because they think this is what is expected of them, and in such cases some distracting task can be used, and the test then repeated. The reflex is not invariably found in OBD, but if it is positive this is strong evidence for OBD, as false positives are rare (Jenkyn *et al.*, 1977; Koller *et al.*, 1982). One study found it to have a significant correlation with cognitive impairment in demented patients (Tweedy *et al.*, 1982). If a grasp reflex is present, a "magnetic apraxia" may also be found, in which the patient attempts to grasp any object he sees moving within his reach.

The *snout reflex* consists of a reflex protrusion of the lips in response to a tapping of the upper or lower lips. This reflex was elicited in 15% of the "normal" population in the 40 to 50 year age range, and this percentage increased to 33% in the 60 to 70 year age group (Jacobs and Gossman, 1980). Its value is unclear as it has been found to be one of the two primitive reflexes (the other being the grasp reflex) that correlate with the degree of cognitive impairment in demented patients (Tweedy *et al.*, 1982). However this finding was not confirmed by Jenkyn *et al.* (1977). Koller *et al.* (1982) found the presence of the reflex correlated with increasing age irrespective of whether cognitive impairment was present or not.

The *palmomental reflex* is produced by firm outward stroking of the thenar eminence which results in contraction of the ipsilateral mentalis muscle (the muscle which connects the lower incisor fossa to the skin of the chin). This is manifest externally by a lateralised puckering of the skin of the chin. The frequency with which this reflex is found in the "normal" population, depends on the strength of the stimulus (Reis, 1961). It has been found in 20% of a cognitively intact population aged between 20–30 years, and in this study its incidence progressively increased to 61% in cognitively intact 80 to 90-year-olds (Jacobs and Gossman, 1980), though it is more commonly found in those with OBD (Jenkyn *et al.*, 1977; Tweedy *et al.*, 1982).

It was such inconsistent findings that led Tweedy *et al.* (1982) to conclude that "cortical disinhibition signs appear to be manifestations of a process that proceeds independently of the disorders that result in dementia". In assessing the significance of these reflexes account should be taken of the type of reflex, the age of the patient, any other evidence for the presence of OBD, how pronounced the reflex is, and whether it can be consistently elicited on subsequent occasions. A poorly sustained palmomental reflex is a frequent finding in the "normal" population, but a definite grasp reflex correlates quite closely with cerebral disease. The value of the snout reflex appears to lie somewhere between the other two. The role played by factors such as ECT and drug treatment, in producing these reflexes in a particular case, can be evaluated by testing the patient on several occasions after the treatment has been discontinued, as well as taking into account the other variables.

The concept of neurological immaturity as a cause of these reflexes in the young has also been used by some to explain the presence of "soft neurological signs" in certain psychiatric patients. These signs will be mentioned further in the next section.

3.7 MINIMAL BRAIN DYSFUNCTION

The term *minimal brain dysfunction (MBD) is usually used to refer to a syndrome of hyperactivity, impulsiveness and attentional deficit*, sometimes referred to as Strauss's syndrome, after the author who initially related it to brain damage (Strauss and Lehtinen, 1947). Since then this concept has been extended by some authors to include other behavioural and neurological phenomena, some of which are listed in Tables 3.6 and 3.7 (Kaufman, 1981). The physical findings are sometimes referred to as "soft" neurological signs (SNS), because they do not have the clear clinical significance of "hard" signs such as an extensor plantar (Babinski) response. Kaufman (1981) suggests that the diagnosis of MBD should not be made when the patient is intellectually retarded.

Rutter (1978) has emphasised that for any disorder to have significance it must have more than just characteristic features, it must also have certain implications in terms of factors such as cause or prognosis. The findings which indicate MBD is a significant entity include, if one concentrates mainly on the components of Strauss's syndrome, the evidence for its genetic association with alcoholism, hysteria, and antisocial behaviour (Morrison and Stewart, 1973); its association with unsocialised aggressive behaviour, both in early life (Stewart *et al.*, 1980) and in adult life (Cantwell, 1979); the finding of a similar picture in children with unequivocal brain disease (Gross and Wilson, 1974); and its response to stimulant medication, which can significantly reduce the behavioural problems associated with MBD (Barkley, 1977).

However, the evidence against MBD being a valid clinical entity includes the poor intercorrelation between different methods of measuring hyperactivity, whether using the observation or questionnaire approach; the interrater variability (Nichols and Chen, 1980) and lack of consistency over time (McMahon and Greenberg, 1977), in the identification of SNS; the failure to statistically extract a "hyperactivity" factor when analysing such data (Rutter, 1982); the absence of SNS in children with unequivocal brain damage, and their presence in children with no evidence of brain damage (Rutter *et al.*, 1970); and the evidence that a beneficial response to stimulant treatment can be found in children suffering from other disorders (Sroufe, 1976), and even in normal

Table 3.6 Functional manifestations (history) of minimal brain dysfunction

LEARNING DISABILITIES

Perceptual difficulties: spatial relationships; arithmetic and other abstractions

Memory impairment

Dyslexia

Writing abnormalities: poor form, sloppiness; mirror writing

BEHAVIOURAL DISTURBANCES

Hyperactivity: purposeless, constant physical activity; persistence at home, neighbourhood, and school; (occasional underactivity)

Short attention span: inability to focus and maintain attention; easy distractability

Personality difficulties: emotional lability; impulsivity; aggressiveness; low frustration threshold; friendlessness

MOTOR DIFFICULTIES

Clumsiness in athletics; poor performance in fine motor tasks; speech abnormalities (dysarthria)

From D. M. Kaufman (1981) *Clinical Neurology for Psychiatrists* (New York: Grune and Stratton). Reproduced by permission.

Table 3.7 Physical findings (soft signs) of minimal brain dysfunction

REFLEX ALTERATIONS

Hyperactive deep tendon reflexes

Unsustained clonus

"ABNORMAL" MOVEMENTS

Choreiform

Mirror (synkinetic)

Associated

INCOORDINATION

Gross motor activities: skipping, hopping, throwing

Fine motor skills: buttoning, transferring; drawing, writing; general clumsiness

Speech impediments

Ocular movements

CONFUSION OF LEFT VERSUS RIGHT

Ambidexterity

Left-handedness

IMPAIRMENT OF SPECIAL SENSES

Poor visual acuity, diplopia

Deafness

From D. M. Kaufman (1981) *Clinical Neurology for Psychiatrists* (New York: Grune and Stratton). Reproduced by permission.

children (Rapoport *et al.*, 1980). In addition there is a substantial overlap between hyperactivity and conduct disordered behaviour (Stewart *et al.*, 1980), and it has been convincingly argued (Rutter, 1981) that what family studies indicate is that the inherited tendency is for antisocial, rather than hyperkinetic, behaviour.

There does appear to be a subgroup of children who show a pervasive hyperactivity in all situations, in contrast to those children with situational hyperactivity, e.g. seen only at school or at home. It is this pervasive group that has been found to be particularly prone to show evidence of cognitive impairment; a low non-verbal IQ; attentional deficits that remain when the child is reassessed after an interval; and a poorer prognosis, with their disordered behaviour persisting into adolescence (Campbell *et al.*, 1977; Roff *et al.*, 1972; Rutter, 1982). It seems likely that *many of the children diagnosed as hyperactive in the United States belong to the situational group, and would be diagnosed as conduct disordered in Britain* (Rutter, 1982). Such a difference in interpretation would explain the low frequency with which hyperactivity is diagnosed in British children who are referred to psychiatric clinics (about 1%), compared to a similar population in the United States (about 50%).

Clinically the patient's history may suggest that he has MBD. He may have required special tuition at school, or had difficulty in his interpersonal relationships due to impulsive aggressive behaviour. During the interview he may exhibit restlessness, inattentiveness, choreiform movements or abnormalities of speech. On examination he may be left handed. Reading, writing or constructional difficulties may be found. Impaired vision or hearing may be present.

One example of the kind of simple test that may prove useful in eliciting neurological "soft" signs, is the patient's skill at finger/thumb coordination. Using each hand in turn he is asked to touch the tip of each finger to his thumb, as fast as possible, and in sequence. He is told to repeat the sequence over and over again until told to stop. He should then be observed for clumsiness, synkinetic movements (associated movements of other muscles not necessary for performance of the task), mirror movements of the opposite hand, or motor impersistence (repeatedly stopping before being told to do so). These and similar tests can be easily and quickly evaluated and can be fitted into a standard neurological examination as a matter of routine. Some authors would include EEG abnormalities, usually involving immature patterns or non-specific changes, as part of the MBD syndrome (Kaufman, 1981).

"Soft" signs have been frequently found in patients with emotionally unstable character disorders, and schizophrenia (Quitkin *et al.*, 1976). It is difficult to control for the various possible factors contributing to the development of such signs, but they have been found in 65.5% of a series of schizophrenic patients before they received neuroleptic drugs (Rochford *et al.*, 1970).

Adults showing features of MBD in their history or on examination, sometimes respond atypically to stimulant drugs in the same way as hyperactive children tend to, i.e. they show a beneficial response with relaxation, a reduction in restlessness, and an improvement in mood and concentration. They may develop abnormal responses to other drugs, e.g. the neuroleptics and anti-depressants.

What is clear is that *MBD is not synonymous with brain damage*, and the features of the syndrome may persist into adult life. The variability in prognosis in different patients showing the feature of this disorder may well reflect the fact that MBD may be due to many different causes (Amado and Lustman, 1982).

3.8 HYSTERIA AND MALINGERING

Hysteria is a controversial topic and when the term is used in clinical psychiatry it usually either refers to certain behavioural traits (hysterical personality type) or a type of neurotic disorder produced by the mechanism of dissociation. *Dissociation primarily involves a " 'narrowing' of the field of consciousness, which serves an unconscious purpose and is accompanied or followed by a selective amnesia"* (ICD 9, 1978). The DSM III avoids using the term "hysterical" and refers to the histrionic personality disorder. It includes the hysterical neuroses in the category of Dissociative disorders (psychogenic amnesia, psychogenic fugue, multiple personality, depersonalisation, and somatoform disorders or hysterical conversion). Though the DSM III includes depersonalisation in the former category, it is a disorder that is found in many different conditions and as it does not involve the impairment of memory that is typically found with hysterical dissociation, it is considered elsewhere (Section 13.3). This "typical" memory impairment specifically involves emotionally disturbing events *(psychogenic amnesia)* and may be associated with wandering behaviour *(psychogenic fugue)*, with or without the patient assuming a new identity during the fugue. Rarely the disorder may involve the patient assuming one or more different personalities at different times *(multiple personality)*.

The *hysterical personality* traits involve behaviour that is excessively dramatic and immature, emotional lability, and an inability to form consistent, mature, interpersonal relationships. Sexual difficulties are usually present, most commonly frigidity (Merskey and Trimble, 1979). It is important not only to identify the personality disorder, but also to make allowances for the way it may colour the features of other complicating psychiatric disorders, e.g. depression may be masked because of the patient's emotional superficiality, or he may react to organic disease in a misleadingly histrionic manner (Trimble and Grant, 1982). A patient with a histrionic personality appears to be at an increased risk of developing a hysterical conversion disorder, so do those with passive–immature dependent personalities, but the majority of patients with these disorders do not have a premorbid histrionic personality type (Merskey and Trimble, 1979).

Symptoms and signs are regarded as *hysterical conversion phenomena* if they *are involuntarily produced as a result of a psychological conflict or need*. They involve the voluntary nervous system in contrast to psychosomatic disorders which, though they can also result from psychological stress, tend to involve the autonomic nervous system. In recent years the more obvious conversion phenomena, such as aphonia, are less often seen, and less clear cut disorders that are more difficult to objectively evaluate, such as backache, are now more common. When the disability specifically impairs the patient's ability to continue his normal work, and the work involves fine coordinated movements of the hands, the term "occupational neurosis" has been used to describe it (Bannister, 1973).

Often an element of doubt remains as to the true nature of the illness and this tempts the physician to overinvestigate such patients. This situation is further complicated when organic disease coexists with a conversion disorder, and this association is not uncommon. It was found in 61 of 89 neurological patients who had been diagnosed as suffering from hysterical conversion disorders in Merskey and Buhrich's study (1975). Slater and Glithero (1965) found neurological disease eventually became evident in 22 of 66 neurological patients originally given the diagnosis of hysteria (with no concurrent organic diagnosis), over an 8-year follow-up period. Such evidence supports those physicians who feel that the diagnosis of hysteria is a cloak for ignorance.

To avoid such errors Merskey (1979) recommends that certain features should be looked for before making a diagnosis of hysteria, emphasising that it should be a diagnosis based on positive findings and not one made just by the exclusion of organic disorders. Four of Merskey's cardinal features of hysteria are as follows:

1. The presence of a typical dissociative disorder, e.g. psychogenic amnesia.
2. Evidence of a precipitating psychological event.
3. The absence of any evidence for an organic cause.
4. The presence of definite signs of functional illness, e.g. agonist and antagonist muscle contraction, when attempting to move a paralysed limb.

Some psychological stress typically precedes the development of a hysterical disorder, but it may not be obvious. Though a causative stress should be looked for, its absence need not prevent a diagnosis of hysteria being made as a working hypothesis on which a trial of treatment can be based.

The presence of some form of "gain" is implicit in the previous definition of hysterical conversion, but as this gain is unconscious it may be difficult to identify and can be a misleading sign. Some degree of gain may appear to be present in disorders that are entirely organic in origin. Two types of gain are recognised. Firstly, there is *primary gain, where the conversion disorder acts as a means of keeping the precipitating psychological stress out of conscious awareness*. This gain has a symbolic value which is a representation of and, to a certain degree, a solution to the underlying psychological conflict (DSM III, 1980). Secondly, there is *secondary gain*, which does not have the same symbolic value and merely *provides an escape from a situation the patient wishes to avoid*.

La belle indifférence may or may not be present. It refers to *an attitude of unconcern exhibited by the patient which, in the physician's opinion, is inappropriate in the light of the apparent seriousness of the illness.* As people can react in different ways to any particular disorder, this sign tells the doctor more about the patient's way of reacting to illness, than the cause of the illness. In fact in one study, far from being indifferent, patients showing la belle indifférence were found to be exhibiting high levels of autonomic activity, when their galvanic skin responses were examined (Lader and Sartorius, 1968).

In Table 3.8 the author lists certain features that are characteristically found on examination of the patient with neurological abnormalities that are psychological (i.e. hysteria or malingering) in origin. These features will help in separating what is psychogenic from what is organic in origin. For a detailed and erudite discussion of this aspect of the neurological examination the reader is referred to De Jong (1970).

The psychogenic abnormality will conform to the patient's view of how the body works and will often vary from that which would be expected in an organic disorder. This may be obviously naive, e.g. sensory loss involving the ventral aspect of the trunk only. In the classical conversion sign the impairment will have a symbolic quality, e.g. loss of vision as a result of witnessing an emotionally traumatic event. Problems arise when the patient has had medical experience and has a sophisticated knowledge of the nervous system and its disorders.

Table 3.8 Features indicating the psychological aetiology of physical "signs"

1. Conforms to the patient's knowledge of anatomy.
2. Symbolically represents the underlying psychological conflict and offers escape from the conflict.
3. Absent or less incapacitating, when the patient is not being examined.
4. They are incompatible with an organic disorder.
5. Day to day variation in their type and severity.
6. Can be altered by suggestion.
7. Can be removed by the use of intravenous amytal or hypnosis.

When the patient is not being formally examined and he is unaware he is being observed, he may be seen to function in a manner incompatible with his claimed disability. This is more characteristic of malingering. If a spouse, or some other cohabitee, is tactfully questioned, a history of such variable behaviour may be elicited, e.g. a long suffering wife may be only too aware that her husband is more than capable of using his paralysed arm when it suits him.

During the neurological examination an emphasis should be laid on those objective findings which cannot be voluntarily controlled and are incompatible with an organic deficit, e.g. normal tendon reflexes in an apparently immobile flaccid arm, or the ability to carry out finger-thumb opposition smoothly and efficiently with the eyes closed, despite an apparent loss of all sensation in the hand.

The neurological signs will tend to vary in distribution and quality, from day to day, and repeated examinations will be necessary to reveal this. It may be possible to influence the signs by suggestion. On examining part of the body where sensation is clearly normal, the physician might assume a perplexed expression and say "I would have expected numbness here". Re-examination later may reveal that loss of sensation has appeared in this area!

Psychogenic deficits may not be clear cut and weakness will be present rather than total paresis. This limits the value of many tests but I will mention three signs of use in identifying hysterical conversion phenomena, Mannhoph's, Hoover's, and the "Yes–No" sign (De Jong, 1970). The *"Yes–No" sign* is for the very naive patient and involves asking for a "yes" or "no" response when testing for loss of sensation: a "no response indicating that he cannot feel the examiner's touch, despite being tested with his eyes closed and with irregular time intervals between the applications of the stimulus! *Mannhoph's sign* depends on the response of the patient's autonomic nervous system when a painful stimulus is applied to an area where anaesthesia is claimed. Perception of the pain is indicated by an increase in the pulse rate of over 10 beats/minute. *Hoover's sign* can be used in assessing a unilateral leg weakness that is psychogenic in origin. When someone attempts to lift a leg that is weak due to organic disease, it is usual for him to press down with the contralateral heel. The examiner places his hand under the heel of the contralateral leg and the absence of this pressure, when the patient "attempts" to lift the "weak" leg, is Hoover's sign, and indicates that he is not really trying to lift the leg.

Table 3.9   Comparison of hysterical neurosis, malingering and Munchausen's syndrome

	HYSTERICAL NEUROSIS	MALINGERING	MUNCHAUSEN'S SYNDROME
SEX PREDOMINANTLY AFFECTED	F	M	M
PRECEDING STRESS	+	+	−
PREMORBID PERSONALITY	Passive-dependent-immature, or histrionic	Often maladjusted	Grossly disturbed
CONSCIOUS MOTIVATION	−	+	+ (Element of compulsion)
GAIN	Avoidance and/or solution of psychological conflict	Material — usually financial	Less obvious, involves assumption of the patient role and deception of medical staff
SELF-INJURY	−	−	+
AFFECT	Anxious or la belle indifférence	Defensive and angry	Defensive and angry

Malingering refers to the conscious production of symptoms or signs in order to mimic physical illness. In some cases this is for obvious gain (often financial), but in others the gain may be less obvious. Malingering is sometimes present in association with hysterical phenomena but *it is difficult to be sure to what extent a behaviour is conscious or unconscious, unless the patient is caught in the act of "faking" or admits to it.* However, hysteria is not a disease entity but a behaviour that can be found in many neuropsychiatric settings, and often coexists with malingering behaviour. Table 3.9 compares the features of disorders resulting from the voluntary and involuntary production of symptoms. There are different types of hysterical disorders, and at one extreme is the premorbidly stable well-adjusted person who develops a conversion disorder in response to stress. At the other extreme are conditions such as *Briquet's hysteria.* This disorder is mainly found in young women and involves a chronic fluctuating illness with somatic complaints involving many different body systems, leading to the patient "shopping around" among different doctors in different specialities, obtaining numerous medications and sometimes being subjected to repeated surgery. This disorder usually starts in adolescence, occurs mainly in females, has a poor prognosis, and is genetically associated with alcoholism and psychopathy (Cloninger and Guze, 1975). It has been estimated to be present in 2% of a consecutive series of female patients undergoing medical investigation (Trimble, 1981a).

Briquet's hysteria overlaps to a degree with *hypochondriasis, "a marked fear of the occurrence of physical disease or (a) markedly recurring belief that they have got a disease".* Both types of patient are excessively concerned with their bodily health and are resistant to doctors' reassurances that they are physically well. Merskey (1979) used the term hysterical hypochondriasis to describe those patients who, in addition to being hypochondrical, showed motor conversion symptoms and appeared to exhibit a certain degree of satisfaction, despite their physical problems. He was in effect describing many of the features of Briquet's hysteria. Unlike other hypochondriacal patients they did not consistently show the characteristic fear of physical disease found in hypochondriasis.

Munchhausen's syndrome is an unusual disorder, involving malingering, and found in patients who are severely disturbed personalities and who repeatedly feign illness in order to gain admission to hospital. Their "gain" is not obvious and appears to involve a compulsive need to deceive medical staff. The feigning behaviour may involve a degree of self-mutilation, e.g. swallowing razor blades to produce haematemesis. These patients will often undergo surgery and other unpleasant procedures as part of their deception. The more mundane malingerer who has a more concrete objective in producing his symptoms and is trying to gain some advantage for himself, will usually try and avoid self-injury and unpleasant medical procedures. The DSM III discriminates between malingering, the voluntary production of symptoms or signs directed towards a clear goal, and factitious disorders, where the goal is less clear, e.g. deception of the medical staff.

Certain neurological conditions may superficially resemble psychogenic disorders. These include, among others, organic brain disease producing an inappropriate affect (dysprosody), and denial of illness (anosognosia). Diagnostic problems may arise with neurological disorders that pursue an episodic course with remissions and exacerbations, e.g. multiple sclerosis, and acute intermittent porphyria.

CHAPTER 4

Psychological Testing and Brain–Behaviour Relationships

4.1 INTRODUCTION

"Neuropsychology is a field of study that proposes a model relating brain dysfunction/damage to observable empirically described behavioural deficits" (Crockett *et al.*, 1981). The patient's behaviour is evaluated by a process that involves the use of standardised neuropsychological tests. When the test results are compared with the results of other methods of investigation there may be differences in the conclusions they suggest, such as the site of a cerebral lesion. This is because the test behaviour correlates to a variable and often unpredictable degree with information provided by procedures which evaluate other aspects of nervous system function, such as the EEG (the electrical activity of the brain) and the CAT head scanner (gross brain structure). Also, test performance is prone to be affected by constantly changing variables, such as the patient's affective state, which can influence the results in different ways at different times.

Because of an increasing awareness of the alterations in brain structure and function that can accompany psychiatric disorders, partly due to the advent of new techniques such as computerised (CAT) and position emission tomography (PETT) scanning, certain theories on brain–behaviour relationships will also be discussed and the first half of the chapter will be concerned with this area. There are a wide variety of test procedures currently in use in neuropsychology and the author will concentrate discussion in the second half, on the Halstead–Reitan Neuropsychological Test Battery and the Wechsler Adult Intelligence Scale (WAIS), with the intention of helping the doctor understand and interpret neuropsychological test results. The WAIS is not a specialised neuropsychological test but is probably the commonest test of intelligence used in adults, and it is advisable for the clinical psychiatrist to have a working knowledge about it. Also the effects of brain disorders on the WAIS subtests will be used to illustrate certain neuropsychological principles. For more detailed information on neuropsychology and the test procedures involved, the reader is referred to Lezak (1976), Walsh (1978), and Filskov and Boll (1981).

The neuropsychological examination can involve using a standardised battery of tests such as the Halstead–Reitan battery or the Luria–Nebraska battery, or by using tests that are tailored to the clinical problem involved. These approaches may be combined and the initial results obtained on a basic set of tests can be used to indicate if further testing is needed, and if so, what specific tests should be used.

When a patient is given a particular psychological test he may reach his goal by a number of routes or, conversely, he may fail for a number of reasons. Because of this, his interaction with the psychotechnician, the manner of his performance, the strategies used and his response to failure or success, must all be noted. This information may increase the clinical value of his test results.

4.2 BRAIN–BEHAVIOUR RELATIONSHIPS

To facilitate the understanding of the varieties of abnormal behaviour that may develop in association with damage localised to different areas of the brain, they will be discussed in the light of some of the current views on brain–behaviour relationships. It should be emphasised that the brain functions as an integrated whole, and any separation of function that is described, should be regarded as relative rather than absolute.

The dominant hemisphere of the brain is primarily concerned with the production and comprehension of verbal language, logical and analytical thinking, and skilled movements. Disease of this hemisphere, usually the left, characteristically results in the aphasias and the apraxias. In the light of current research on the role of the right hemisphere (see below), it is necessary to be more specific about the role of the left hemisphere in controlling speech. It is concerned primarily with the semantic (meaning) and syntactic (grammatical structure) aspects of *propositional speech*, that is to say *speech which makes a specific statement* (Ross, 1981). The term apraxia is a loose one which covers a wide spectrum of disorders, some of which may be the result of damage to the non-dominant hemisphere.

The non-dominant hemisphere is primarily concerned with visuo-spatial skills and appears to have a dominant role in attention to, and awareness of the body and its surrounding space. The attentional role mainly involves the contralateral side of the body and space (Watson *et al.*, 1981). Lesions of this side of the brain classically produce the agnosias. Recent evidence indicates that this side of the brain also has an important role in the perception of and the communication of affect by means of non-verbal behaviour and prosodic variations in speech (Heilman *et al.*, 1975; Ross, 1981; Tucker *et al.*, 1977). Variations of prosody (rhythm, melody, etc.) can communicate emotional meaning, irrespective of the actual words used. Non-verbal behaviour, involving body posture and facial expression, is also a potent means of communicating emotion.

The cortex of the brain is the most highly specialised part of the central nervous system and it integrates, refines and coordinates motor and sensory functions,

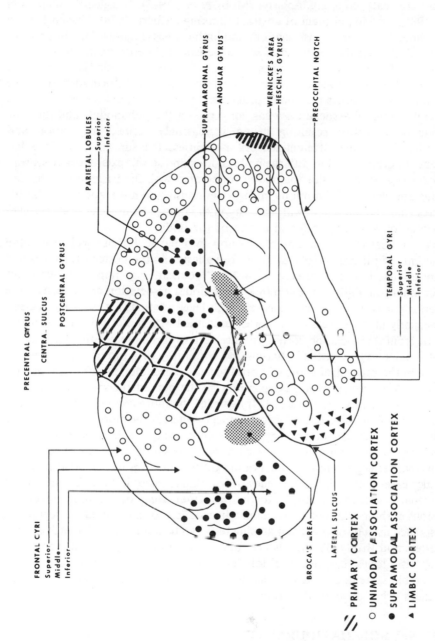

Figure 4.1 Diagram of dominant cerebral hemisphere

PARIETAL LOBULES
Superior
Inferior

SUPRAMARGINAL GYRUS
ANGULAR GYRUS

WERNICKE'S AREA
HESCHL'S GYRUS

PREOCCIPITAL NOTCH

PRECENTRAL GYRUS
CENTRAL SULCUS
POSTCENTRAL GYRUS

TEMPORAL GYRI
Superior
Middle
Inferior

FRONTAL GYRI
Superior
Middle
Inferior

BROCA'S AREA

LATERAL SULCUS

⫽ PRIMARY CORTEX

○ UNIMODAL ASSOCIATION CORTEX

● SUPRAMODAL ASSOCIATION CORTEX

▲ LIMBIC CORTEX

at levels of varying complexity. However, subcortical disease can, by interrupting the connections between the cortex and subcortical structures, produce deficits of a "cortical" type, e.g. aphasia (Mohr *et al.*, 1975), "neglect" (Watson *et al.*, 1981), and impairment of abstract thinking (Albert, 1978). The cortex can be divided into primary, association, and limbic areas (Figure 4.1). The primary cortex deals with the reception of somatosensory afferents (postcentral gyrus), auditory afferents (Heschl's gyrus), visual afferents (calcarine fissure region), and the initiation of motor efferents (precentral gyrus). Information from the primary sensory areas is initially processed by the unimodal cortex, and then several unimodal association areas converge on the polymodal, and then the supramodal cortex, resulting in an increasingly refined integration and coordination of the different sensory modalities. The supramodal cortex has extensive communication with the limbic cortex and so this exteroceptive sensory information from outside the body is integrated with the basic drives (sexual, eating and drinking), emotions, memory engrams and motivation. The limbic cortex has connections with the hypothalamus, from which it receives information about the internal milieu of the body.

The clinical manifestations of a lesion in a particular site will reflect the functions of the area involved. Therefore a lesion in the postcentral gyrus will manifest itself as a relatively "low level" deficit, e.g. impaired two-point discrimination ability. A lesion in a supramodal association area, such as the inferior parietal lobule, can cause a "high level" deficit, e.g. sensory neglect.

Similarly in those areas of the cortex concerned with motor behaviour-damage to the frontal association cortex will interfere with the more refined aspects of motor behaviour, e.g. the initiation and continuity of a motor act, whereas a lesion in the precentral gyrus will produce a localised deficit in muscle power, the muscle group(s) involved depending on the part of the gyrus affected. In keeping with this view, Luria (1973) regarded the more complex motor deficits as resulting from prefrontal cortical damage, whereas the more mundane motor behaviours, such as motor dexterity, were impaired in premotor cortical lesions.

When lesions occur in areas where cerebral lobes adjoin, there will be clinical signs that reflect an impaired integration of the functions of the adjacent lobes. In such cases there will be a tendency for overlap to occur in the different clinical syndromes specifically related to the particular areas of the brain involved. Lesions in these adjacent areas can produce deficits of cross-modal integration. Tests such as auditory–visual matching tests can be used to identify such deficits (Butters and Brody, 1968). Also certain circuits in the brain are not confined to specific lobes, e.g. temporal lobe epilepsy usually results from a lesion in the limbic system, a system which is not confined to the temporal lobe but includes other areas of the brain, such as the frontal lobe.

4.3 NEUROBEHAVIOURAL CONSEQUENCES OF FRONTAL LOBE DISEASE

Phylogenetically, the frontal lobes are the most recently developed part of the nervous system, and this is reflected in the subtlety of the clinical consequences of lesions in this area of the brain. Such lesions commonly produce changes in cognition and/or personality (Stuss and Benson, 1982). Personality change may be the only clinical sign, particularly if the orbitofrontal part of the lobe is involved. Lesions in the dorsolateral part of the lobe tend to produce cognitive deficits as well, but even then they may have no obvious effect on intellectual functioning as assessed by standard psychological tests, such as the WAIS. *The personality change associated with orbitofrontal lesions has been described as being of the "pseudopsychopathic" type, and the "pseudo-depressed" type is associated with dorsolateral lesions*, though it is more common to see elements of both types following damage to the frontal lobes (Blumer and Benson, 1975).

The frontal lobe is concerned with the control of different levels of motor behaviour (including speech). Motor activity is affected by lesions of the precentral gyrus (primary motor area), premotor area (just anterior to the primary area), and the dorsolateral part of the frontal lobe. The different functions of these areas have been clarified by investigation of patients with localised lesions caused by surgery. Lesions in the dorsolateral area have been produced by surgery for epilepsy (Stuss and Benson, 1982), and in the orbitofrontal area by leucotomy surgery for psychiatric disorders (Kelly, 1976).

Overlap is seen in the cognitive deficits associated with lesions in these two areas, and the interference effect and impaired sorting behaviour, especially, appear to be associated with lesions in either area (Stuss and Benson, 1982). *Interference refers to the inability to select appropriate information from the memory store due to interference from inappropriate memories. Sorting behaviour involves the ability to make conceptual shifts.* The latter can be assessed by tests such as the *Wisconsin Card Sorting Test*, in which the patient is given four stimulus cards which are laid out in front of him. Each card is in some way different from the others. He is then given a series of cards and asked to match each to whichever of the stimulus cards he thinks is conceptually similar. The examiner changes the particular concept he is using, e.g. shape, colour, etc., once the subject has correctly identified it (the examiner uses "yes" or "no" comments only, to indicate whether the correct concept is being used). The number of correct responses within the time limit will indicate the degree of conceptual flexibility. However, the mechanisms by which these deficits arise may differ according to which part of the frontal lobe is involved (Drew, 1974).

Table 4.1 shows the different disorders that can result from impairment of frontal lobe function. Dysfunction of the primary motor cortex will cause *upper motor neurone weakness*, and if this involves the contralateral hand it will cause impairment in the rate of finger tapping. Though this sign is of limited value in localisation, other than indicating the side of the lesion (Reitan, 1964). An early clinical sign in some frontal lobe tumours is a contralateral upper motor neurone (UMN) type of facial weakness that is only seen with reflex facial movements, e.g. smiling.

Buccolinguo–facial apraxia (inability to blow out a match to command) is commonly associated with motor aphasia and may be an important sign in aphemia. *In aphemia the patient can read and write without difficulty, but is mute.* He can communicate by writing (this is an uncommon type of aphasia,

Table 4.1 Neurobehavioural consequences of frontal lobe disease

LEFT HEMISPHERE	EITHER/BOTH HEMISPHERES	RIGHT HEMISPHERE

	Contralateral
	  upper motor neurone weakness,
	  motor slowing,
	  voluntary conjugate gaze impairment,
	  limb-kinetic apraxia	

	Perseveration Impersistence Verbal/action separation Interference effect Impaired sorting	
	Personality change	
	?Amnesia	
Verbal —————	Decreased fluency —————————	Non-verbal
Motor aphasia —— Aphemia	Impaired language—————————	Aprosody
Buccolinguo- facial apraxia		?Motor inattention

and particularly unusual as the patient may carry a notebook around with him in order to communicate) but, apart from the apraxia and a transient right hemiparesis at the onset, may have no neurological signs (Benson, 1979). It is due to a lesion undercutting Broca's area.

With lesions further forward more subtle effects on motor behaviour are seen, such as aprosody. A more specific deficit of *motor aprosody*, analogous to motor aphasia, has been linked to lesions of the right frontal lobe (Ross, 1981).

Anterior to the precentral gyrus is the frontal eye field area. An epileptic discharge in this area may produce deviation of the eyes to the opposite side. A lesion here will impair voluntary gaze to the opposite side of the body and may cause a failure of inhibition of visual fixation (the *Doll's Head Eye phenomenon*). The inability to voluntarily look laterally, which probably has a survival value in less developed primates, is controlled by this area of the brain. However, impairment of voluntary conjugate lateral gaze is more commonly seen in the acute stages of lesions in the internal capsule interrupting the frontal–mid-brain connections, but recovery is usual (Brodal, 1969). Though unable to look voluntarily to the contralateral side, if the patient is asked to look at a slow-moving object his eyes will move with the object even if it moves to the contralateral side: this is because a reflex movement of the eyes is involved. This deficit demonstrates the differential effects on voluntary and involuntary (reflex or emotional) motor behaviour, that can result from a cerebral lesion, and may cause a degree of clinical confusion. This is especially true when the involuntary ability persists while the voluntary ability is lost, giving the impression that the patient is in "control" of his disability. The reverse impairment is seen with lesions of the occipital eye fields, where voluntary conjugate eye movements remain intact, but involuntary movements are impaired. However, in such cases there are usually visual field or other defects also present.

Impaired fluency of motor behaviour can involve speech, writing or non-verbal behaviour. Verbal fluency can be tested by asking the patient to say, in a limited period of time, as many different words as he can beginning with a certain letter. Using such a test, Perret (1974) found that the performance of patients with left frontal lesions was significantly inferior to that of patients with lesions in the right frontal lobe or elsewhere in the brain. All his patients with organic brain disease (OBD) performed worse than a healthy control group. Using words beginning with the letter S, normal controls have been found to produce an average of 14 words/minute (Cutting, 1978b). In Cutting's study male chronic alcoholics, who are prone to develop frontal lobe damage (Lishman, 1981), averaged 7 words/minute. This test may also reveal impersistence or perseveration. Fluency of production of drawings may also be impaired, but this appears to be mainly seen with right frontal lesions (Jones-Gotman and Milner, 1977).

Flexibility of motor behaviour is often impaired and this can be tested in two ways, one involving writing and the other involving hand positions. To test the former the patient can be asked to write a connected sequence of alternating characters, such as *02 02* (Luria and Homskaya, 1964). The impaired patient is unable to continue changing the form of the letters he writes and begins to make errors and perseverate, repeating one letter over and over again. One of the author's patients, with right frontotemporal damage due to a subarachnoid haemorrhage, performed this test normally, but in her history she described a tendency to "make extra loops" in her letters when she was tired and trying to write. An example of this phenomenon in writing is shown in Figure 4.2, which demonstrates perseveration of o's, r's, etc.

Repetitive hand positions can be used to test flexibility of motor behaviour. In one test the patient is asked to strike on the table with the flat of his hand, the edge of his hand, and his fist, in "sequence". Some patients who make errors in hand positioning are still able to correctly name the hand positions in sequence (thus saying "palm, edge, fist") at the same time. This demonstrates the phenomenon of *"verbal/action separation"*, whereby the patient understands the errors he is making and can say what he should be doing, but is unable to stop his incorrect motor behaviour. This can be understood as a disorganization of motor activity which is dependant on the participation of speech for its control (Luria, 1973), and is particularly associated with left sided lesions. In some patients verbalising what they should be doing may improve their motor performance, and this effect has been associated with lesions in the posterior part of the frontal lobe, in contrast to the more anterior lesions where the improvement is not seen (Luria and Homskaya, 1964).

Whereas the patient can continue to verbalise correctly he may cease the accompanying motor behaviour before being requested to do so. Such motor

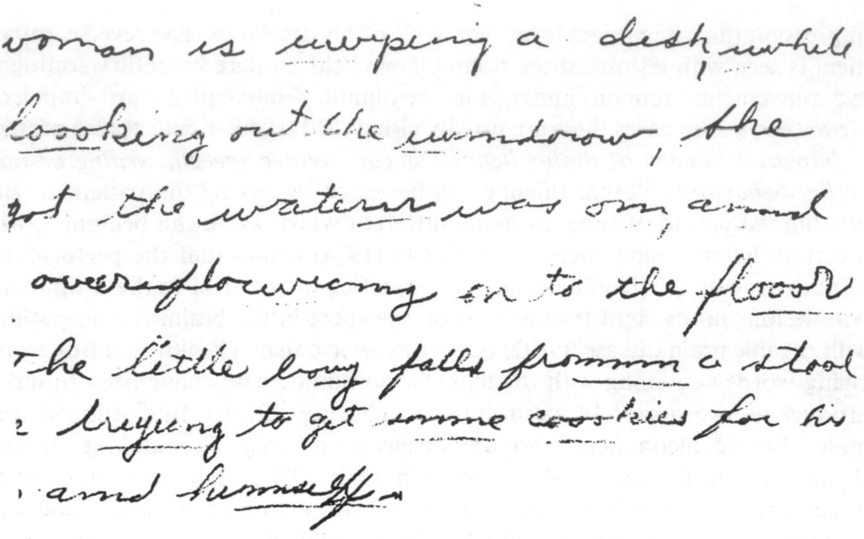

Figure 4.2 Perseveration in writing. From Benson (1979); reproduced by permission of Churchill Livingstone Inc.

impersistence may obstruct the examination of the patient, as the physician must constantly repeat his instructions. This lack of flexibility and associated perseveration may be seen at the cognitive level and be revealed in tests such as the Picture Arrangement, Block Design and Digit Symbol WAIS subtests, and the Wisconsin Card Sorting test.

Damage to the frontal lobe has been associated with *impairment of abstract thinking, memory and intellectual ability*. Whether or not abstract thinking is impaired is not clear. There is some controversy over what abstract thinking involves and how to test for it, and Stuss and Benson (1982) reviewed the evidence relating it to frontal lobe damage. They conclude that the basic ability to abstract may not be affected, but that it may appear to be so because of cognitive deficits such as an inability to describe abstract thought and a lack of flexibility in changing mental sets. Hecaen and Albert (1975) suggested that the memory impairment seen in patients with frontal lobe damage is more apparent than real, in effect a *"pseudo-dysmnesia"* or *forgetting to remember*, which is presumably due to factors such as interference and impaired motivation. Orbitofrontal lesions have no significant effect on standard tests of intelligence, and dorsolateral lesions do so only on occasions (Girgis, 1971; Stuss and Benson, 1982).

4.4 NEUROBEHAVIOURAL CONSEQUENCES OF PARIETAL LOBE DISEASE

The functions of the parietal lobe are varied and complex. It has a major role receiving somatosensory information from the rest of the body and processing it, integrating the various sensory modalities required for different functions. It also evaluates the spatial relationships between the body and objects in external space, and between objects in external space. There is a close functional relationship between the parietal and occipital lobes of the brain. Clinical signs of parietal lobe disease are listed in Table 4.2. It should be noted that the experience of pain is not perceived at the cortical level.

Table 4.2   Neurobehavioural consequences of parietal lobe disease

LEFT HEMISPHERE	EITHER/BOTH HEMISPHERES	RIGHT HEMISPHERE
	Contralateral lower quadrantanopsia	
	Impaired light touch perception and localisation, two-point discrimination, perception of position sense and passive movement	
	Spatial disorientation	
Motor ———————— (ideomotor or ideational)	Apraxia ————————————	Constructional Dressing
Sensory aphasia ———— Agraphia Alexia Acalculia (tested verbally)	Impaired language ————	Aprosody
	Asterognosis	
	Finger agnosia Right-left disorientation	
	Sensory inattention	
		Anosognosia

The post-central gyrus receives sensory afferents via the thalamus, and lesions in this cortical area result in a failure to appreciate and localise light touch, failure to perceive two point discrimination, and an inability to perceive posture and passive movement. These signs may be clinically inconsistent and difficult to elicit reliably.

If the patient closes his eyes and stretches out his arms horizontally, the arm contralateral to the damaged hemisphere may tend to drift. This phenomenon of *"parietal drift"* may be a result of impaired postural sense but is not a finding confined to lesions of the postcentral gyrus or the parietal lobe, and it may be seen as a result of lesions elsewhere in the hemisphere, e.g. as a result of limb weakness.

A particularly interesting sign seen in parietal lobe disease is *anosognosia* or *denial of illness*. This is seen, for example, when the patient with a left hemiparesis denies or appears to be unaware of his disability, and may produce a false explanation for why he is unable to effectively use the weak part of his body. Parietal lesions may cause the patient to ignore (or neglect) exteroceptive sensory information from his body and environment. This neglect may involve the contralateral side of the visual field (unilateral spatial neglect) and may affect his ability to read and write. Figure 4.3 shows an example of this phenomenon in a sample of writing from a patient with a right parietal lesion. Spatial neglect is shown by the enlarging left margin and the upward slant of the writing.

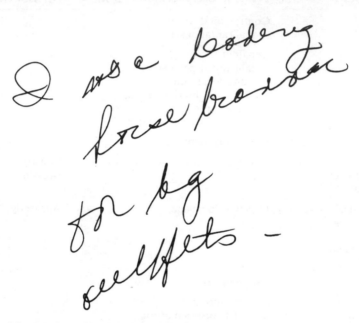

Figure 4.3 **Neglect of the left spatial field in writing. From Benson (1979); reproduced by permission of Churchill Livingstone Inc.**

Watson *et al.* (1981) proposed a functional model to explain the phenomenon of neglect and the pathological and clinical features that have been associated with it (see Figure 4.4). This model will now be considered, as it helps in the understanding of certain aspects of brain function and the possible mechanism by which anosognosia develops. It shows the exteroceptive sensory input (ESI) passing via the thalamus to the postcentral gyrus, and then to the association cortex, including the inferior parietal lobule. Sensory input also passes to the mid-brain reticular formation, which maintains tonic arousal via its extensive connections with the cerebral cortex, and also acts to modulate sensory input through its connections with the thalamus.

The inferior parietal lobule (IPL), the posterior cingulate gyrus (PCG), and the prefrontal area (PFA) including the superior temporal sulcus, all form an

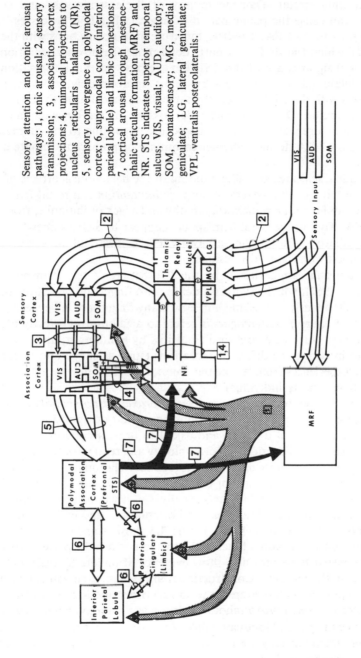

Sensory attention and tonic arousal pathways: 1, tonic arousal; 2, sensory transmission; 3, association cortex projections; 4, unimodal projections to nucleus reticularis thalami (NR); 5, sensory convergence to polymodal cortex; 6, supramodal cortex (inferior parietal lobule) and limbic connections; 7, cortical arousal through mesencephalic reticular formation (MRF) and NR. STS indicates superior temporal sulcus; VIS, visual; AUD, auditory; SOM, somatosensory; MG, medial geniculate; LG, lateral geniculate; VPL, ventralis posterolateralis.

Figure 4.4 Sensory attention and tonic-arousal pathways. From R. T. Watson et al. (1981). Arch. Neurol., 38, 501–506. © 1981 American Medical Association; reproduced by permission

interconnecting circuit. Damage to any of these structures, and even the thalamus, can cause the phenomenon of neglect. The IPL processes ESI and then passses it to the PFA. The IPL, by virtue of its connections with the limbic system, of which the PCG is a part, determines the novelty, emotional and motivational significance of the ESI. On the basis of this information it can then modulate the level of sensory input appropriately, by virtue of its connections with the PFA, which has a feedback mechanism to the mid-brain and the thalamus. On this model it is possible to see by what mechanism habituation to a repeated stimulus can occur. According to the characteristics of the ESI the PFA decides whether to initiate or prepare to initiate a motor response.

This model facilitates an understanding of the behavioural effects of lesions in different parts of this system. A *sensory inattention* can result from lesions of the IPL, and a *motor inattention*, apathy and a lack of initiative, from lesions of the PFA. The two cerebral hemispheres appear to differ somewhat in their roles as mediators of attention and awareness, neglect and anosognosia being more common with right sided lesions.

Finger agnosia can be tested by the "In-between" test (Kinsbourne and Warrington, 1962), which involves touching two fingers on one of the patient's hands simultaneously and asking him how many fingers are in between (his eyes are closed of course). *Astereognosis* refers to a failure to correctly identify a familiar object (such as a coin or a ring) just by handling it, and indicates an inabilty to integrate the different sensations (such as shape and texture) that the patient experiences from feeling the object, though he may be able to describe each of these aspects individually.

Qualitative differences in *constructional apraxia (visuo-spatial agnosia)* may be seen according to whether the lesion is on the left or right side of the brain. If the patient is shown a design and asked to draw a copy of it, the patient with a left parietal lobe lesion will draw slowly and tend to produce a coherent, correctly orientated drawing, with the spatial relations of the parts being preserved, but with an absence of detail. The patient with a right-sided lesion will tend to produce a drawing energetically, but it will be grossly disorganised with impairment of spatial relations and orientation, and with the addition of incorrect lines (Warrington, 1969). Figure 4.5 shows some of these differences in construction using Koh's blocks. When there is a right parietal lesion, the patient's constructions may also show evidence of unilateral neglect involving the details on the left side. Constructional apraxia is often associated with an inability to put one's clothes on in the correct order and in the correct manner, the so-called *dressing apraxia*, though this is a less common phenomenon.

Lesions of the parietal lobe cause different cognitive deficits that overlap with each other and are usually not found as isolated phenomena. These *"disorders of spatial orientation"* (Walsh, 1978) include an impairment in the patient's ability to recall the arrangement of the constituent parts of a familiar area (topographical disorientation), e.g. his home or country (geographical disorientation). Such deficits can be tested for by asking the patient to draw

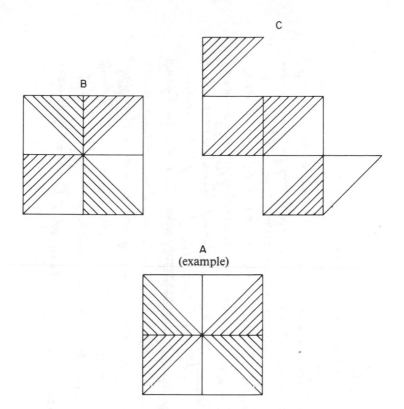

Figure 4.5   Constructional apraxia with left (B) and right (C) parietal lobe lesions

a simple map of his house or country, and mark on it the position of the most important areas.

The patient may be unable to draw or write down the details of familiar routes, or, if he can do this, he may nevertheless get lost in familiar surroundings. This emphasises the difficulty of identifying the fundamental deficits that underly such clinical phenomena. Other factors that may contribute to and confuse the clinical picture include visual inattention (visual cues on the left side of visual space being ignored) and memory impairment.

The patient's ability to perceive the relative spatial relationships between objects, or between the patient and objects in his visual field, may be impaired. Though such an impairment may be found in association with topographical disorientation, such an interrelationship is not essential (Gilliatt and Pratt, 1952). De Renzi and Faglioni (1967) devised a simple test to evaluate the patient's ability to orientate objects in relation to each other. The test involves the patient being shown a sheet of paper with a number of crosses drawn on it, which he then has to copy, while maintaining the spatial relationships between the crosses. Similarly, in the final part of the Halstead Tactual Performance test the patient is required to use tactile and kinaesthetic cues to draw a form board he has

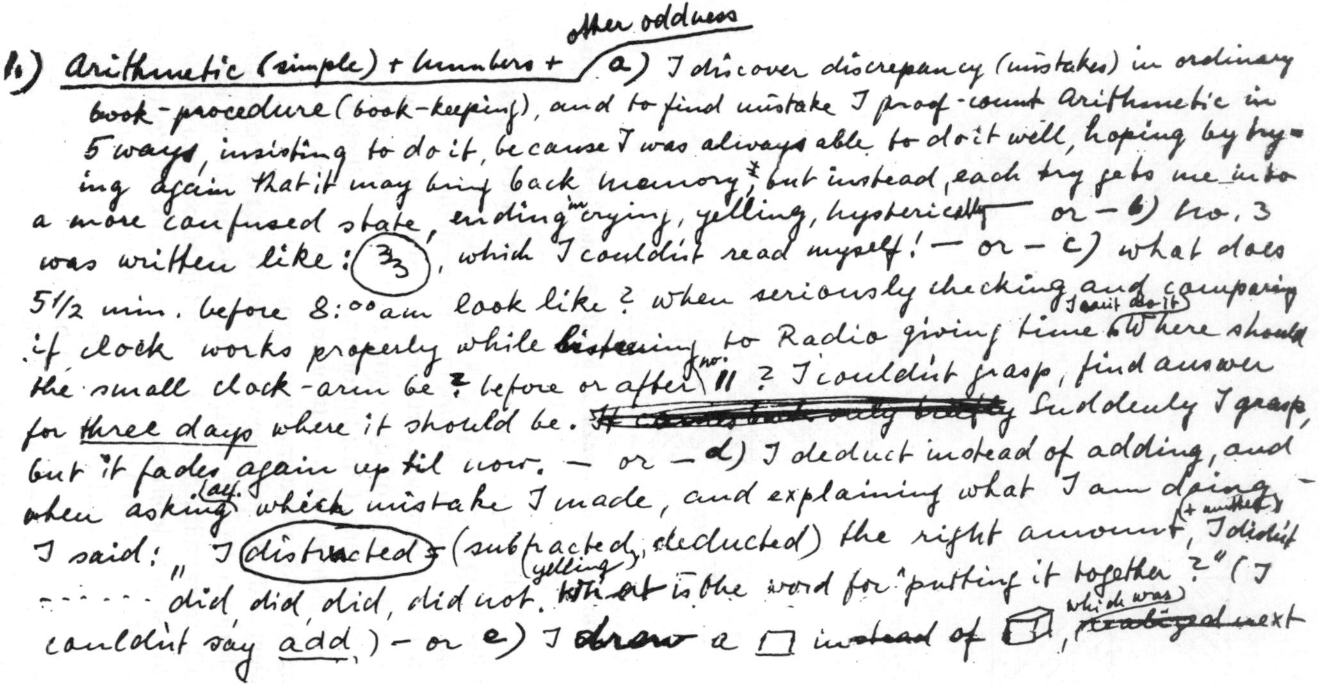

other oddness

b) <u>Arithmetic</u> (simple) + numbers + a) I discover discrepancy (mistake) in ordinary book-procedure (book-keeping), and to find mistake I prof-count Arithmetic in 5 ways, invisting to do it, because I was always able to do it will, hoping by try-ing again that it may bring back memory; but instead, each try p.to me into a more confused state, ending=trying, yelling, hysterically; — or — b) no. 3 was written like: (33), which I couldn't read myself! — or — c) what else

5½ min. before 8:00 am look like? when seriously checking and I sent doits.... it clock works properly while listening to Radio giving time (or here about the small clock-arm be ? before or after 11? I couldn't grasp, find answer for three days where it should be. Suddenly I grasp. but it (adds again up til now — or — d) I deduct instead of adding; and when asking which mistake I made, and explaining what I am doing, I said: " I (distracted) (subtracted, deducted) the right amount, instead — or — e) I observe 2 ☐ instead of ☐, I... did did, did, did not, What is the word for putting it together?" (I couldn't say add.) — or — e) I observe 2 ☐ instead of ☐,

Figure 4.6 Sample of writing by brain damaged patient

touched but never seen, and he is scored on the accuracy with which he reproduces the relative positions of the holes. The latter has little value as a means of localising a cerebral lesion.

Reversal of spatial relationships is also a sensitive test and if the patient is asked to draw a diagram copying a simple arrangement of sticks, difficulty in reversing the arrangement of the sticks in the drawing has been found to be particularly indicative of parietal lobe lesions (Butters and Barton, 1970).

The left hemisphere controls the production of language and a sensory aphasia tends to accompany left sided parieto-temporal disease, whereas there is evidence that the perception of emotion expressed by means of non-verbal behaviour and variations in prosody, appears to be controlled by the right parieto-temporal region.

Gerstman's syndrome consists of right–left disorientation, finger agnosia, acalculia, and agraphia without alexia. It has been associated with a lesion of the left angular gyrus, and though there may be a tendency for these signs to occur together, the lesions involved are usually extensive and the evidence to support the localising value of the syndrome is limited (Walsh, 1978). Damage to the optic radiations can cause a *contralateral lower quadrantanopsia.*

Figure 4.6 is a sample of writing from a 58-year-old woman who sustained severe brain damage after being struck by a car; 12 months later she developed epileptic seizures and then a compulsion to write excessively (hypergraphia). Her primary language was German which explains some of the syntactic errors in her writing. This writing sample demonstrates perseveration in writing (the number 3—line 6); difficulty in analysing spatial relationships (reading the time—line 7); dyscalculia (deducting instead of adding—line 11); paraphasia—"distracted" instead of "subtracted"—line 13); and constructional difficulties (attempting to draw a cube—line 15).

4.5 NEUROBEHAVIOURAL CONSEQUENCES OF TEMPORAL LOBE DISEASE

The temporal lobe processes information from all sensory systems, though it mainly mediates auditory perception, olfaction and visual perception. It forms part of the limbic system with its medial structures and thus integrates exteroceptive sensory information from all modalities, with memory, emotional and motivational functions. The consequences of lesions in this part of the brain are listed in Table 4.3.

The primary projection area for auditory afferents (Heschl's gyrus) receives information from both sides of the body, but predominantly from the contralateral side, and the termination of auditory afferents in the gyrus is arranged according to the tone level they carry (tonotopically). A lesion in this area does not produce clinical deafness, but it elevates the auditory threshold and this may be identified by specialised testing.

Lesions of the dominant temporal lobe will interfere with the analysis of verbal auditory material, whereas the contralateral lobe analyses non-verbal auditory

Table 4.3 Neurobehavioural consequences of temporal lobe disease

LEFT HEMISPHERE	EITHER/BOTH HEMISPHERES	RIGHT HEMISPHERE
	Contralateral upper quadrantanopsia, elevation of auditory threshold	
	Personality change	
	"Hippocampal" global amnesia	
Non-rhythmic ————	Modality specific impairment of auditory perception————————	Rhythmic
Verbal————————	and memory ————	Non-verbal
Sensory aphasia ————	Impaired language ————	Aprosody

material. This means that a lesion in the right lobe will result in an impaired performance in the interpretation of pitch and rhythm, which can be tested for by the Seashore Rhythm test (part of the Halstead–Reitan battery). *It is this separation of function which underlies the preservation of the ability to sing that is found in some markedly dysphasic patients.* A lesion on the other side will impair performance on the Speech-Sounds Perception subtest of the Halstead–Reitan battery.

The temporal lobe has a major role in the formation of memories, and the memory disorders seen in temporal lobe disease can be divided into those which are modality specific and those which are global. *Damage to the left temporal lobe interferes with memory in the verbal modality, whereas memory for non-verbal material will be predominantly impaired with lesions to the right lobe. In contrast, with bilateral damage to the hippocampi (which may result from herpes encephalitis), the memory defect is global, involving both verbal and non-verbal modalities.* Global amnesia is characterised by a normal immediate memory, but difficulty in learning new material and an impaired ability to recall it after an interval of 5 minutes or longer. When patients with hippocampal memory deficits are tested they will acknowledge that they were given information to remember and freely admit that they cannot remember it. They may also spontaneously complain of difficulties with their memory.

The global amnesia seen in Korsakoff's psychosis, where the damage (usually the result of thiamine deficiency caused by chronic alcoholism) is to the mamillo-thalamic region, is qualitatively different. In this memory deficit, the patient will not only have difficulty in recalling information given to him 5 minutes beforehand, but may also deny the information was ever given. He may deny that he has any problems with his memory and, in contrast to the "hippocampal" patients, those with Korsakoff's psychosis confabulate.

Confabulation was defined by Berlyne (1972) as the "falsification of memory occurring in a clear consciousness in association with an organically derived amnesia". When a patient is unable to produce a correct memory on request he can either say "I don't know" or produce a "false memory". The former response may be seen in mild confabulators, but it is less frequent in severe confabulators, who show a tendency to perseverate incorrect responses (Shapiro *et al.*, 1981). The combination of perseveration, a failure to inhibit incorrect responses and a failure to monitor one's own performance, are not only found in confabulation, but also in association with frontal lobe disorders. It has been suggested that the memory deficit interacts with frontal lobe dysfunction, to produce confabulation (Stuss *et al.*, 1978). Usually confabulation is transient, but it can be prolonged for years and the difference in course between it and the amnesia suggests that they are due to different underlying mechanisms.

Evidence for damage to the prefrontal area of the brain has been found in chronic alcoholic patients (Tarter, 1980) and as this region is involved in the mediation of attention (Watson *et al.*, 1981) this may go some way to explain the lack of awareness these patients exhibit towards their memory disorder. Also the sequence of stored long-term memories tends to be affected and the temporal relationship of past events becomes disrupted, but the latter impairment does not explain the confabulation (Talland, 1961), and neither does disorientation for time (Mercer *et al.*, 1977).

These disorders of global memory involve verbal and non-verbal material, but memory for motor behaviour may be relatively intact (Brooks and Baddeley, 1976), which can provide an alternative strategy for bypassing the amnesia. Unfortunately there are no really good tests of memory. One of the more popular tests is the *Wechsler Memory Scale,* which contains seven subtests and is designed to elicit general information about the patient, current affairs, orientation, immediate and short-term verbal memory, and immediate visual memory. These test results tend to correlate closely with IQ and if there is a marked discrepancy between the patient's memory quotient and his IQ, a memory deficit is indicated.

The left temporal lobe being on the language dominant side, a lesion in Wernicke's area will produce a fluent sensory aphasia, and a lesion on the other side may produce aprosody. Involvement of the optic radiations can produce a *contralateral upper quadrantanopsia*.

Temporal lobe epilepsy has been found to be associated with certain types of psychopathology and the development of certain personality traits, and this relationship is discussed further in Chapter 7.

4.6 NEUROBEHAVIOURAL CONSEQUENCES OF OCCIPITAL LOBE DISEASE

The ococipital lobe is primarily concerned with vision and the consequences of occipital lobe lesions are shown in Table 4.4. The optic radiations terminate in the primary visual cortex in such a way as to maintain the spatial relationships of the visual percepts. Complete lesions of the primary cortex will produce cortical blindness and if they are unilateral they will cause a contralateral hemianopsia. If they are more focal they will cause a scotoma (a localised irregular visual field defect) which may be unnoticed by the patient and only found on careful visual field testing.

Those fibres in the optic radiations which subserve central vision (originating from the macula of the retina), pass to the tip of the occipital pole and are often spared in the visual field defects that develop with occipital lobe lesions. The presence or absence of macula sparing is a finding which may help to localise the site of a lesion producing a visual field defect.

Cortical blindness may be associated with anosognosia (Anton's syndrome), and the patient may fabricate reasons for his inability to see. In such conditions the pupillary reflexes are characteristically preserved and when the visual defect is the result of a vascular accident, recovery of vision is usual. However, exclusion of functional blindness can be made by means of the menace reflex (eye blinking in response to a sudden threatening movement towards the patient's eyes), the optokinetic reflex (jerky eye movements when looking at a rapidly moving sequence of objects), and the EEG (preservation of alpha rhythm), all of which are only impaired in true blindness.

Table 4.4   Neurobehavioural consequences of occipital lobe disease

LEFT HEMISPHERE	EITHER/BOTH HEMISPHERES	RIGHT HEMISPHERE
	Contralateral homonymous hemianopsia	
	Cortical blindness	
	Scotoma	
	Prosopagnosia	
	Impaired visual object fixation and field scanning	
Visual object agnosia		
Simultanagnosia		
Colour agnosia		
Alexia		

Efferents from the primary visual cortex are processed via the association areas so that all aspects of a visual object are integrated. This results in the perception of the "whole" object. Failure of this process results in *simultanagnosia (only one aspect of the object, e.g. colour or shape, can be appreciated at a time)*.

Visual object agnosia refers to a failure to recognise familiar objects, though they can be recognised by other senses such as touch. Failure to recognise may be due to a field defect, simultanagnosia, or a defect in the integration of visual perception and memory. In practice there are usually visual field or other defects complicating the agnosia.

In prosopagnosia there is a failure to recognise familiar faces (sometimes including the patient's own face) and it is often associated with colour agnosia and simultanagnosia. Damasio *et al.* (1982) proposed a functional model that would explain the pathological and clinical features associated with proso-pagnosia. Though this is an uncommon condition this model provides an understanding of the higher cortical mechanisms involved in processing visual information. According to it, facial recognition involves afferents carrying the visual percept, passing to the primary visual cortex, after relaying in the lateral geniculate bodies. This information then passes via the inferomedial association areas of the occipital lobe (in the lingual and fusiform gyri) to the rostral temporal cortex, and then to the hippocampal formation. The latter connects extensively with the limbic system and the other association areas of the brain, and by this route the initial stimulus pattern can evoke the appropriate memories in other modalities, and hence recognition of familiar patterns. The occipital association areas appear to be crucial for this process, though it seems that it can be carried out even when only one of the occipital lobes is intact. Post-mortem evidence indicates that bilateral damage is probably necessary for prosopagnosia to develop (Damasio *et al.*, 1982). It may be that this part of the brain is not specific for facial recognition, but that it appears so because the perception of familiarity is particularly important in relation to facial patterns and in eliciting the appropriate behavioural response.

A lesion of the occipital lobe can interfere with the ability of the eyes to scan the visual field and to direct attention to specific details in that field. This disturbance of visual fixation may result in *Balint's syndrome, i.e. an inability to visually localise objects in space, an inattention to objects in the periphery of the visual field, and an inability to fixate objects.* There may be difficulty in following a moving object visually, though voluntary eye movements are preserved, in contrast to the defect seen with lesions of the frontal eye fields.

Certain visual disorders are associated with damage to one particular side of the brain, as in the case of *word blindness* (the left side) *where the patient can speak and write normally, but cannot read (alexia without agraphia).* The right occipital lobe tends to deal with the spatial relationships of visual stimuli.

The posterior cerebral artery supplies the visual cortex of the occipital lobe, the medial aspects of the temporal lobe, and the posterior cingulate gyrus. Involvement of the latter may underlie the association between anosognosia and cortical blindness. If the medial temporal structures are involved, following occlusion of the posterior cerebral artery, a global memory deficit may occur, and ischaemia in this area is probably the cause of transient global amnesia (Alexander, 1982).

4.7   THE WECHSLER ADULT INTELLIGENCE SCALE (WAIS)

This is the commonest test of intelligence used in adults and is composed of 11 subtests which are listed in Table 4.5. The "Hold" tests are those tests which are most resistant to the effects of aging and organic brain disease (OBD), and the "Don't Hold" tests are those where performance is most likely to deteriorate

Table 4.5   The WAIS subtests

WAIS "HOLD" SUBTESTS (McFie, 1975)
*Vocabulary (V): The definition of each of a series of words.
†Picture Completion (PC): The identification of the missing part in each of a series
   of pictures.

WAIS "DON'T HOLD" SUBTESTS (McFie, 1975)
†Block design (BD): The copying of a series of designs using multicoloured blocks.
†Digit Symbol (D.Sym): Learning to match specific symbols with specific numbers.
*Digit Span (D.Span): The maximum number of digits that can be repeated
   forwards, + the maximum number of digits that can be repeated backwards. In
   each case repetition is immediate.
†*Arithmetic (A): The solution of a series of arithmetical problems (writing is not
   allowed).

OTHER WAIS SUBJECTS
†Object Assembly (OA): The completion of a series of jigsaw puzzles.
*Information (I): A series of questions testing general knowledge.
*Comprehension (C): The patient indicates his behaviour under certain
   circumstances that require judgement, abstract thought and social awareness.
†Picture Arrangement (PA): The arrangement of several pictures in the correct
   order to demonstrate a logical progression of events (in other words to tell a
   short story). The test is repeated with several different groups of pictures.
*Similarities (S): The identification of similarities between pairs of words.

---

*Tests mainly measuring verbal abilities. All other tests predominantly measure non-verbal abilities.
†Tests involving a time limit.

as a result of these factors. The distribution of tests into these two groups was
originally suggested by Wechsler (1944). McFie (1975) modified Wechsler's
Deterioration Quotient (DQ) formula as follows:

$$DQ = \frac{(\text{``Hold'' subtests total} \times 2) - \text{``Don't Hold'' subtests total}}{\text{``Hold'' subtests total} \times 2} \times 100$$

If the DQ is greater than 20%, this indicates a significant impairment of
mental efficiency and suggests organic brain disease is present. *Neither
Wechsler's nor McFie's formula were very effective at separating those patients
with OBD from those without.* The WAIS in general is not a very effective means
of identifying OBD, but for the purposes of this discussion it will be used as
a model to demonstrate how OBD may affect psychological test results.

Generally speaking the verbal subtests involve a short duration stimulus and
are thus sensitive to the effects of poor attention and memory impairment, as
well as to disorders of the dominant cerebral hemisphere. These tests tend to
involve "well-learned" material, and are thus relatively resistant to the effects
of OBD. In contrast the non-verbal tests involve a more prolonged stimulus and
are less impaired by disorders of attention, memory and language, but they
are sensitive to OBD as they tend to involve learning new material. Performance
on these tests is also impaired by motor slowing as they are time limited, unlike

Table 4.6 Factors influencing the WAIS subtest scores

	V	PC	BD	D. Sym	D. Span	A	OA	I	C	PA	S
Thought Disorder		+							+	+	+
Abstract thinking						+			+		+
Judgement and and planning			+				+		+		
Memory					+	+					
Attention and concentration				+	+	+					
Premorbid intellectual level	+ +	+				+		+ +	+		+ +
Social ability									+	+	
Socio-economic background	+					+		+	+		
Culture	+							+	+		

V, PC, BD = "Hold" tests*
D. Sym, D. Span, A = "Don't Hold" tests*

*McFie (1975).

the verbal tests (except for the arithmetic subtest). They are also affected by motor incoordination, disease of the non-dominant hemisphere, and depression of mood. Psychiatric patients tend to be more difficult to test than non-psychiatric patients, and their results are more difficult to interpret. Table 4.6 shows some of the factors which influence performance on the various WAIS subtests.

The verbal subtest scores are combined to produce a total, the Verbal Intelligence Quotient (VIQ), and the non-verbal subtests are combined to produce a non-verbal Performance IQ (PIQ). A composite Full Scale IQ (FSIQ) is also produced by combining all the test results. A score of 100 FSIQ points represents the mean for the normal population. As the standard deviation (SD) = 15 points, 68% of the normal population will be expected to have full scale IQ scores between 85 and 115 points. 2 SD below the mean = 70 IQ points, and marks the statistical cut-off point between normal intelligence and mental retardation. However, there is evidence that these figures are becoming less valid, as the population norms show a tendency to change over time, and so it is necessary to produce an updated version of the test.

The effects of lateralised cerebral lesions on the sub-tests of the WAIS will tend to reflect the differentiation of cerebral functions into those involving verbal and those involving non-verbal processes. In clinical practice the functions of each cerebral hemisphere are not so easily, nor so reliably, separated. Hence, dominant (left) hemisphere lesions tend to produce a reduction in verbal IQ, and non-dominant (right) hemisphere lesions produce a reduction in performance IQ. In practice, assessing the clinical significance of a verbal–performance IQ

(V–P) discrepancy is complicated by several factors. In the normal population, a FSIQ above the average level (100 FSIQ points) tends to be associated with a VIQ that is superior to the PIQ, more often than the reverse. This relative superiority of verbal ability decreases with the FSIQ. Wechsler (1944) demonstrated that as the FSIQ decreases from 120 to 75 points, the proportion of patients with a PIQ that is greater than their VIQ, increases from 21% to 74%. In general terms a PIQ greater than VIQ discrepancy of 15 points or greater, is more likely to be clinically significant, than the reverse discrepancy. This is because of the greater sensitivity of the performance subtests to the effects of other variables, as well as OBD, though in either case the chances of the difference being clinically significant will tend to increase with the size of the discrepancy and the pattern of variability in the subtest scores.

This V–P separation is further complicated because certain functions which appear to be non-verbal, such as recognition of faces, may in fact be mediated verbally, to a certain degree, if the faces are well known to the patient. This may be due to the attachment of a verbal label to the face. Certain occupations may have the effect of increasing verbal or non-verbal skills. Journalism may have the former effect and, conversely, certain artistic occupations may tend to elevate performance IQ scores. Alternatively, a particular neuropsychological profile may influence a person's choice of career.

Timed tests tend to be sensitive to brain damage and so performance IQ will tend to be reduced under these and other circumstances, such as aging, where speed of response is reduced. As such factors interfere with the significance of a WAIS V–P IQ difference, other confirmatory evidence must be looked for, if cerebral disease is suspected. The scores on certain subtests may be helpful in this respect. Some subtests are resistant to OBD and reflect premorbid intellectual level (the Vocabulary and Information subtests) as shown in Figure 4.6. Also a poor premorbid intellectual endowment may affect the clinical presentation of certain psychiatric disorders, e.g. mentally retarded patients who become depressed may develop a picture of pseudodementia.

4.8 THE HALSTEAD–REITAN BATTERY

Modern neuropsychological testing favours the use of combinations of tests, as are found in the Halstead–Reitan and the Luria–Nebraska batteries (Lezak, 1976; Walsh, 1978). These batteries incorporate several tests aimed at evaluating different aspects of brain function, and performance on those tests that evaluate left hemisphere function, can be correlated with other tests such as those screening for aphasia and sensory perception on the right side of the body, in order to provide a comprehensive evaluation of different functions subserved mainly by this side of the brain. Other tests can be used to assess right hemisphere functions.

It is normal procedure to include other tests with the basic Halstead–Reitan battery (which is shown in Table 4.7). These tests include an assessment of grip strength; sensory perception in different modalities, on the two sides of the body;

a screening test for aphasia (the Modified Halstead–Wepman Aphasia Screening Test); a test for constructional apraxia; the Wide Range Achievement Test (WRAT) for learned skills in arithmetic, spelling and word recognition; the WAIS; and the MMPI (Boll, 1981).

In the normal course of events, scores on WRAT should be comparable to the person's WAIS IQ. A difference of 10 points or more between the two tests is likely to be clinically significant (Golden, 1979). If the WRAT score is the lower, a learning disability should be considered; and if it is higher, adult-onset brain damage should be considered, as these tests are remarkably stable in the face of organic brain disease. However, certain of the WRAT subtests may be affected by focal lesions, e.g. the arithmetic score may be decreased by a lesion of the angular gyrus.

Table 4.7   The Halstead neuropsychological test battery

TEST	PROCEDURE	BEHAVIOUR UNDER TEST
Category test	A series of visual stimuli are each classified under a number from 1 to 4 according to some aspect of the stimulus.	Learning Concept formation
Tactual Performance test	Fitting of different shaped blocks into the appropriate holes in a board, using touch only. Alternate hands, then both. Then the board is drawn from tactile memory only, without ever being seen.	Learning Memory Motor speed Psychomotor coordination Tactile and kinaesthetic sense
Finger Oscillation test	Rapid tapping on a lever, alternate hands.	Motor speed
Rhythm test	Comparing pairs of rhythmic beats for similarity or difference.	Attention and concentration Non-verbal auditory perception
Speech-Sounds Perception test	Identification of nonsense phonemes from choice of written alternatives.	Auditory-verbal perception Auditory-visual coordination Attention and concentration

Further discussion of the clinical uses of all these tests can be found in Filskov and Boll (1981), and Golden (1979); on the use of the MMPI, in Dahlstrom *et al.* (1972), and Graham (1977); and on the use of the WAIS, in Matarazzo (1979) and Zimmerman and Woo-Sam (1973).

4.9   OTHER TESTS

The Minnesota Multiphasic Personality Inventory (MMPI) is a questionnaire which evaluates a patient's personality characteristics. A criticism of the MMPI, of relevance to neuropsychiatry, is that it does not tell the clinician anything about *change* in personality, unless the test is used on more than one occasion, before and after the change. Also, the questions asked may fail to identify certain attitudes which are evident from more direct questioning. Despite limitations of these types, the MMPI can still provide helpful information in neuropsychiatric evaluation, if interpreted in the context of the total clinical problem.

   The MMPI consists of 566 questions which present the patient with a series of statements to which he answers "yes" or "no". His subsequent responses are classified into a series of scales (see Table 4.8) which can be helpful, not only in assessing his current attitudes, but also in relation to his performance on the rest of the test battery.

Table 4.8   The MMPI scales

MMPI VALIDITY SCALES
L   Identifies tendency for patient to present himself in a good light.
F   Abnormal responses are present (may be acutely disturbed or "faking bad").
K   Identifies defensiveness, use of denial, and poor insight.

MMPI CLINICAL SCALES
Hs   (hypochondriasis) Excessive concern over bodily health.
D   (depression) Depressed mood and outlook.
Hy   (hysteria) Multiple somatic complaints of probable psychogenic origin.
Pd   (psychopathic deviate) Social maladjustment in several areas of behaviour.
MF   (masculinity–femininity) Sex determined attitudes.
Pa   (paranoia) Suspicious and defensive.
Pt   (psychasthenia) Obsessive–compulsive tendencies.
Sc   (schizophrenia) Social withdrawal, disorders of thinking and perception.
Ma   (hypomania) Hypomanic symptoms.
O   (social introversion) Tendency to avoid decisions and social interactions.

   The cut-off point between normality and abnormality on the MMPI is taken as 70, and scores above this level are regarded as abnormal. However, it is the patient's score profile that is more important than any of his individual scores. A hysteria score greater than 70 would suggest that the patient has a tendency to develop physical symptoms in response to stress situations. In interpreting such a score, allowance must be made for other factors, as non-psychiatric patients who have chronic physical illness tend to develop elevation of their hypochondriasis, hysteria and depression scores. If high scores are obtained on the hypochondriasis and hysteria scales, with a relatively low score on the depression scale, this being called the Conversion V Triad, and these three scores are greater than other scores on the MMPI, the presence of conversion symptoms is strongly suggested. A low depression score under these circumstances reflects the patient's tendency to dissociate himself from his (physical) illness and may be manifest clinically as "la belle indifférence". Raised hypochondrasis and hypomania scores may be seen in OBD, and are clinically associated with somatic complaints, overactivity and denial of disability. High scores have also been found to statistically differentiate malingerers from authentic patients seeking compensation, after a head injury (Heaton *et al.*, 1978).

There have been attempts to use the MMPI to assess organic brain disease, and Wiggins *et al.* (1971) devised a series of content scales, one of which was designed to identify organic symptoms. A high score on his "ORG" scale indicated a tendency to report neurological symptoms, somatic symptoms of a functional type, impairment of judgement, memory and concentration, and periods of behaviour for which the patient was amnesic. These patients also tended to show an inability to understand what they read and, if they were psychiatric patients, they were more likely to exhibit anxiety and impaired concept formation.

Watson and Thomas (1968) devised an Organic Sign Index (OSI) which was the product of the total depression, masculinity–femininity, and schizophrenia subscale scores, minus the combined scores on the psychopathic deviate and hypomania scales. A score of under 40 favoured the diagnosis of organic brain damage, whereas a score of over 40 favoured the diagnosis of schizophrenia. However, *the MMPI cannot effectively differentiate process schizophrenic patients from those with OBD* (Filskov and Leli, 1981).

The MMPI may be helpful provided its limitations are kept in mind and it is interpreted in association with the relevant clinical details, the results of neuropsychological tests and other investigations.

Unstructured tests such as the Rorschach, where the patient has to provide responses to a series of ambiguous stimuli (ink-blots), may reveal a poverty of information when administered to patients with OBD. Those responses which are produced tend to be concrete and accompanied by a degree of perplexity. Such behaviour is also found in other psychiatric disorders though, and tests of this type have little real value in neuropsychiatric assessment.

4.10   CLINICAL USES OF NEUROPSYCHOLOGY

Table 4.9 shows how neuropsychological testing may help in identifying and localising organic brain disease. More than one of the methods listed in this table are often used in combination.

Pathognomonic signs are those signs, such as gross motor weakness or constructional apraxia, which are unequivocally abnormal, when present. Though they may be scored as present or absent, there is a high threshold to their being scored present, in order to ensure the clinical significance of a positive finding. Because of this, less pronounced deficits may be incorrectly scored as absent.

Table 4.9 Methods of neuropsychological evaluation

1. Pathognomonic neurological signs.
2. Lateralised motor and sensory differences.
3. Functionally related cognitive deficits.
4. Statistical analysis of the pattern of test results.
5. Comparison of results to statistical norms.

Valuable information can be provided by finding differences between the motor and sensory functions of the two sides of the body. Such *lateralised motor and sensory differences* are independent of developmental, emotional, cultural and educational variables. Motor tests of this type include grip strength, using a hand dynamometer, and the Finger Oscillation test, which measures the rate at which a lever can be depressed (allowing for a 10% superiority of the dominant over the non-dominant hand).

Other ways of using neuropsychological test results include looking for *functionally related cognitive deficits*, such as those involving verbal functions. If they are found, they will indicate dysfunction in the dominant cerebral hemisphere. Those cognitive deficits involving non-verbal functions will implicate the non-dominant hemisphere.

Another way of looking for clinically significant interrelationships between test results may be found by subjecting them to *statistical analysis*. In some cases the patient's test results may be *compared to statistical norms* found in different control populations, such as those without organic brain disease (OBD), those with generalised OBD, or those with localised OBD. This process can be used to indicate statistically the chances of a particular patient belonging to one of the control groups, e.g. 15% of a non-brain-damaged population had superior scores to the patient on this test. Interpreting information like this underlines the difficulty that is encountered in evaluating the clinical significance of test results when the normal population will also show a wide variation in scores on the same tests, e.g. evaluating the clinical significance of a discrepancy between the WAIS verbal and performance intelligence quotients in a particular case.

Table 4.10 lists the possible clinical uses to which neuropsychological testing can be put. Obtaining a test profile at an early stage in the patient's illness can be invaluable in cases where there is a suspicion that a progressive brain disease is present. Obtaining a baseline implies testing will be repeated at a later date, and serial testing may not only help to clarify whether an organic component is present, but may indicate the rate at which deterioration or improvement is occurring. This can help in the assessment of the efficacy of a particular treatment, as well as the patient's prognosis. It may also enable a retrospective diagnosis to be made. For example, in depressive pseudodementia a successful trial of treatment can result in an improved cognitive performance, compared with previous test results.

If OBD is present the pattern of scoring on psychological testing may indicate a long-standing cerebral impairment, possibly perinatal in origin, in contrast

Table 4.10   Clinical uses of neuropsychology

1. Identification of organic brain disease.
2. To obtain baseline levels of cognitive functioning for comparison with later test results.
3. To clarify if cognitive impairment is of recent onset or long-standing.
4. Rate of progress or recovery of cognitive deficits.
5. Areas of deficit and preservation of cognitive functions.
6. To identify the site(s) of brain damage.
7. The assessment of response to treatment.
8. To differentiate organic from functional disorders.
9. To ascertain the relative contributions of organic and functional factors.

to the findings when cerebral disease is of more recent onset. The Halstead Category test, and the Tactual Performance test (the accuracy with which the spatial arrangement of the holes in the Sequin–Goddard Form Board, are reproduced from memory), are two procedures which are particularly prone to be impaired by OBD of recent onset. In addition, the patient's history of educational and occupational achievements, taken with his scores on the Wide Range Achievement Test, will indicate his premorbid cognitive level, and provide further evidence for cognitive impairment being of relatively recent onset.

Charting the areas of deficit and preservation in a patient's cognitive skills is important in helping him to learn how to bypass his deficit and take advantage of his preserved skills during treatment, rehabilitation and vocational guidance. For example, a patient with motor aphasia may be helped in speech therapy by using melodic intonation, provided his right hemisphere is relatively undamaged (Sparks and Holland, 1976). Also identifying the areas of deficit may give some indication of the aetiology of the lesion, as is the case when a global memory deficit of the type associated with bilateral hippocampal damage is found.

The clinician's assessment of the patient's response to treatment may be helped by serial psychological testing. By this method it is possible to monitor the cognitive recovery of a patient with post-traumatic brain damage. A failure to make the progress expected in such a case may be due to the patient developing depression. The onset of such a complication may be indicated not only by his clinical signs, but by monitoring his performance on a personality inventory, such as the Minnesota Multiphasic Personality Inventory (MMPI). The MMPI can be used as part of a neuropsychological test battery because of its well validated ability to objectively evaluate a patient's attitudes and opinions. The differentiation of functional from organic disorders will be mentioned in the next section.

4.11   PSYCHIATRIC DISORDERS

Numerous factors can affect neuropsychological test performance in a psychiatric patient, including his mental state. However, emotional disturbance has not been shown to significantly impair test performance, but studies looking at such a relationship would require the patient to be able to complete his testing, and so would exclude anyone who is too disturbed to do this. So testing is not particularly helpful in those cases where a patient is acutely disturbed and the physician is attempting to ascertain the cause, organic or otherwise, of the disturbance. In such cases it is helpful to identify "hard" organic signs clinically, e.g. aphasia.

Using psychological testing to separate the "organic" from the "non-organic" psychiatric patients has been generally successful, except in two groups. Chronic or process schizophrenic patients frequently score in the "organic" range on such tests and this is more marked the greater the chronicity and severity of the schizophrenic illness. Such impairment has been found to be closely associated with cerebral atrophy in many studies (Luchins, 1982). The second group of patients who score in this range are the elderly "non-organic" group, and this may be partly due to undiagnosed dementia or to an "organic" contribution to their illness (Heaton and Crowley, 1981).

When trying to clarify whether or not a patient is suffering from an organic disorder, a particular problem in a suspected case of pseudodementia, a non-organic aetiology will be suggested by: an inconsistency between the patient's report of his deficits and his performance on psychological testing; the patient's pattern of score failures not being understandable on the basis of cerebral pathology; and an inconsistency in the findings on testing when compared with those from the history or examination. It may also be helpful to observe the patient's response to his poor performance—the demented patient usually being relatively unconcerned (unless a catastrophic reaction develops), whereas the depressed patient either exaggerates and draws attention to his failure, or refuses to cooperate. Inconsistencies may be found in non-organic cases, when the results of testing at a later date are compared to the patient's original scores. Findings such as these must be taken into account with other variables, such as the patient's current social situation and his premorbid personality, as well as factors related to the test situation, such as the competency and skill of the person administering the test. In cases where there is some doubt about the significance of the test results, an expert neuropsychological opinion should be sought. In many cases organic and non-organic factors will both be present. Then the difficult task of assessing the relative contributions of each, must be undertaken.

Testing psychiatric patients may be further confused by treatment variables. Those drug effects which may interfere with the results include sedation and akathisia (disturbance of concentration and attention), anticholinergic effects (disturbance of memory), akinesia and extrapyramidal rigidity (motor speed and response). Where possible it is advisable to allow such side effects to subside and to avoid any sudden changes in treatment, such as an increase or decrease in drug dosage, before carrying out detailed neuropsychological testing. This is particularly important because some tests cannot be repeated for several months, once they have been administered, to avoid a "learning effect".

The effect of electroconvulsive treatment (ECT) on brain function has not been extensively studied, but the current state of knowledge indicates that marked deficits of memory are commonly present in the first few days after treatment (Heaton and Crowley, 1981). These defects are more in the area of delayed recall, rather than short-term learning. Retrograde amnesia (loss of memory for events occurring up to several years before treatment) occurs also. Verbal and visuo-spatial memory are relatively more affected after ECT is applied to the dominant and non-dominant hemispheres, respectively. There is no convincing evidence that significant memory deficits remain after a period of a few weeks following the end of ECT treatment. However, it is possible that patients with pre-existing organic brain disease may acquire further irreversible cognitive damage, and clinical impression supports this assumption.

CHAPTER 5

Neuropsychiatric Aspects of the EEG

5.1 INTRODUCTION

The electroencephalogram (EEG) recorded from the scalp measures the electrical activity of the cerebral cortex subjacent to the recording EEG electrodes. However, a subcortical midline pacemaker (probably diencephalic) produces the rhythmical activity seen in the normal EEG tracing, and so subcortical lesions, by interfering with this activity, can also cause changes in the EEG tracing. Also, the reticular activating system (RAS) acts on the pacemaker and its arousal causes desynchronisation of the EEG, and so a lesion in the RAS pathway may affect the EEG recording. Thus cortical lesions and lesions remote from the cerebral cortex can both cause EEG abnormalities.

A barrier of bone and tissue separates the electrodes from the brain and interferes with the sensitivity of the EEG. The EEG tracing can be affected by alterations in the electrical potential of this extracerebral tissue, e.g. as a result of eye movements. In view of this barrier between the electrodes and the brain, and the fact that the EEG reflects electrical activity in the cortical gray matter, it is not surprising that the EEG recording can be normal in the presence of significant intracranial structural abnormality. It also reflects and is sensitive to changes in the cerebral metabolism and blood flow. Ingvar *et al.* (1976) demonstrated a close correlation between EEG frequency indices and the cerebral oxygen uptake, and the gray matter cerebral blood flow, and hence, the metabolic activity of the brain tissue.

EEG recordings can be made using a bipolar technique, where the active and indifferent electrodes are both attached to the scalp; or a monopolar technique, where the active scalp electrode is compared with a "neutral" electrode, which is often attached to the ear lobe.

The neonatal EEG is characterized by delta activity, which has a frequency of less than 4 cycles per second (c/s). As the central nervous system matures this activity becomes gradually replaced by faster rhythms, with the theta rhythm (4–7 c/s) becoming the dominant activity at the end of the first year of life. The alpha rhythm (8–13 c/s) then becomes progressively more prominent, after making its initial appearance, in the majority of children, by the age of 3 years.

Eventually the normal adult EEG pattern becomes established and is characterized by a predominance of the alpha rhythm in the parieto-occipital regions, when the EEG is recorded with the patient awake and his eyes closed. This rhythm has a voltage of 30–50 microvolts (μV). There may be a lesser degree of precentral beta activity (greater than 13 c/s), and minimal theta activity.

In the first two decades of life the EEG undergoes changes that reflect the maturational changes that are occurring in the nervous system, and during this period the EEG is more difficult to interpret. However, even 10–15% of healthy adults show mild abnormalities in their EEG tracings which usually consist of generalised asynchronous (i.e. onset in different electrodes at different times) slow waves (less than 8 c/s), an abnormally low amplitude (less than 20 μV) of all activity, or an excess of fast (greater than 13 c/s) activity. The more marked these changes are, the more likely they are to reflect an underlying cerebral disorder.

In the EEG's of healthy subjects over the age of about 60 years, changes tend to be quantitatively different, with abnormalities being seen of a similar type to those found in younger, neurologically immature patients, except for the occurrence of temporal slow wave activity as a normal variation in some elderly patients (Klass and Daly, 1979). Other age related changes include a slower, less responsive alpha rhythm, more marked beta activity, and an increase in generalised slow waves.

Overbreathing is a way of activating epiletic discharges in the EEG tracing. It acts by lowering the level of carbon dioxide in the blood, which results in cerebral vasoconstriction and, in the normal EEG tracing, causes paroxysmal delta activity to appear. The normal paroxysmal slow wave response is most marked in the young and becomes less pronounced with increasing age. In the predisposed, it may precipitate a cerebral dysrhythmia of the 3 c/s spike and wave type; or cause an enhancement of pre-existing generalised slow wave activity; or precipitate asymmetrical slow wave activity. Other conditions which reduce cerebral metabolism, notably hypoglycaemia and anoxia, will also enhance the hyperventilation response, making it more intense and prolonged.

Overbreathing may be a useful diagnostic test in some psychiatric patients as it is commonly found in association with anxiety states, and can cause depersonalisation, perceptual distortions, and other symptoms which, when occurring paroxysmally, may mimic a temporal lobe seizure. This combination has been called the *Hyperventilation syndrome (HVS)*. If the patient develops all his symptoms and signs as a result of overbreathing, and they are unaccompanied by an epileptic discharge, this strongly suggests a diagnosis of HVS. In cases of HVS it is necessary to look for some precipitating factor that may be amenable to treatment, such as a specific phobia.

Newer techniques that measure cerebral electrical potentials may be of even more value in neuropsychiatry. These techniques include videotelemetry, computer analysis of the EEG (CEEG), and the measurement of evoked potentials. The computer can be used to analyse the frequency and amplitude distributions in a way that is not possible using the traditional visual reporting technique. *Telemetry is a technique which enables the patient to move about, while his EEG is recorded from a radiofrequency transmitter.* It involves using EEG electrodes attached to the patient's scalp and miniature battery powered amplifiers. Prolonged recordings of many hours can be carried out in this way and can be combined with videotape recording (videotelemetry) of the patient's activity, so both the EEG and the video recording can be viewed on the same screen, and clinico-electrical correlations made. *Brain evoked potentials are "the electrophysiologic responses of the brain to repeated presentation of discrete sensory stimuli"* (Rappaport, 1982), and this technique shows some promise as a means of exploiting correlations between neurophysiological and neuropsychological variables in a way that will help in the diagnosis of certain neuropsychiatric disorders.

For a more extensive discussion of the clinical aspects of the EEG the reader is referred to Klass and Daly (1980) and Spehlman (1981).

5.2 THE USES OF THE EEG IN NEUROPSYCHIATRY

Table 5.1 indicates those ways in which the EEG may be helpful in neuropsychiatry. Table 5.2 lists those disorders which are often associated with certain characteristic, but not pathognomonic, EEG patterns.

The EEG is particularly valuable in the diagnosis of seizure disorders, toxic-metabolic encephalopathies, encephalitis, Creutzfeldt–Jacob disease, and focal

Table 5.1   The uses of the EEG in neuropsychiatry

AS A BASELINE

DIAGNOSIS OF
          Epilepsy
          Hyperventilation syndrome
          Delirium (especially hepatic coma)
          Encephalitis (especially due to herpes simplex)
          Dementia (especially Creutzfeldt–Jacob disease, subacute sclerosing
            panencephalitis, Huntington's chorea)
          Sleep disorders
          Tumours (especially if rapidly progressing)
          Drug use (especially barbiturates)
EXCLUDE ORGANIC DIAGNOSIS IN
          Pseudodementia
          Pseudoseizures
          Post-traumatic syndrome
          Other conditions (stupor, catatonia)
MONITOR PROGRESS AND TREATMENT IN
          Delirium
          Drug and alcohol withdrawal
          Epilepsy with or without psychiatric complications
          ?Psychopathy
          ?Schizophrenia

progressive mass lesions, e.g. a subdural haematoma. *The EEG may be normal in the presence of a slowly progressing space occupying lesion.* Though it is, in general, a helpful investigation for localising such lesions. It may provide information of prognostic significance in some disorders, e.g. a good prognosis is indicated in cerebral infarction when the vascular episode is associated with little change in the EEG, or the resulting EEG abnormality recovers rapidly.

Table 5.2   Typical EEG patterns

DIAGNOSIS	EEG PATTERN	FURTHER COMMENTS
Creutzfeldt–Jacob disease (see Figures 5.1 and 5.2	Periodic, generalised, repetitive, bilaterally synchronous triphasic waves (1–2 c/s). Can be caused by a sensory stimulus.	Rapid dementing illness due to a slow virus, with widespread neurological impairment and myoclonus. Typical EEG pattern develops late in illness.
Subacute sclerosing panencephalitis (see Figure 5.3)	Periodic, generalised, repetitive, bilaterally synchronous slow discharges (2 c/s).	Rapidly fatal dementing illness, usually in those under 20 years of age. Myoclonus accompanies discharges. Due to measles virus.
Hypsarrhythmia (see Figures 5.4 and 5.5)	Continuous, generalised, high amplitude, irregular slow waves and multi-focal spike discharges.	Found in diffuse cerebral disorders. Usually leads to brain damage or death in infancy. Multiple seizures and myoclonus usually present.
Hepatic coma (see Figures 5.6 and 5.7)	Rhythmical or runs of medium to high amplitude broad triphasic waves (2 c/s), in a bilateral synchronous and symmetric fashion.	In liver failure it indicates a poor prognosis. Found in other metabolic disorders.
Petit mal epilepsy or generalised absences (see Figure 5.8)	Symmetrical, synchronous 3 c/s spike and wave discharge.	Autosomal dominantly inherited epilepsy of childhood, usually ceases with adulthood.
Cerebral hemisphere infarct (see Figure 5.9)	Localised high voltage complexes, recurring regularly (periodic lateralised epileptiform discharges).	Associated with impaired consciousness, seizures and focal neurological deficits. EEG pattern characteristically seen in herpes simplex encephalitis. Also seen with tumours.

98

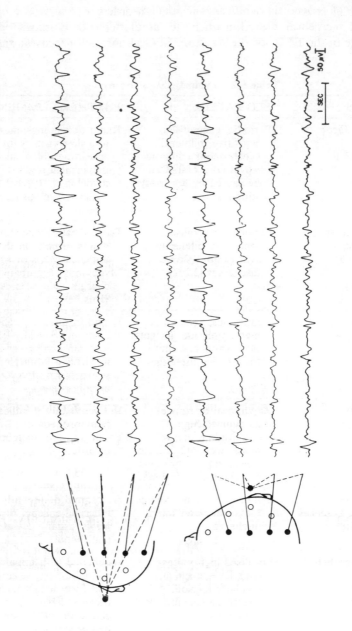

Figure 5.1 EEG in Creutzfeldt–Jacob disease. From Spehlman (1981); reproduced by permission of Elsevier Biomedical Press

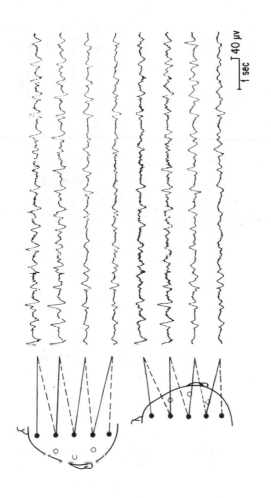

Figure 5.2   EEG in Creutzfeldt–Jacob disease. From D. W. Klass and D. D. Daly (1979). *Current Practice of Clinical Electroencephalography.* © **1979 Raven Press, New York; reproduced by permission**

100

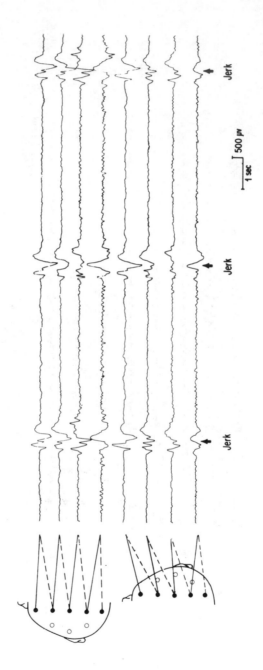

Figure 5.3 EEG in subacute sclerosing panencephalitis. From D. W. Klass and D. D. Daly (1979). *Current Practice of Clinical Electroencephalography.* © 1979 Raven Press, New York; reproduced by permission

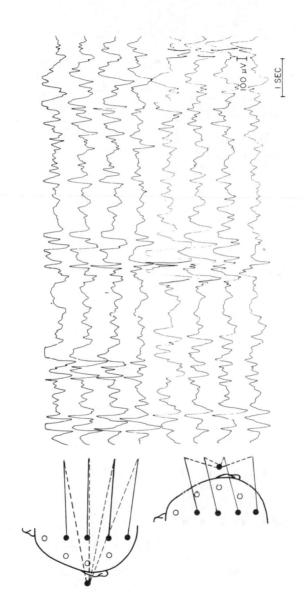

Figure 5.4 EEG showing hypsarrhythmia. From Spehlman (1981); reproduced by permission of Elsevier Biomedical Press

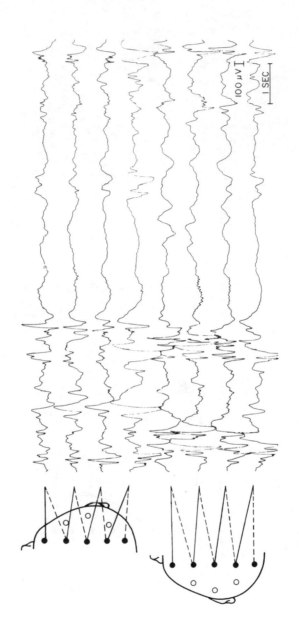

Figure 5.5 EEG showing hypsarrhythmia. From Spehlman (1981); reproduced by permission of Elsevier Biomedical Press

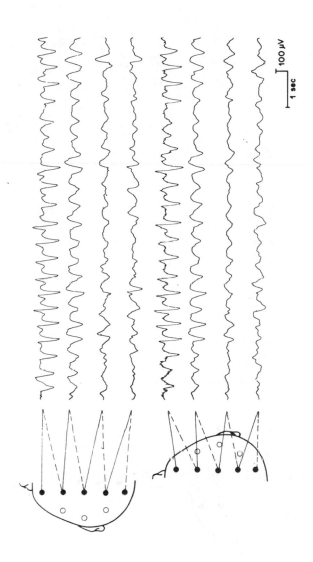

Figure 5.6 EEG in hepatic encephalopathy. From D. W. Klass and D. D. Daly (1979). *Current Practice of Clinical Electroencephalography.* © 1979 Raven Press, New York; reproduced by permission

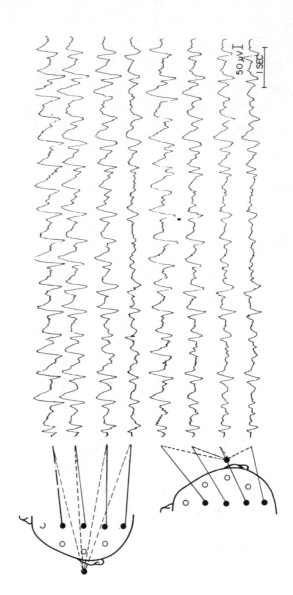

Figure 5.7 EEG in hepatic encephalopathy. From Spehlman (1981); reproduced by permission of Elsevier Biomedical Press

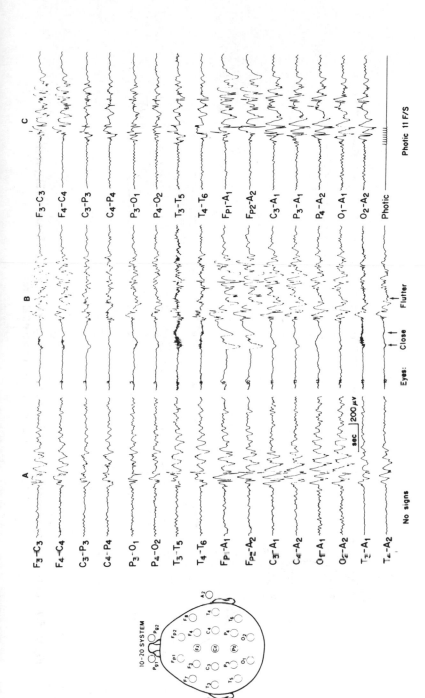

Figure 5.8 EEG in petit mal epilepsy. From D. W. Klass and D. D. Daly (1979) *Current Practice of Clinical Electroencephalography.* © 1979 Raven Press, New York; reproduced by permission

106

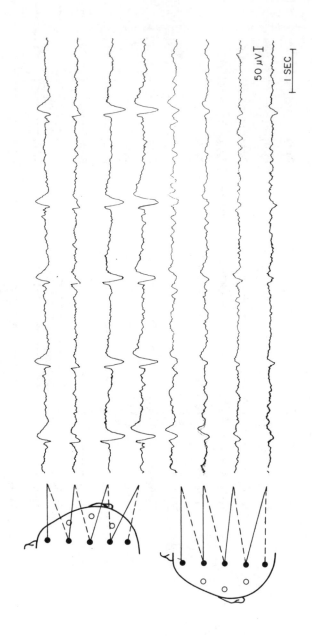

Figure 5.9 EEG showing periodic lateralised epileptiform discharges. From Spehlman (1981); reproduced by permission of Elsevier Biomedical Press

Such recovery is also helpful in differentiating an infarct from a malignant tumour (Lishman, 1978).

Those EEG features which usually indicate underlying cerebral abnormality, when found in recordings from adults who are alert, but at rest, include spike and sharp waves, slow waves, and a reduction in amplitude (compared with previous recordings). However, epileptiform activity may be found in 2% of asymptomatic individuals (Zivin and Ajmone-Marsan, 1968) and this emphasises that epilepsy is a clinical diagnosis primarily, and the EEG tracing alone is not diagnostic. This is particularly true of petit mal epilepsy, where the 3 c/s spike and wave discharges are accompanied by clinical seizures in only 25% of cases (Metrakos and Metrakos, 1961).

The important role of the EEG in delirium (Chapter 9) and dementia (Chapter 10), are discussed elsewhere.

The baseline EEG

A high percentage of EEG's requested by psychiatrists are within normal limits. This does not mean that the investigation has been wasted, as it still provides a baseline against which later EEG's on the same patient can be compared, as well as helping to screen out certain conditions. In the early stages in dementia and in mild cases of delirium, EEG abnormalities may be absent or minimal. Minimal changes may not be regarded as abnormal in the absence of a previous EEG on the same patient, for comparison. It is particularly useful in the assessment of patients taking phenytoin, in whom slowing of the alpha rhythm is an early sign of intoxication and may precede clinical signs.

Some patients on psychotropic medication may be at risk of developing seizures because of pre-existing neurological damage, a family history of epilepsy, or a previous history of seizures (due to drug ingestion or some other provoking event). In such cases it may be advisable to try and anticipate the development of seizures by monitoring the patient's EEG's when potentially epileptogenic medication is required.

5.3 EPILEPSY

The diagnosis of epilepsy is greatly facilitated if the EEG is carried out during a seizure, when spikes (pointed waves, 20 to 70 msec in duration) and/or slow waves, can be seen in a focal or generalised distribution, depending on the seizure type. Unfortunately, recording during a seizure is usually not possible and the diagnosis of epilepsy must be made with the help of inter-ictal EEG's only. Findings of particular significance, in such an EEG, are paroxysms of spike and wave activity, generalised spikes, focal spikes or sharp waves (pointed waves 70 to 200 milliseconds in duration), or localised sharp or slow wave complexes. *A normal inter-ictal EEG is quite compatible with a diagnosis of epilepsy, and does not rule it out.* If the diagnosis is seriously being considered, the EEG should be repeated and provocative techniques, such as hyperventilation and photic stimulation, can be used to increase the chances of identifying an epileptogenic focus. Hyperventilation acts by causing hypocapnia, which produces cerebral vasoconstriction and, in the normal EEG tracing, causes paroxysmal delta activity to appear. As has been mentioned, a variety of symptoms and signs, called the Hyperventilation syndrome, may accompany this decrease in cerebral blood flow. It is also helpful in intensifying paroxysmal discharges, and may even precipitate a focal discharge in the predisposed patient.

Photic stimulation, produced by a light source flashing at varying frequencies into the patient's eyes, may provoke epileptic activity and can also produce paroxysmal low amplitude spike and slow wave discharges in non-epileptic patients. In the latter cases there will not be a clinical seizure associated with these discharges. Both photic stimulation and hyperventilation are particularly effective at precipitating petit mal (3 c/s spike and wave) epileptic discharges and, in addition to an "absence" of a few seconds duration, the patient may show the clinical feature of eyelid fluttering. Occasionally brief limb movements or alterations of muscle tone are seen.

The use of activating procedures such as a post-prandial recording, sleep deprivation and/or the administration of an epileptogenic agent (e.g. chlorpromazine), may be helpful in provoking a latent abnormality in the EEG. The inter-ictal EEG is more likely to be abnormal if the patient is drowsy or asleep. King et al. (1982) found two such recordings quite adequate for identifying an epileptic focus on the inter-ictal EEG, but their patients had experienced frequent seizures and had had at least one clinical seizure within 2 weeks prior to the EEG recordings. When seizures are less frequent an abnormal EEG may be more difficult to obtain. Where temporal lobe epilepsy is suspected, electrodes can be placed closer to the temporal lobes via the nasopharyngeal route, or by inserting sphenoidal electrodes into the face below the zygomatic arch (in order to reach the region of the foramen ovale). The latter procedure is more uncomfortable, but the resultant EEG tracing is more reliable and less subject to artifactual interference than the nasopharyngeal recordings.

"Epileptic equivalent"

Though it is accepted that epilepsy should be primarily a clinical diagnosis, there are a group of patients who, in addition to having paroxysmal EEG abnormalities, experience episodic phenomena of a type that are found in temporal lobe seizures, but without the typical features of these seizures. The term "epileptic equivalent" will be used here to describe these phenomena, as this term has been used by Betts et al. (1976) in association with "symptoms of a similar nature (to those of an epileptic seizure) occurring in patients without clinical epilepsy."

These patients experience psychic phenomena including depersonalisation, derealisation, disorientation, hallucinations, and dissociative states, e.g. multiple personality and religious possession experiences (Davies and Neil, 1979;

Ervin *et al.*, 1955; Hill, 1952; Marinacci, 1963; Mesulam, 1981; Tucker *et al.*, 1965). The features of these disorders overlap with those found in certain non-organic disorders, especially those produced by hyperventilation. As over-breathing can produce seizure discharges in the EEG in certain patients, the boundaries between epilepsy and the Hyperventilation syndrome are seen to be far from clear.

A number of these "borderline" patients show a response to anticonvulsant treatment, but this should not be taken as evidence that these are true epileptic phenomena. It may be that the response in these cases is related to the mood normalising properties of such drugs (Post *et al.*, 1982; Reynolds, 1982). To confirm the presence or absence of true epilepsy may require videotelemetry.

5.4 ENCEPHALITIS

Headache and drowsiness with pyrexia, usually with other neurological signs, will be present in most cases of encephalitis. However, psychiatrists see a selected population of patients and are particularly likely to see those cases of encephalitis where psychiatric symptoms predominate (Himmelhoch *et al.*, 1970). In such cases an abnormal EEG may be one of the few indications of the organic aetiology of the disorder. In the acute phase of encephalitis, patients typically show a polymorphonuclear leucocytosis in the blood, and their CSF may show an elevated pressure with an increase of protein and mononuclear cells, but a normal sugar and chloride content.

Herpes simplex is the commonest cause of sporadic encephalitis (HSE) and, because of its propensity for attacking the structures of the limbic system, it can present with psychiatric symptoms, though the severe inflammatory reaction quickly causes neurological features to develop. The EEG may show a rather striking periodic lateralised epileptiform discharge (PLED) pattern (Figure 5.9). Such a pattern is particularly characteristic of HSE when the discharges are bilateral and independent. PLED's are found in many neurological conditions and are clinically associated with a depressed conscious level, focal neurological signs and recurrent focal seizures (Klass and Daly, 1979).

5.5 SLEEP DISORDERS

Sleep is sometimes used as a provocative procedure during an EEG recording and it will occasionally reveal an epileptic focus when waking records have been normal. It is particularly useful in localising the site of the ictal focus in patients who have TLE. Alternatively, an EEG recording can be made after a patient has been deprived of a night's sleep and this may activate an epileptic focus.

Monitoring a patient's sleep EEG may be helpful in the diagnosis of the compulsive sleep attacks of narcolepsy, when rapid eye movement (REM) activity typically occurs within minutes of the onset of sleep, instead of occurring 70 to 90 minutes later, which is the normal pattern. Early onset REM activity is also seen in sleep apnoea, when monitoring the patient's respirations during sleep will help to confirm the diagnosis. The significance of REM onset in sleep depends on it occurring during a period of normal night-time sleep, and its presence or absence during brief daytime sleep episodes, is not of the same diagnostic value.

A sleep latency (the time required to fall asleep) of less than 5 minutes during daytime sleep, is abnormal and is found in Narcolepsy and the Kleine–Levin Syndrome.

5.6 DRUG AND ELECTROCONVULSIVE THERAPY (ECT)

Organic treatment in psychiatry may also affect the EEG, and Table 5.3 shows some of the EEG effects commonly seen as a result of drugs used therapeutically in psychiatry (Klass and Daly, 1979; Spehlmann, 1981). Most antidepressants and most major tranquillisers (especially the sedative group), are epileptogenic. This epileptogenic activity is indicated in Table 5.3, where these drugs are shown to induce paroxysmal activity in the EEG, lowering the seizure threshhold. The monoamine oxidase inhibitors (MAOI) have variable effects on the EEG. Non-barbiturate anticonvulsant drugs, when taken in the therapeutic doses, tend to have little effect on the EEG. In the author's experience, lithium is particularly

Table 5.3   Common effects of psychiatric drugs on the EEG

DRUG	Increased slow activity (under 8 c/s) Non-paroxysmal	Paroxysmal	Decreased alpha activity (8–13 c/s)	Beta (over 13 c/s) Increased	Decreased
Barbiturates (and primidone)				+	
Benzodiazepines (and other sedatives)				+	
Amphetamines				+	
Propoxyphenes				+	
Phenothiazines	+	+			+
Tricyclic antidepressants	+	+			
Anticholinergic agents			+		
MAOI	+				
Opiates	+		+	* +	
Phenytoin	+		+		
Psychotomimetics (LSD-25, mescaline, psilocybin)			+		
Lithium	+	+			

*Chronic morphine use.

likely to cause diagnostic problems, producing focal paroxysmal and non-paroxysmal EEG abnormalities. Cannabis, in modest doses, has no significant effect on the EEG.

Fast activity on the EEG may be the first indication that the patient is taking covert barbiturates, and it is this group of drugs, and most of the other sedative drugs, which cause physical dependence and can cause seizures when withdrawn. The EEG recording taken from patients before starting to withdraw these and other psychotropic drugs, including alcohol, may be helpful in predicting an impending convulsion, which will be indicated by the presence of slow waves, spike, or spike and wave discharges (Itil, 1982). Such discharges may only be revealed by photic stimulation. Such a finding would need to be taken into account when managing the patient in such withdrawal states. When an abnormal EEG is caused by drug ingestion, covertly or otherwise, it may take a while to return to normal following abstinence (up to 2 weeks in the case of the benzodiazepines).

The persistence and severity of EEG changes caused by ECT increases with the number of treatments used. In 80–90% of patients, these abnormal EEG tracings will resolve within a month following the cessation of the course of ECT treatment. Two patterns of abnormality are usually seen. The first involves a generalized slowing of the EEG pattern, which may be regular or irregular. This is most marked on the left side of the brain with bilateral ECT, but when unilateral ECT is used the slowing will be most marked over the treated hemisphere (Weiner, 1980). The second pattern involves bilaterally synchronous runs of frontally predominant theta activity.

5.7 PSYCHIATRIC DISORDERS

As 10–15% of the clinically normal population have EEG patterns that show some abnormality, it is important to take into account the patient's clinical history and other findings on examination and investigation, when interpreting the clinical significance of such EEG abnormalities. In general there is a higher incidence of EEG abnormalities found in a psychiatric population, compared with the "normal" population, but the frequency of such abnormalities is more common in certain psychiatric disorders, notably psychopathy and catatonic schizophrenia.

EEG abnormalities are particularly frequent in those adults with aggressive psychopathic disorders and were found in 65% of the persistently aggressive patients in Hill and Watterson's study (1942). In such patients the EEG abnormalities usually involve posterior temporal slow wave foci, bilateral rhythmic theta activity in the central and temporal regions, and alpha variants. Alpha variants are rhythms that are faster or slower than the alpha rhythm, but have the same characteristics as the alpha rhythm in terms of distribution and responsiveness to eye opening (Hill, 1952).

Such findings are regarded as normal when present in the EEG's of younger patients, and it has been suggested that in the adult they reflect the temporo-limbic immaturity which underlies the aggressive, impulsive and impaired learning behaviour of the psychopathic personality. Genetic factors may be of importance in the aetiology of this dysrhythmia, because the relatives of these patients show a high incidence of similar EEG abnormalities, but mainly if they are also prone to episodes of irritability (Hill and Watterson, 1942). These immature patterns become less marked with age and this tends to be clinically associated with a maturing of their behaviour patterns. *A diagnosis of epilepsy should not be made on the basis of acute outbursts of aggressive behaviour in patients whose EEG's show these immature patterns.*

There is a raised incidence of EEG abnormalities in schizophrenia and they involve spikes, spike and waves, paroxysmal slow waves, and fast activity, with a reduction in alpha activity. As in aggressive personality disorders there is a preponderance of EEG abnormalities in the temporal lobe areas, compared with other areas of the brain. The incidence of EEG abnormalities in schizophrenia varies from 5 to 80% (Abenson, 1970), depending on the type of schizophrenia, and being most common when catatonic features are present.

The clinical state of the patient at the time of the recording also influences the EEG, and low amplitude slow activity has been found to be present in catatonic stupor, disappearing with the resolution of the stupor. Unlike the findings in aggressive psychopaths, schizophrenics do not show an immature type of pattern and the EEG abnormalities do not have a tendency to become less marked with increasing age (Hill, 1952).

Davies and Neil (1979) found that schizophrenic patients who show paroxysmal abnormalities, whether or not the EEG abnormality develops before or during treatment, have a tendency to show the clinical features which have been associated with minimal brain dysfunction. They show impaired impulse control, irritability, and a poor response to phenothiazines, when compared to schizophrenic patients without such EEG abnormalities. Itil *et al.* (1966) found that the presence of high voltage slow waves was a poor prognostic sign, and Itil (1982) recommends that these patients be particularly carefully evaluated for the presence of some other cerebral disorder which might be responsible for the EEG slowing.

The *B mitten EEG pattern* consists of sharp transients (a term used to describe any wave or complex which stands out from the background activity), which are formed by the last waves of the frontal sleep spindle followed by a higher voltage

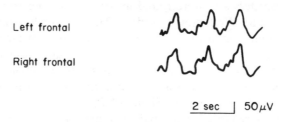

Left frontal

Right frontal

2 sec | 50 μV

Figure 5.10   The B-mitten EEG pattern

slow wave (thus giving the appearance of a mitten as shown in Figure 5.10). It occurs bilaterally and synchronously over the anterior areas of the brain, and is best seen in monopolar recordings. It seems that the thalamus may play an important role in the development of this abnormality, as it has been particularly associated with the EEG's of patients with thalamic tumours. It has been associated with reactive, as opposed to process, schizophrenia (Struve *et al.*, 1972). The B mitten is found during stages 3 or 4 of sleep, and its significance is disputed. More recent work has suggested a relationship between this finding and depression in psychotic illness (Struve and Klein, 1976).

EEG abnormalities are more frequent is schizophrenia than in the affective psychoses, though there is no significant qualitative difference in the EEG findings between the two groups. Itil and Fink (1966) found that depressed patients who have low voltage fast activity on their EEG are particularly at risk of developing an anticholinergic psychosis, when treated with drugs that have an anticholinergic action. As might be expected, a slow EEG has been shown to predict a sensitivity to sedative drugs (Itil, 1982).

CHAPTER 6

Cranial Computed Tomography
In Neuropsychiatry

6.1 INTRODUCTION

No book on diagnosis in neuropsychiatry would be complete without mention of Computerised Axial Tomography of the head (CAT head scanning). This is an investigatory technique which has had a major impact on neurology and neurosurgery (Gawler *et al.*, 1976), though its value in psychiatry remains less obvious. This technique was first described by Hounsfield (1973). CAT head scanning involves using x-rays and a computer, to reconstruct an image of a "slice" of the brain at a predetermined level, usually parallel to the orbitomeatal line. This produces a picture showing the brain in remarkable detail. The sensitivity of the scanner is such that it can discriminate between gray and white matter in the nervous system.

Before looking at a CAT head scan, certain points should be kept in mind. Though its accuracy in detecting abnormalities is over 90%, it has difficulty in demonstrating lesions in the posterior fossa, the pituitary fossa region and other areas at the base of the brain. This is because the close proximity of high density (bone) and low density (air) areas causes the formation of artefacts.

Interpretation of the scan pictures can be interfered with by, among other factors, sex and age-related differences in the size of certain structures, e.g. the third ventricle (which is particularly relevant if the measurement of brain parameters is being considered). The ventricles and cerebral sulci tend to become larger with increasing age, and this is particularly marked in those over the age of 60 years (Meese *et al.*, 1980).

The resolution that the scanner is capable of varies with different machines, and small lesions may not be visualised. This is important in conditions such as temporal lobe epilepsy, where a small tumour at a critical site may be responsible for the seizures. Some abnormalities may not be easily seen because they may be of the same density as the surrounding brain tissue, e.g. a subdural haematoma. In such cases the lesion may be revealed by causing displacement of normal and easily identifiable brain structures. Certain structures may be

Table 6.1 Some variations of normality and abnormalities visible on the CAT head scan

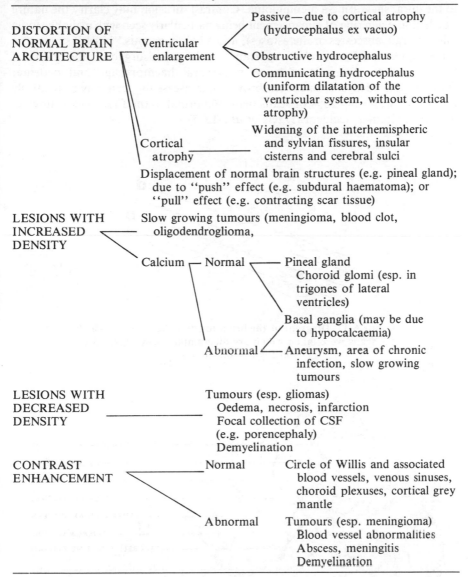

DISTORTION OF NORMAL BRAIN ARCHITECTURE

Ventricular enlargement
- Passive—due to cortical atrophy (hydrocephalus ex vacuo)
- Obstructive hydrocephalus
- Communicating hydrocephalus (uniform dilatation of the ventricular system, without cortical atrophy)

Cortical atrophy — Widening of the interhemispheric and sylvian fissures, insular cisterns and cerebral sulci

Displacement of normal brain structures (e.g. pineal gland); due to "push" effect (e.g. subdural haematoma); or "pull" effect (e.g. contracting scar tissue)

LESIONS WITH INCREASED DENSITY

Slow growing tumours (meningioma, blood clot, oligodendroglioma,

Calcium
- Normal
  - Pineal gland
  - Choroid glomi (esp. in trigones of lateral ventricles)
  - Basal ganglia (may be due to hypocalcaemia)
- Abnormal — Aneurysm, area of chronic infection, slow growing tumours

LESIONS WITH DECREASED DENSITY

Tumours (esp. gliomas)
Oedema, necrosis, infarction
Focal collection of CSF (e.g. porencephaly)
Demyelination

CONTRAST ENHANCEMENT
- Normal — Circle of Willis and associated blood vessels, venous sinuses, choroid plexuses, cortical grey mantle
- Abnormal — Tumours (esp. meningioma) Blood vessel abnormalities Abscess, meningitis Demyelination

visible due to calcification, especially the pineal gland and the choroid glomi in the posterior horns of the lateral ventricle.

Table 6.1 shows some of the principle abnormalities, and variations of normality, that may be seen on the CAT scan. Abnormalities such as ventricular enlargement or cortical atrophy may be generalised or focal. The site of a particular abnormality may indicate its origin, e.g. atrophy of the temporal pole

116

as a sequel to a closed head injury; or its nature, e.g. the proximity of a tumour to the dura, suggesting a meningioma. Contrast infusion may clarify the nature of a lesion, e.g. a ring of enhancement being particularly seen with a glioblastoma (also in brain abscesses or metastases), and a homogeneous "blush" suggesting a meningioma. Of particular importance to the neurosurgeon is the ability of the scanner to discriminate between cerebral haemorrhage and oedema, following a head injury. But in cerebrovascular disease the scan may be relatively unreliable, with only 50% of scans being abnormal in the first week following a cerebrovascular accident (Davis *et al.*, 1975).

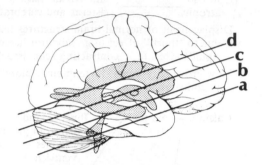

Figure 6.1   Diagram of the brain to show the levels at which the scans were taken which are diagrammatically represented in Figures 6.2 to 6.5

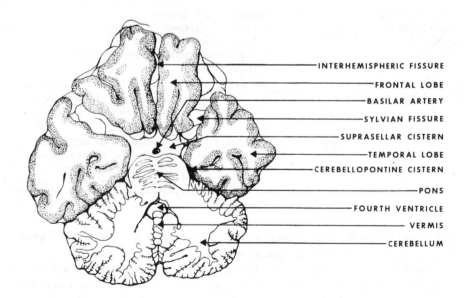

INTERHEMISPHERIC FISSURE
FRONTAL LOBE
BASILAR ARTERY
SYLVIAN FISSURE
SUPRASELLAR CISTERN
TEMPORAL LOBE
CEREBELLOPONTINE CISTERN
PONS
FOURTH VENTRICLE
VERMIS
CEREBELLUM

Figure 6.2   Section of the brain at level a

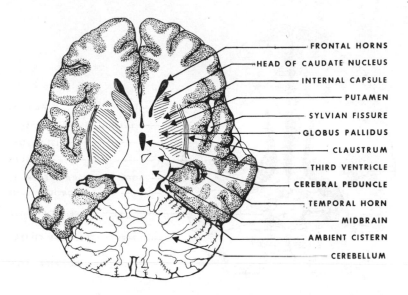

Figure 6.3   Section of the brain at level b

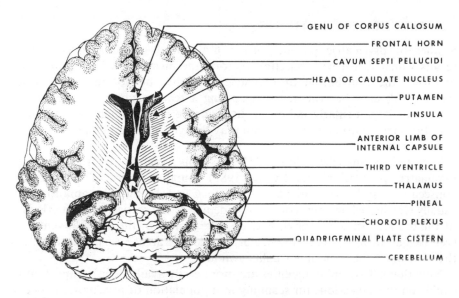

Figure 6.4   Section of the brain at level c

Figures 6.2 to 6.5 show, diagrammatically, sections of the brain as they would be seen on brain scans taken at different levels. The levels are indicated on Figure 6.1. Most of these structures labelled would be visible on a scan but their clarity and the consistency with which they are seen depends on the brain under examination and the resolution of the scanner.

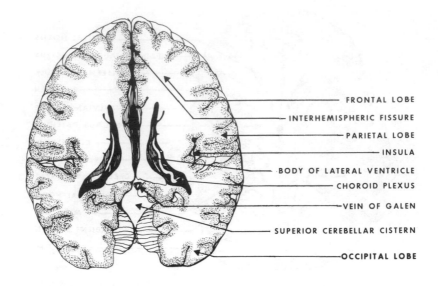

FRONTAL LOBE
INTERHEMISPHERIC FISSURE
PARIETAL LOBE
INSULA
BODY OF LATERAL VENTRICLE
CHOROID PLEXUS
VEIN OF GALEN
SUPERIOR CEREBELLAR CISTERN
OCCIPITAL LOBE

Figure 6.5   Section of the brain at level d

6.2   PSYCHIATRIC PATIENTS

Studies of psychiatric patients, using CAT head scanning, have yielded results which varied with selection factors; the mean age of the population involved; the distribution of diagnoses, whether or not they were institutionalised; and the criteria for regarding a scan as normal or abnormal. The latter is particularly important as evidence is accumulating that subtle variations from normality on the scan may be significant, especially in chronic schizophrenia.

Tsai and Tsuang (1981) found 25% of scans were abnormal in a selected psychiatric population, but Evans (1982) found a figure of 74% in 100 consecutive psychiatric patients subject to CT scanning. The abnormalities usually seen in such patients consist of widening of the cortical sulci and fissures of the brain (cortical atrophy), and/or enlargement of the cerebral ventricles (ventricular atrophy). The presence of low density areas, usually infarcts, are the next most common abnormality found.

Now that CT scanning facilities are more easily available it is important to decide on the indications for scanning in a population of psychiatric patients. Tsai and Tsuang's study suffered from a low number of patients in certain subgroups, but they found that there was no significant difference between cognitive, neurological or EEG abnormalities, in predicting abnormal scan results ($27.5 \pm 1.5\%$ of patients, in each case). All those patients under 40 years of age who had no history of any significant head injury in the past, were found to have normal scans if they were normal on physical and mental examination, even if their EEG's were abnormal.

Bradshaw *et al.* (1983), Feussner *et al.* (1981) and Larson *et al.* (1981), found that *focal neurological findings predict abnormal scan results.* Larson *et al.* (1981) found that six of their 123 patients with psychiatric disorders had significantly abnormal scans with focal findings. All the other abnormal scan results (55 cases in all) involved either atrophy, incidental focal abnormalities, or were false positive. However, Holt *et al.* (1982) found that the scan result significantly helped the psychiatrist in the evaluation of the patient's case, in 25 of the 99 psychiatric patients who were scanned. Only 11 of these cases had abnormal results, and this study indicates how a negative scan can be of value in clarifying a clinical problem.

In an effort to identify subtle changes in brain structure, a variety of techniques have been used, including linear measurements, e.g. the width of the third ventricle, and ratio measurements, of which the best known is Evan's Index.

$$\text{Evan's Index} = \frac{\text{Distance between the tips of the frontal horns of the lateral ventricle}}{\text{Maximum width of the skull measured between the inner tables of the skull}}$$

The technique of planimetry has been used to measure brain tissue and cerebral ventricular areas. Other techniques are in the process of being developed, such as the computer manipulation of scan data in order to measure the volume of brain structures (Jernigan *et al.*, 1982a). Despite these techniques some workers (Jacoby *et al.*, 1980a) still find visual evaluation of the cerebral sulci and ventricles a very effective means for evaluating cerebral atrophy. In some studies measurements of the absorption coefficients of different areas of the brain have been used as a means of assessing brain density, in an attempt to obtain data with clinical implications (Bondareff *et al.*, 1981).

6.3 SCHIZOPHRENIA

Cerebral atrophy

CAT head scanning in chronic schizophrenic patients has supported the neuropsychological evidence that there is a subgroup of patients with this diagnosis who have organic brain disease (Heaton and Crowley, 1981). Scanning has demonstrated an apparent excess of cerebral atrophy (ventricular dilatation and/or cortical atrophy) among schizophrenic patients compared to age-matched "normal" controls. However, not all studies have confirmed this relationship (Jernigan *et al.*, 1982a). The evidence for such a subgroup is particularly strong as it has come from several centres (Golden *et al.*, 1980a,b; Johnstone *et al.*, 1976; Nasrallah *et al.*, 1982; Okasha and Madkour, 1982; Weinberger *et al.*, 1979a,b), and they constitute about 50% of a population of chronic schizophrenic patients (Luchins, 1982). Cerebral atrophy has also been found in acute schizophrenia (Nyback *et al.*, 1982; Weinberger *et al.*, 1982), but is less frequently found in such cases, with an incidence of about 20% (Luchins, 1982).

These cerebral changes have been shown to consistently correlate with: neuropsychological impairment (Famuyiwa *et al.*, 1979; Golden *et al.*, 1980a,b; Johnstone *et al.*, 1976; Rieder *et al.*, 1979); "negative" symptoms, e.g. motor retardation, loss of affect, etc. (Andreasen *et al.*, 1982b); resistance to the antipsychotic action of neuroleptics (Weinberger *et al.*, 1980a); and a history of maladjustment in childhood (Weinberger *et al.*, 1980b). There has been a notable failure to find any consistent correlation between cerebral atrophy and the duration of illness, duration of hospitalisation, or degree of exposure to neuroleptics or other forms of treatment (Golden *et al.*, 1980a,b; Weinberger *et al.*, 1979a,b).

Correlation has been found for cerebral ventricular size, between healthy siblings, but there is even greater correlation between monozygotic twins. When one of the siblings has schizophrenia there is no correlation, and the affected sibling will usually have the larger ventricles (Reveley *et al.*, 1982; Weinberger *et al.*, 1981). Apart from indicating that cerebral ventricular size is under genetic control, to a certain degree, this provides further evidence for a subgroup of schizophrenic patients with enlarged cerebral ventricles. The significance of this abnormality remains unclear. Whether it is part of the schizophrenic process or an epiphenomenon, e.g. the result of treatment, remains to be seen.

Cerebellar atrophy

Atrophy of the cerebellum, particularly the vermis, has been found in the CAT head scans of schizophrenics, by Heath *et al.* (1979). The significance of this finding is not clear, though the presence of neurological soft signs, which are particularly found in schizophrenics with poor premorbid adjustment (Quitkin *et al.*, 1976), may be the consequence of cerebellar dysfunction. In the normal person there is evidence that the cerebellum acts to inhibit hippocampal activity and stimulate the septal region, both structures being implicated as being important in the mediation of emotional experience and the control of emotional behaviour. It is on the basis of evidence such as this that cerebellar stimulation has been used in the treatment of epilepsy (Cooper *et al.*, 1976), and chronic psychosis (Heath, 1975). Impairment of cerebellar function may explain some of the features of schizophrenia, and this in turn implicates cerebellar disease as an aetiological factor in this illness, but more work is necessary in this area.

Reversed cerebral asymmetry

In the normal human brain the right frontal and left occipital areas are larger than the same areas on the contralateral sides. This asymmetry has been found to be present even in the foetal brain. Reversal of this asymmetry, with relative enlargement of the left frontal and right occipital areas, has been found in certain conditions, notably early infantile autism, delayed speech acquisition, developmental dyslexia, left-handedness (especially if there is a family history), and schizophrenia (Luchins *et al.*, 1982). It has also been associated with a low verbal IQ in some patients, and a better prognosis when present in patients who have developed aphasia.

This finding in schizophrenic patients cannot be explained on the basis of cerebral atrophy and, in fact, tends not to be found in those patients who have cerebral atrophy. This may indicate that schizophrenic patients with abnormal brain scans can be divided into two groups, those with cerebral atrophy, and those with reversed asymmetry. However, carefully controlled studies have failed to confirm these findings (Andreasen *et al.*, 1982; Jernigan *et al.*, 1982b). This may be because there is a third schizophrenic subgroup with no abnormalities evident on brain scanning, or that the aforementioned abnormalities are due to experimental error, i.e. artifacts of the measurement techniques used.

It has been suggested (Luchins *et al.*, 1982) that this finding supports the hypothesis that schizophrenia is related to a disturbance of the function of the cerebral hemisphere dominant for propositional language. This disturbance could be caused by whatever process causes gross brain disease (cerebral atrophy) in one group of patients and by an abnormality of cerebral lateralisation (reversed asymmetry) in another group. The low verbal IQ, in the latter group, is further support for this theory.

The evidence suggests that reversed asymmetry may reflect a long-standing alteration in brain structure, possibly of perinatal origin. A genetic link between the HLA–A_2 antigen and schizophrenics with this reversed asymmetry, but not those with normal asymmetry (Luchins *et al.*, 1981), has been found, but not confirmed.

6.4   AFFECTIVE DISORDERS AND DEMENTIA

Patients with affective disorders have a lower incidence of abnormal scans than schizophrenic patients. As a group their brain scans do not differ significantly from normal controls, but there is preliminary evidence of one subgroup that may differ. A group of elderly patients with depression of late onset, involving endogenous features, have been shown to have enlarged ventricles (Jacoby and Levy, 1980b) and a higher mortality on follow-up 2 years later, when compared with a group of elderly depressives with relatively smaller sized ventricles (Jacoby, 1981).

Another unconfirmed study involved assessment of the density of the centrum semi-ovale, as a means of discriminating between patients with pseudodementia and those with true dementia, the latter group being found to have the lower density (Naeser *et al.*, 1980). Other studies have provided evidence indirectly supporting this finding. Bondareff *et al.* (1981) found that senile dementia patients had lower frontotemporal brain tissue densities than healthy controls. Also, Naguib and Levy (1982a) found an association between a poor prognosis in senile dementia and a low density of brain tissue in the right parietal region. This is in keeping with their other findings, that the presence of aphasia, apraxia and agnosia were also associated with a poor prognosis, in contrast to those patients with senile dementia who did not show these features.

In view of the large number of demented patients in the older age groups, it is difficult to decide who to scan and who not to. Bradshaw *et al.* (1983) found that the chances of finding a potentially remediable lesion were increased if those demented patients exhibiting focal neurological signs, papilloedema, headache or speech disorders, were scanned, in preference to those without these features. Further analysis of these data by Manu (1983) revealed that women, patients in the 65 to 74 year age range, and patients with ataxia, seizures, disorientation or mental confusion, were also more likely to have significant findings on their CAT brain scans.

6.5   REVERSIBLE CEREBRAL "ATROPHY"

The safety and ease with which the scanner can be used facilitates sequential scanning in patients and has led to the realisation that what appears to be "cerebral atrophy" on one scan, may not be present on later scans of the same patient, i.e. the "abnormality" may be reversible. Such reversible changes have been found in patients treated with adrenocorticotrophic hormone or steroids, in patients with Cushing's disease, and in anorexia nervosa. In these cases the scan changes were found to be reversible after the appropriate treatment had been instituted, which either involved discontinuation of the drug or correction of nutritional deficiencies (Bentson *et al.*, 1978; Heinz *et al.*, 1977; Okuro *et al.*, 1980). This "atrophy-like" appearance may be caused by fluid passing into the intravascular spaces due to a low level of serum proteins, secondary to malnutrition and/or protein catabolism. Fluid retention may also be a contributory factor in some cases.

A similar phenomenon has been found in patients with alcoholic brain damage. Cerebral atrophy has been demonstrated in alcoholic patients even as young as in their third decade, and may have antedated the drinking in some cases (Bergman *et al.*, 1980). However, it is more marked in older alcoholics with a longer drinking history. It is associated with cognitive deficits, but the correlation between impaired cognition and cerebral atrophy is not close. In general this atrophy tends to be most marked in the frontal regions. Follow-up studies of alcoholic patients with repeated scanning and psychological testing, after abstinence from alcohol for about 1 year, has demonstrated that this atrophy, and the cognitive deficits, can be partially reversed (Lishman *et al.*, 1980; Tarter, 1980). This raises the question: what is the neuropathological basis of this "atrophy"? One possibility is that chronic alcohol use leads to a reversible loss of neuronal dendritic spines (Riley and Walker, 1978), but this question remains to be answered.

6.6   POSITRON-EMISSION TRANSAXIAL TOMOGRAPHY (PETT) BRAIN SCANNING

By using rectilinear scans to detect gamma ray emitting radionuclides from the brain of a patient who has been administered a radioisotope, it is possible to quantitatively reconstruct the distribution of cerebral radioactivity, with the help of a computer (Ter-Pogossian *et al.*, 1975). With the development of the technique of computerised transaxial tomography, this process was refined so that "slices" of the brain could be reconstructed to show regional cerebral blood flow (rCBF) and metabolism. Short-acting positron emitting isotopes were used, e.g. intravenous ^{18}F fluro-deoxyglucose or inhaled oxygen-15. Though the resolution of these scans is inferior to the more advanced CAT head scanners, they have the advantage of demonstrating brain function pictorially, whereas the CAT scanner can only demonstrate the structure of the brain.

The initial results of PETT scanning the brains of psychiatric patients have shown that in contrast to "normal" controls, schizophrenic patients tend to have a reduction in frontal blood flow (see Buchsbaum *et al.*, 1982). This "hypofrontal" pattern has been demonstrated in previous studies of rCBF, using less sophisticated techniques, and has been associated with those patients showing disorders of motor activity (Franzen and Ingvar, 1975; Ingvar and Franzen, 1974).

6.7   NUCLEAR MAGNETIC RESONANCE (NMR) TOMOGRAPHY OF THE BRAIN

Lauterbur (1973) was one of the first people to describe the technique of NMR imaging. It employs radiofrequency excitation of hydrogen nuclei in human tissue, in the presence of a magnetic field. This results in the formation of an electric current that is detected by a receiver placed around the patient. The strength of the current depends on the number of protons that are produced by this excitation, and the rate of recovery of the hydrogen nuclei.

As with CAT head scanning the computer is used to reconstruct "slices" of the patient's brain. So far the advantages found over the CAT scanner are that artefact formation is less of a problem, ionising radiation is not used, the posterior fossa of the brain can be visualised more clearly, and grey and white matter differentiated more clearly (Doyle *et al.*, 1981). The latter is particularly striking and is due to grey matter containing relatively more hydrogen, in the form of water, whereas in white matter the hydrogen is bound to large molecules to a greater extent (hence the former has a darker appearance on the NMR head scan).

NMR tomography promises to be superior to CAT head scanning in identifying white matter disease, e.g. demyelination (Young *et al.*, 1981), and promises to be an exciting advance in the area of brain imaging.

CHAPTER 7

Personality Change, Epilepsy and Head Injury

7.1 INTRODUCTION

A common clinical problem faced by the neuropsychiatrist is evaluating and identifying the cause(s) of a patient's change in personality. This change may have occurred in a person with a normal well-adjusted premorbid personality, or someone who was already suffering from some premorbid disturbance of personality functioning. By personality I am referring to the person's *"natural and acquired impulses, and habits, interests, and complexes, the sentiments and ideals, the opinions and beliefs, as manifested in his relations with his social milieu"* (Drever, 1964). Certain behavioural traits (enduring patterns of behaviour) will be present and should be identified, though it must be borne in mind that they will always be liable to some variability as a result of different environmental influences.

Before an individual can be regarded as having undergone a change in personality, it is preferable for him to have attained an age (usually in the second or third decade of life) when his behaviour is characterised by certain traits, and his nervous system no longer has the "plasticity" of immaturity which will allow it to compensate for the effects of any acute neurological insult, and thus complicate the assessment of any subsequent behavioural changes. The DSM III does not specify any age limitations in its criteria for the diagnosis of Organic Personality syndrome, but makes reference to the need for there to be "significant" changes in behaviour, for this diagnosis to be made in the child. *The criteria for the Organic Personality syndrome consist of a specific organic factor causing a personality change involving either emotional lability, impaired impulse control, marked apathy, or a tendency to suspiciousness.* Adequate criteria for the diagnosis of any of the other Organic Mental Disorders, or for an Attention Deficit Disorder, must be absent.

In the assessment of such cases it is necessary to interview a "secondary" informant to obtain reliable information about the patient's premorbid personality and to identify any events in the patient's history that may constitute adequate cause for the change in personality. The nervous system functions as

124

a coordinated structure and no single part of it functions in isolation, but certain areas have different functions. In focal disease of the brain the clinical features of the behavioural change may indicate the area of the brain involved. These specific syndromes will now be described. The relevant sections in the chapter on Neuropsychology are intended to complement the following clinical descriptions. Where appropriate, reference will be made to the behavioural effects of seizures originating from certain areas in the brain (Lishman, 1978; Marsden, 1976b).

7.2 FRONTAL LOBE SYNDROME

Personality change, often with a relative absence of neurological or cognitive defects, is particularly associated with frontal lobe lesions and there is evidence that it involves features from one or both of two particular clinical syndromes. These syndromes are called the "pseudo-psychopathic" and the "pseudo-depressed" (Blumer and Benson, 1975).

The *"pseudo-psychopathic" syndrome* refers to a change in personality in which the individual behaves in a socially disinhibited manner. He is impulsive, self-centred and emotionally immature. These changes may involve a tendency to facetious humour or "witzelsucht" (Oppenheim, 1889). Depression or elation may appear, and they may alternate. However, the mood changes tend to be rather shallow and may not reflect the patient's subjective mood (Hecaen and Albert, 1975). The elation may involve a child-like quality, called "moria" by Jastrowitz (1888). Disinhibition may occur and is a particular problem when it involves behaviour of an aggressive or sexual type. Overactivity occurs and behavioural outbursts may be seen, and can involve extreme violence. Judgement, foresight and the finer aspects of social behaviour, such as tact and politeness, are impaired. Paranoid or grandiose tendencies may also be seen.

The "pseudo-psychopathic" syndrome has been particularly associated with damage to the orbitofrontal part of the frontal lobe. Cognitive, language and motor deficits are not a feature of lesions localised in this area (Stuss and Benson, 1982). This part of the frontal lobe appears to have an important role as a modulator of behaviour, inhibiting impulsive and socially inappropriate actions, and modulating emotional behaviour. By controlling sexual or aggressive impulses, for example, according to the circumstances and the potential consequences of the behaviour, a person is more able to act in a socially aware and emotionally mature manner. The refined aspects of normal adult behaviour requires that such controls are present. The frontal lobe is able to carry out this function and produce the appropriate behaviour, by virtue of its connections with the limbic system, which enable it to evaluate the intended actions in relation to the stored memories of previous experiences and their consequences.

One of the first reported examples of this type of personality change was Phineas Gage, whose case was reported by Harlow (1868). Gage developed the syndrome after an accident at his work which resulted in a metal bar passing through the frontal lobes of his brain. He subsequently exhibited features of both the "pseudo-psychopathic" and "pseudo-depressed" personality type.

The *"pseudo-depressed" syndrome* involves a reduction in the quantity and quality of motor behaviour, resulting in apathy, impersistence, lack of flexibility in switching motor sets, loss of initiative and spontaneity. A loss of libido and a reduction in emotional responsiveness, may also be seen. These patients show a slowing of thought and motor activity that can give the appearance of depressive psychomotor retardation; however, there is an "empty indifference" in their ideation, in contrast to the morbid preoccupations of the truly depressed patient. This picture may progress to a stage of akinetic mutism, when a progressive frontal lobe lesion is present.

This syndrome has been associated with damage to the dorsolateral region of the frontal lobe (Stuss and Benson, 1982) and, in contrast to orbitofrontal lesions, some degree of intellectual impairment is not uncommon, though it may not be evident on routine psychological testing. The prefrontal cortex has a role in controlling the level of arousal and motor behaviour, according to the emotional and motivational significance of the sensory information it receives from the inferior parietal lobule (Watson *et al.*, 1981). A lesion of this part of the frontal lobe will, therefore, produce a relative lack of motor response (a motor inattention) to incoming sensory information, irrespective of the nature or importance of this information. In this context the development of the clinical features of apathy and loss of initiative (the capacity to act in an independent way), is understandable. A lesion disconnecting this part of the frontal lobe from its afferent or efferent connections could produce a similar picture, and damage to these pathways can cause a "sub-cortical" dementia, a condition which is clinically similar to the "pseudo-depressed" syndrome.

The two types of frontal lobe syndromes are not mutually exclusive, and features of both often coexist, particularly when the lesion is poorly localized, e.g. the result of a closed head injury. In such cases the clinical picture may be one of transient shallow mood swings, occurring against a background of persistent apathy.

Such behavioural changes usually do not develop *de novo*. *The patient's premorbid personality will influence the subsequent behavioural manifestations of frontal lobe damage.* Disinhibition will result in more serious problems if the patient exhibited aggressive traits in his premorbid personality, than if he was stable and well adjusted. This is one reason why careful evaluation of the patient's premorbid personality is a necessary prerequisite in order for the operation of orbitofrontal leucotomy to produce a good result (Kelly, 1976).

If epileptic attacks occur and the discharge involves the primary motor cortex, focal motor seizures will occur which may remain localised or may spread with a Jacksonian march, the movements reflecting the spread of the epileptic discharge from the initial ictal site to adjacent areas of the motor cortex. Such an attack may culminate in a grand mal convulsion if the discharge spreads to the opposite side of the brain. If the ictal focus is in the premotor area, the seizure may cause the head and eyes to turn to the opposite side (an adversive aura). Dysphasia may occur if the left lobe is involved. Elevation of one arm, followed by turning of the head towards the arm, is typically seen when a seizure discharge originates in the contralateral supplementary motor area (anterior to the central sulcus on the medial aspect of the hemisphere). The site of the initial seizure discharge may be indicated by a post-ictal impairment of function (Todd's paralysis) at the site of origin of the seizure discharge. This may involve a transient contralateral focal weakness or dysphasia.

If the lesion is in the orbital area, a temporal lobe seizure may occur. This usually involves a sudden brief episode of impaired consciousness, which may be followed by a short period of automatic behaviour. An unusual aura involving a subjective disturbance of thinking with a feeling of thoughts intruding into the mind or thoughts becoming crowded, may be experienced (Lishman, 1978). Transient episodes of being only able to think about a single idea have been described and such experiences do not always appear to be the result of an epileptic discharge, but are sometimes regarded as a form of "epileptic equivalent". Also, other paroxysmal disorders may occasionally occur, involving hallucinations or disorientation (Hecaen and Albert, 1975).

Table 7.1   Causes of the frontal lobe syndrome

Alcohol	Chronic abuse.
Blood vessel	Subarachnoid haemorrhage from an anterior cerebral artery or anterior communicating artery aneurysm.
	Giant aneurysm.
Degenerative	Pick's dementia, subcortical dementia.
	Hydrocephalus (communicating, obstructive, normal pressure).
Metabolic	Hepatic encephalopathy.
Growth	Primary, e.g. meningioma.
	Secondary.
Infection	Abscess, herpes simplex encephalitis, syphilis.
Injury and	Trauma (especially closed head injury).
post-operative	Stereotactic psychosurgery (tractotomy, limbic leucotomy).

Causes of the frontal lobe syndrome

Table 7.1 shows the conditions that tend to preferentially involve the frontal lobes.

Chronic alcohol abuse can cause a generalised dementia, though the cerebral damage has a particular propensity to affect the frontal lobes of the brain (Lishman, 1981). This may explain some of the cases of frontal lobe personality change that have been described in patients who have a history of hepatic encephalopathy (Murphy *et al.*, 1948).

Frontal lobe personality change in the relative absence of intellectual impairment is a common sequel to *subarachnoid haemorrhage* (SAH) from either an anterior cerebral or anterior communicating artery aneurysm. The majority of the blood supply to the brain comes from the anterior, middle and posterior cerebral arteries. Because they are connected at the Circle of Willis, an interruption of the blood flow in one of these arteries will have neurobehavioural results which will be influenced by the patency of this interconnecting system.

One important vessel that arises directly from the internal carotid artery is the anterior choroidal artery and it supplies the basal ganglia, thalamus, amygdala, internal capsule and the hippocampal formation. The anterior cerebral artery, through several branches, supplies the orbitofrontal region, the medial surfaces of the frontal and parietal lobes, the paracentral lobule, the frontal convexity and parts of the cingulate gyrus, corpus callosum and fornix (Walsh, 1978).

SAH from an anterior cerebral or anterior communicating artery aneurysm may result in a deterioration, but it can also cause an *improvement* in the patient's personality. In 17% of one series of 81 cases, the patients' relatives felt his behaviour had improved (Storey, 1970). This improvement seemed to be partly due to a "leucotomy effect" in those who had had obsessional traits in their premorbid personalities. Their obsessional traits became less marked and they were more affectionate and understanding in their relationships with others, exhibiting less irritability and more vitality. Personality change without intellectual impairment was particularly associated with right sided lesions. Occasionally frontal lobe damage may result from a bleeding aneurysm in a site remote from the frontal lobe (Levin *et al.*, 1982).

Giant cerebral aneurysms are an uncommon finding, but Bull (1969) described six cases (27% of his series of aneurysms at the base of the brain) presenting primarily with dementia. Two were diagnosed as frontal lobe tumours, and another caused a subfrontal mass. One of these was from the middle cerebral artery and another from the carotid bifurcation. Neurological signs were slight (papilloedema and UMN facial weakness in both), but plain skull radiographs were abnormal. Anterior cerebral aneurysms can affect the frontal lobes by pressure and ischaemia, and physical examination may reveal an audible cranial bruit.

There is a particular tendency for the frontal horns of the cerebral ventricles to enlarge more than other areas of the ventricular system in *hydrocephalus*, whether it is obstructive or communicating in type. This probably causes disturbance in frontal lobe function and would explain the development of features such as apathy, inertia and incontinence of urine, which are sometimes prominent in these conditions (Ojemann *et al.*, 1969).

Frontal lobe tumours which progress slowly tend to be relatively silent, especially if they involve the right frontal lobe. They may present as a dementia or as a change in personality. Slow growing meningiomas as particularly found in the orbito-frontal region and may produce clinical manifestations for years before they become clinically overt (Hunter *et al.*, 1968). Tumours of the anterior part of the corpus callosum tend to spread to involve the frontal lobes, but in these cases a rapidly progressive dementia occurs in association with the "frontal lobe" personality change (Schlesinger, 1950).

Bacterial or viral infections may affect this region of the brain. A *frontal lobe abscess* is usually the result of frontal sinusitis or a fracture of the frontal bone. After the initial illness the abscess may develop insidiously, with few neurological signs (Gates *et al.*, 1950). *Syphilitic inflammation* of the brain has a propensity for involving the frontal lobes and it has been described as presenting with personality change, such as a shallow affect, in addition to the other features of General Paralysis of the insane (Lishman, 1978). The *herpes simplex virus* is particularly prone to attack the orbito-frontal cortex (Greenwood *et al.*, 1983).

The orbito-frontal region and the temporal lobes are particularly vulnerable to *closed head injury*, and post-traumatically a subtle personality change, e.g. a more outward-going attitude, may be the only change noted (Levin *et al.*, 1982). It should be emphasised that brain damage resulting from a severe closed head injury is unlikely to be focal in type, and will involve several areas of the brain, including the subcortical pathways that mediate arousal and other processes that are essential for the efficient performance of higher cortical functions. So the clinical picture in such cases will be complicated by a variable degree of subcortical damage.

Psychosurgery has been used to produce selective frontal lobe damage for therapeutic purposes. The consequences of such surgery have, indirectly, increased our knowledge of the neurobehavioural role of the frontal lobes. Frontal lobectomy, sparing the orbito-frontal region, has been used to treat epilepsy (Stuss and Benson, 1982). Leucotomy surgery, aimed at interrupting the fronto-limbic connections, has produced extensive orbito-frontal damage in the past, when the freehand technique was used, but more recent operations using stereotactic techniques have minimal side effects. Stereotactic surgery refers to the use of certain techniques, such as a rectangular frame—the Leksell frame—which attaches to the patient's head. This allows the surgeon to identify his target point with great accuracy and hence produce only a small localised lesion in the brain. The two operations used on the frontal lobe (Kelly, 1976) are the tractotomy (cutting the fibres overlying the posterior orbital cortex) and the limbic leucotomy (aimed at the lower medial quadrant of the frontal lobe, usually with an additional lesion in the anterior cingulate gyrus).

Ström-Olsen and Carlisle (1971) followed up 150 patients who had had a stereotactic tractotomy and found 56% of the previously depressed, 50% of the obsessional, and 41% of the anxious patients, had benefitted, with only 11% of the whole series having developed personality changes, notably a tendency to be irritable, over-talkative and outspoken. These changes in personality were not troublesome.

Certain symptoms have been found to respond to a limbic leucotomy. This operation can produce a significant decrease in anxiety, depression and obsessional symptoms, as well as reducing the distress they cause. When a sample of these patients were evaluated after the initial post-operative month, some exhibited mild personality changes with a tendency to be impulsive, outspoken or lethargic, but these effects were mild (Kelly, 1976). The results of these operations are impressive when one considers the severe impairment of most of the patient's pre-operatively and their resistance to other treatment modalities.

Frontal lobe features may be pronounced in both Pick's dementia and the subcortical dementias. These conditions are discussed further in Chapter 10.

7.3 TEMPORO-LIMBIC SYNDROME

Lesions of the anterior pole of the temporal lobe may be "silent", particularly if the right side only is involved, but usually they result in changes in personality and intellect. The clinical signs of temporal lobe disease may be roughly separated into those associated with lesions of the lateral part and those associated with lesions of the medial part. Structures in the latter region form part of the limbic system.

The neurological deficits found with the more lateral temporal lobe disorders are modality-specific memory impairment (verbal memory—left temporal lobe, non-verbal memory—right temporal lobe), modality-specific auditory perception (rhythmic sounds—right temporal lobe, non-rhythmic sounds—left temporal lobe), and visual field deficits (typically a contralateral upper quadrantanopsia). A sensory aphasia and other disorders of language functions can occur, if the posterior part of the dominant lobe is involved.

Hallucinatory phenomena or illusions may occur, and by their nature indicate the site of the lesion in the temporal lobe. Visual hallucinations in a hemianopic field of vision almost always indicate a temporal lobe disorder. Olfactory (smell)

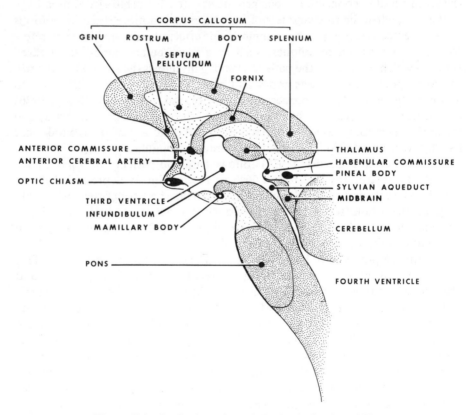

Figure 7.1   Sagittal section of the brain in the midline

or gustatory (taste) hallucinations usually arise from ictal foci in the region of the uncus. These hallucinatory experiences may occur as part of a temporal lobe seizure (TLE). TLE can occur with lesions virtually anywhere in the temporo-limbic region. Other perceptual disturbances seen in TLE are mentioned in Chapter 16.

Figures 7.1, 7.2, 7.3 and 7.4 demonstrate the anatomical relationships of the parts of the limbic system. The structures and tracts involved in this system are listed in Table 7.2. They are situated in the anterior and medial parts of the temporal lobe, the orbital part of the frontal lobe, the diencephalon, the mid-brain and the cingulate gyrus, and certain other gray matter structures. The limbic system is involved, among other things, in the formation of associations between afferent stimuli and emotional tone. This involves the mechanism of conditioned learning, which is mediated by the *"memory circuit"* which consists of the *mamillary body–fornix–hippocampal pathway*. There are three main circuits in the limbic system, the Papez, the Basolateral and the Defence Reaction circuits. (The latter two will be described in Chapter 8.) The *Papez circuit* (Papez, 1937) passes from the *septum*, via the *cingulate gyrus* to the *hippocampus*, via the *fornix* to the *mamillary bodies*, via the *mamillo-thalamic tract* to the *anterior thalamus*, and then back to the *cingulate gyrus*.

The actual anatomical relationship between these structures is demonstrated in Figure 7.2. Papez suggested that sensory information from the cerebral cortex is stored in the hippocampus, and it is then passed on to the hypothalamus, where the emotional feeling that is generated is then passed to the cingulate gyrus. Impulses from the cingulate gyrus passing to the cerebral cortex would then add emotional colouring to any concurrent psychic experiences. Despite the seminal nature of Papez's paper, it is unlikely, in the light of current knowledge, that the cingulate gyrus is the primary receptive site for emotional experience (Boddy, 1978).

The amygdala is a crucial structure in this system and appears to play a major role in connecting the sensory association cortices with the hypothalamus (Bear, 1979a). The amygdala and hippocampi are connected by the cingulate gyrus, the fornix and the stria terminalis, to the hypothalamus, septal nuclei, tuberculum olfactorium and nucleus accumbens. The latter two form part of the dopaminergic mesolimbic system. The nucleus accumbens appears to play a role in mediating pleasure (which is experienced when it is electrically stimulated), and appears to act to "reward" certain behaviours, thus providing positive reinforcement. Conversely, dysphoria is experienced when the hippocampus or amygdala are electrically stimulated in man (Trimble, 1981a). It should be noted that the caudate nucleus is not part of the limbic system.

The clinical features of disorders of the temporal lobe are better understood if one initially considers the *Klüver–Bucy syndrome* (KBS). Klüver and Bucy (1939) observed the behaviour of rhesus monkeys after they had been subjected to a bi-temporal lobectomy (including removal of the amygdalae, unci and hippocampi). These monkeys demonstrated features which appeared to result from the disconnection of the temporal lobes from the diencephalon. In one

Table 7.2 Components of the limbic system

GRAY MATTER STRUCTURES

	Amygdala
AN thal	Anterior nucleus of thalamus
CG	Central gray matter
	Cingulate gyrus
G	Gudden's ventral tegmental nucleus
HAB	Habenular nuclei
	Hippocampal gyrus
	Hippocampal formation
HYPO	Hypothalamus
IPN	Interpeduncular nucleus
MAM B	Mammillary body
NAUTA	Nauta area of lateral midbrain
NUC SEPTUM	Septal nucleus
	Subcallosal gyrus
	Supracallosal gyrus
	Tuberculum olfactorium
	Uncus

CONNECTING TRACTS

AC	Anterior commissure
DBB	Diagonal band of Broca
	Fimbria
	Fornix
	Mamillothalamic tract
MFB	Medial forebrain bundle
	Olfactory stria (medial and lateral)
	Stria medullaris
	Stria terminalis

sense the operation can be said to tame the monkey and *the mnemonic TAMES can be used to remember the features of the syndrome* (see Table 7.3).

The sensory information from the outside world is processed by the temporal lobes and analysed in relation to the memories of previous experience. As a result of this, sexual and other drives are directed towards the appropriate object choices, which have been learnt mainly during the formative years, by the process of conditioning. The sensory experience evokes certain emotions by means of its connection with the limbic system. The diencephalon monitors and controls the internal milieu of the body, via the autonomic and endocrine modalities, and interacts with the appropriate temporal lobe structures to generate the basic drives involving sexual, exploratory, aggressive, eating and drinking behaviour (Bear, 1979a).

The midline limbic structure, the hypothalamus, appears to control the level of drive activity, whereas the temporal lobe, by virtue of its connections with afferent impulses from the outside world and the appropriate memory engrams, influences the choice of the object to which the drive activity is directed. Thus a *disconnection syndrome* develops when these two parts of the limbic system are separated, resulting in drives involving excessive aggressive, exploratory,

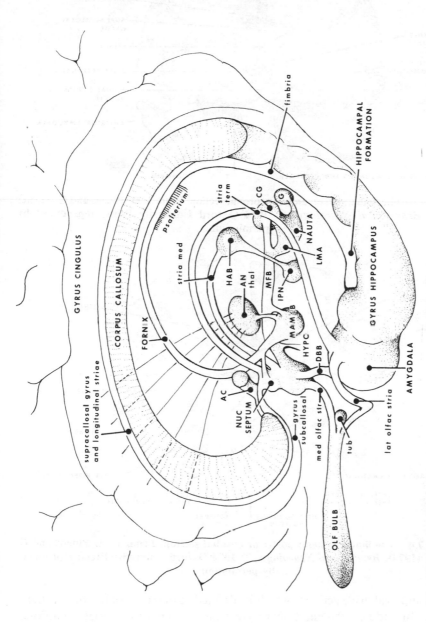

Figure 7.2   The limbic system. From J. H. Pincus and G. Tucker (1974). *Behavioural Neurology*. © 1974 Oxford University Press; reproduced by permission

134

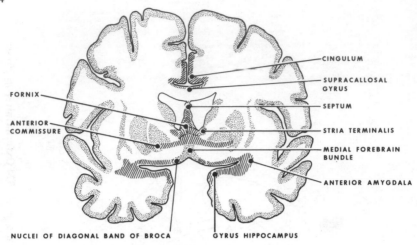

Figure 7.3   The limbic system: anterior coronal section. From J. H. Pincus and G. Tucker (1974). *Behavioural Neurology.* © 1974 Oxford University Press; reproduced by permission

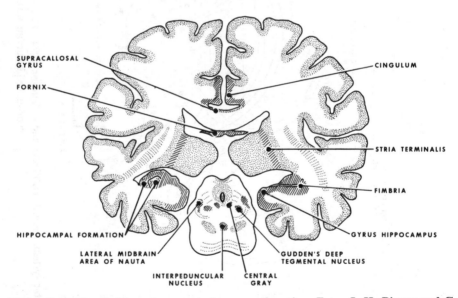

Figure 7.4   The limbic system: posterior coronal section. From J. H. Pincus and G. Tucker (1974). *Behavioural Neurology.* © 1974 Oxford University Press; reproduced by permission

sexual and oral drive activity, which is directed at inappropriate objects (Bear, 1979a). In addition the emotional significance of and appropriate emotional response to environmental stimuli, is impaired, resulting in apathy and indifference. Disconnection from the memory circuits results in failure to recognise familiar objects (visual agnosia).

Table 7.3   Temporo-limbic "disconnection" versus "hyperconnection"

KLÜVER–BUCY SYNDROME ("Disconnection")	INTER-ICTAL PERSONALITY IN TLE ("Hyperconnection")
Tames monkey (apathetic and indifferent to threatening stimuli)	Deepening of emotions
	Dysphoria
Agnosia (visual and auditory)	*Deja vu and other illusions of familiarity or unfamiliarity
Motor activity increased (restless and with a constant switching of attention to any stimulus in the environment. Tends to examine objects with his mouth)	Viscous, circumstantial
Eating excessively (inappropriate object choice)	Anorexia nervosa
Sexual overactivity (inappropriate object choice)	Hyposexuality

*Usually ictal.

Removal of the temporal neocortex and the amygdala appear to be crucial to the formation of the features of the KBS. Bilateral removal of the amygdala can result in all the features of the syndrome developing, except for the agnosia (Wood, 1958), which can be produced by bilateral removal of the temporal neocortex (Bagshaw *et al.*, 1972; Stepien *et al.*, 1960).

In contrast, many of the features of the so-called *inter-ictal personality syndrome of temporal lobe epilepsy* are the opposite of those found in the KBS. Bear (1979b) suggested that recurrent seizure discharges in temporo-limbic structures facilitate the development of new functional pathways, i.e. causes "hyperconnection" in contrast to the "disconnection" syndrome seen in KBS. These pathways may be formed as a result of a "kindling" type of process, induced by recurrent epileptic neuronal discharges which facilitate nervous conduction in certain neuronal pathways (Goddard *et al.*, 1969). This "hyperconnection" would explain why the patient with TLE tends to exhibit certain character traits such as a deepened emotionality, a tendency to dysphoria, and hyposexuality. In addition, he often has difficulty in detaching himself from one particular train of thought and so is unable to switch from one idea to another, resulting in circumstantiality and "viscosity". Table 7.3 contrasts these two syndromes. Anorexia nervosa is not particularly associated with epilepsy, though it has been reported (Szyper and Mann, 1978). *Déjà vu* and similar phenomena are usually encountered during a seizure, whereas the other components of the *"hyperconnection" syndrome* are inter-ictal and are not usually a feature of the seizure itself. The deepening of emotions is a characteristic feature of this syndrome and is diagnostically important, since these patients can show many of the features associated with the schizotypal personality, including magical thinking, paranoid tendencies, circumstantial speech and difficulty establishing interpersonal relationships, but they do not show the schizotypal emotional flattening.

This is a controversial subject, but there is evidence that some patients with epilepsy, particularly TLE (Bear and Fedio, 1977) are prone to develop certain personality traits, notably humourlessness, circumstantiality, dependency, and a sense of personal destiny. When patients with unilateral temporal lobe foci were evaluated by Bear and Fedio, they found that the latter two traits, together with anger and paranoia, were particularly associated with an ictal focus in the left temporal lobe, whereas elation and obsessionalism, and more recently hypergraphia (Roberts *et al.*, 1982), were preferentially associated with right-sided ictal foci. All these aforementioned traits were found to be significantly more common in epileptic patients when they were compared to two non-epileptic populations. One of these populations contained subjects who were physically healthy, the other contained patients suffering from chronic organic disorders not involving the cerebral hemispheres. These differences in personality traits were much less pronounced when patients with TLE were compared to patients with generalised epilepsy. The TLE patients showed a significant increase in the traits of: a sense of personal destiny, dependency, paranoia, and philosophical interests (Hermann and Reil, 1981). The differences are also less pronounced when TLE patients are compared to non-epileptic psychiatric patients (Bear *et al.*, 1982; Mungas, 1982), though Bear *et al.* still found definite differences in affect, thought and behaviour. In patients with epilepsy, other factors may play a role in causing psychopathology. These factors include not only recurrent neuronal discharges, but the type of epilepsy, its social and educational consequences, the presence of brain damage, and treatment factors such as anticonvulsants and neurosurgery (Reynolds, 1983). Aggression in relation to organic brain disease will be discussed in the next chapter.

In conclusion it should be noted that *there is no good evidence for there being any specific "epileptic personality", but that epileptics do appear to show quantitative differences in certain personality traits, when compared to non-epileptics, though these differences are less marked when non-epileptic psychiatric patients are looked at.* However, some differences have been found even then, the differences varying with the type of psychiatric disorder involved.

Causes of the temporo-limbic syndrome

Table 7.4 shows those disorders that tend to preferentially affect the temporo-limbic structures in the brain. R. Post (1975) has demonstrated that *cocaine abuse* can produce three different syndromes in man—a euphoric, a dysphoric, and a schizophreniform picture. The euphoria is associated with hyperactivity, hypersexuality, hyperarousal and anorexia. The dysphoria is associated with apathy, depression, delusions and anorexia. The schizophreniform psychosis involves hallucinations and delusions, anhedonia, stereotyped behaviour and an excessive concern with detail. In some cases there is a progression through these "stages"—euphoria ⟶ dysphoria ⟶ psychosis. In view of the evidence, notably the potent effect of the drug in kindling the limbic system of primates, and the marked affective changes produced by the drug, Post and

Kopanda (1976) have postulated that a limbic kindling process may be involved in man.

Personality change following *subarachnoid haemorrhage* is most common when it is due to rupture of an aneurysm of the middle cerebral artery. This artery passes through the lateral cerebral fissure to supply the orbitofrontal and lateral aspects of the temporal and parietal lobes (Walsh, 1978).

In one study, personality change was found following 63% of 71 cases of middle cerebral artery haemorrhage (Storey, 1970), and it was usually associated with both intellectual and neurological deficits. Few of these patients showed any improvement in personality as a result of their SAH. The changes seen included a tendency to be dependent, emotionally labile and fatuous. Depression and anxiety are particularly likely to occur in those with a premorbid neurotic predisposition.

Table 7.4 Causes of the temporo-limbic syndrome

Drugs	Cocaine abuse.
Blood vessel disease	Subarachnoid haemorrhage from a middle cerebral artery aneurysm.
Degenerative	Dementia of Alzheimer's type, Pick's dementia.
Epileptic	Inter-ictal personality syndrome.
Growth	Primary, secondary, limbic encephalitis.
Hypoxia	Mesial temporal sclerosis.
Injury and post-operative	Trauma (especially closed head injury). Temporal lobectomy.
Infection	Abscess, herpes simplex encephalitis, rabies.

Primary degenerative dementia commonly involves the temporal lobes at an early stage. In *dementia of the Alzheimer's type*, the initial symptoms are usually of memory impairment of gradual increasing severity. This is probably due to the fact that the histopathological changes that characterise this disorder are most frequently found in the temporal cortex, especially the hippocampus (Ball, 1982). In the early stages of *Pick's dementia* it is personality change, rather than memory impairment, that predominates. However, features of the Klüver–Bucy syndrome may be seen at a relatively early stage in the dementia (Cummings and Duchen, 1981).

Temporal lobe tumours produce more mental disturbance and are more likely to produce epilepsy (50% of cases), than those anywhere else in the CNS. With or without epilepsy there appears to be a particular risk of schizophrenia-like psychosis developing, especially when the dominant lobe is involved (Sherwin *et al.*, 1982). In some cases the psychosis may antedate other evidence of a lesion in this area (Torrey and Peterson, 1974). In 100 consecutive TLE patients subjected to temporal lobectomy, Falconer (1969) found that 22% had hamartomas or other small cryptic tumours. The commonest finding was medial temporal sclerosis in 47%, presumably the result of febrile convulsions in childhood damaging the medial temporal structures, which are particularly vulnerable to anoxia at that time.

Carcinoma may affect cerebral function in many ways, not only as a primary tumour or a secondary deposit in the CNS, but also as a remote effect with no tumour cells present in the CNS. Almost any part of the nervous system may be affected indirectly by malignant disease. Histologically the changes often involve a combination of inflammation and degeneration. This is most commonly associated with carcinoma of the bronchus and the tumour may only be found at post mortem. In those cases where the tumour has been resected, remote neurological damage has still occurred later, even in the absence of any evidence of tumour recurrence (Lishman, 1978). Corsellis *et al.* (1968) described several cases of *limbic encephalitis*, where the medial temporal structures were preferentially, and indirectly, affected by carcinoma. Memory impairment was the most prominent symptom. Affective changes, progressive dementia, hallucinations and epilepsy were seen in some cases, and an increase in CSF protein and lymphocytosis, with EEG abnormalities in the temporal region, were frequently found. Progression was not an essential feature in this syndrome. The means by which the tumour produces this effect is unknown. The part of the CNS involved suggests that an opportunistic subclinical herpes simplex infection may be responsible, possibly resulting from an impaired immunological system, due to the tumour.

Anterior temporal lobectomy for epilepsy results in a mild deficit of verbal or non-verbal memory, depending on whether the left or right lobe is removed. Pre-operatively, care must be taken to ensure there is no significant disease of the contralateral lobe, or else a severe and disabling short-term memory deficit and features of the Klüver–Bucy syndrome may result (Greenwood *et al.*, 1983).

The temporal lobe is the commonest site for an *intracerebral abscess*, which usually develops as a complication of a middle ear infection. Neurological signs are often slight and a high threshold of suspicion should be maintained for such a complication (Gates *et al.*, 1950). The signs of infection may not be pronounced as the abscess is walled off by fibrous tissue from the surrounding brain. There is usually an elevated cerebrospinal fluid (CSF) pressure and protein, and a CSF lymphocytosis (Lishman, 1978).

In *herpes simplex encephalitis* the virus tends to attack the orbito-frontal and the inferior and medial temporal structures of the brain, and in cases where affected patients have survived, some have shown features of the Klüver–Bucy syndrome (Greenwood *et al.*, 1983). The *rabies virus* tends to attack the medial parts of the temporal lobe causing episodes of terror, hypersexuality, pharyngeal spasm, hydrophobia and violent rages. The characteristic histopathological findings—negri bodies—are concentrated in the region of the hippocampus (Boddy, 1978). The incubation period following infection, usually via the saliva of a rabid dog, can last up to a year.

7.4 THE "BASAL SYNDROME" AND OTHER ORGANIC DISORDERS

This term had been used to describe the clinical picture that is associated with damage to the diencephalon, mid-brain and orbito-frontal cortex (Lishman,

1978). As the latter region forms part of the frontal lobe *and* the limbic system, there is inevitably some overlap between the characteristic clinical features of lesions in these three areas. Other clinical findings in this syndrome are global amnesia of the Korsakoff type (mammillo-thalamic damage), disorders of thirst, appetite, sleep, temperature regulation and sexual behaviour. The pituitary gland may be involved, producing features of hypopituitarism. Mood swings may be seen with lesions in this region and they may reach psychotic proportions. Transient manic reactions have also been described following operations on the hypothalamus (Lishman, 1978). An epileptic discharge from this area tends to manifest autonomic features, e.g. hyperventilation, flushing, and an urge to urinate or defaecate.

Where the third ventricle narrows to the aqueduct of Sylvius, a small tumour, an area of inflammation or any small lesion, can cause an obstruction to the flow of CSF. This will result in hydrocephalus and raised intracranial pressure which, if acute, clinically causes headache, papilloedema, hypertension and bradycardia, nausea and vomiting. Alternatively the obstruction may be intermittent or more gradual, producing an increasing obstruction to the flow of the CSF, resulting in an insidious and generalised intellectual deterioration.

Because the brain tracts are crowded together in these areas, small lesions can cause relatively widespread neurological disruption. They can cause pseudobulbar palsy (mid-brain) or parietal lobe signs (thalamus). Sometimes such lesions are almost silent, causing just a few clinical signs, such as hypalgesia or analgesia (thalamus) or impairment of conjugate gaze (mid-brain).

Thiamine deficiency can cause damage to the thalamus, mammillary bodies, and the brain adjoining the Sylvian aqueduct and the third ventricle. This is usually secondary to chronic alcoholism, but it can result from disorders of the upper gastrointestinal tract (carcinoma, recurrent vomiting, infections or pure dietary deficiency). The acute stage of this disorder is called *Wernicke's encephalopathy* and clinically involves a confusional state with cranial nerve palsies (the oculomotor and abducens nerves), and impairment of conjugate gaze, due to the damage in the mesencephalic region. Nystagmus and ataxia result from vestibulo-cerebellar damage, and tend to be the neurological signs that remain, often indefinitely, as an indication of the aetiology of any resulting memory deficit. In 84% of patients with Wernicke's encephalopathy, a global memory deficit is left after recovery *(Korsakoff's amnesia)*, and it is the result of mamillothalamic damage (Victor *et al.*, 1971). Memory impairment of this type is frequently seen following *subarachnoid haemorrhage* (SAH) from an aneurysm of the anterior communicating artery (Logue *et al.*, 1968), or it may occur as a result of operative intervention, following the haemorrhage (Lindqvist and Norlén, 1966). In most of these patients the dysmnesia improves with time.

An unusual phenomenon was described by Walton (1953), who found that several of his patients developed their memory impairment after an interval of up to several weeks, following the SAH. This was attributed to the formation of tissue adhesions in the septal region, the dysmnesia improving when the adhesions later resolved. In other cases the adhesions may lead to obstruction of the flow of cerebrospinal fluid and the development of hydrocephalus.

The vertebrobasilar system of vessels supply the brain stem, the cerebellum and the posterior part of the diencephalon. The basilar artery then divides into the posterior cerebral arteries which, directly or via their branches, supply most of the occipital lobe, the inferior surface of the temporal lobe and the posterior part of the hippocampus (Walsh, 1978). In view of the latter it is understandable why occlusion of the posterior cerebral artery can cause a global memory deficit, and why ischaemia in this area is probably the cause of transient global amnesia (Alexander, 1982).

Bull (1969) found an unusually close relationship between *massive aneurysms of the vertebrobasilar system* and dementia (four out of six of his cases). Neurological signs were present in all cases, but plain skull radiographs were normal in all. Two of them clinically mimicked a *third ventricle cyst*, a tumour that is particularly likely to cause mental symptoms and recurrent attacks of weakness (which may cause falling) in the limbs, headache and dizziness (Merritt, 1979).

Tumours most likely to be seen in this area include craniopharyngiomas, pinealomas, and third ventricle cysts. Tumours of the thalamus can be classified into medial and lateral groups on the basis of clinical differences. Lateral lesions cause neurological deficits, such as hemianopsia, hemisensory deficits and hemichorea. Medial lesions cause less obvious abnormalities of mood, memory and personality. The latter tumours are usually gliomas and because of their site of origin they do not usually involve the hypothalamus. The medial syndrome can be regarded as a form of subcortical dementia and shows clinical overlap with other subcortical disorders cause this picture. Other causes of thalamic damage include cerebrovascular disease, post-operative, and idiopathic degeneration.

The shearing forces associated with a *closed head injury* may produce transient or permanent damage to the hypothalamo-pituitary system. The effects of such damage may be clinically subtle. Behavioural disturbance is the commonest neuropsychiatric sequel to head injury in children, and in some cases the clinical features are similar to those seen following encephalitis lethargica (see below).

Though neuropathological changes are diffuse in *encephalitis lethargica*, they are mainly found in the mid-brain and diencephalon, in the acute stage of the illness, and this is reflected in the classical triad of signs — fever, somnolence and opthalmoplegia (Yahr, 1974). Personality change following encephalitis lethargica is particularly seen in the young and includes episodes of over-activity and compulsive antisocial behaviour, aggression, emotional lability and disinhibited behaviour. Self-mutilation and sexually deviant behaviour may occur, and feelings of guilt are frequently present in between these antisocial outbursts. Many patients become progressively more disturbed with time, though others improve around puberty or as a result of developing parkinsonism. There is a relative absence of intellectual deficits (Lishman, 1978).

Whether or not this is an endemic disease, is a moot point. Greenough and Davis (1983) have recently described three children who developed somnolence, lethargy and emotional lability (one child became profoundly depressed and attempted suicide), after a mild viral-like illness. They suggest that these cases may be the result of encephalitis lethargica and recommend that this diagnosis be considered in children who develop chronic emotional and behavioural disturbances with atypical depression.

Meningitis, especially due to tuberculosis, can involve the base of the brain. This may result in the development of communicating hydrocephalus, with or without raised CSF pressure. Obstructive hydrocephalus may be caused by an abscess in the cerebellar region and it is this site, along with the frontal and temporal lobes, that intracranial abscesses most commonly develop. It is usually a complication of a middle ear infection (Gates *et al.*, 1950).

Though damage to the occipital and parietal lobes, the basal ganglia and cerebellum, may produce enduring neurological and psychological deficits, changes in personality are not a characteristic or consistent clinical feature.

7.5 HEAD INJURY

In assessing the neuropsychiatric consequences of a head injury it is necessary to carry out a full history and examination, particularly with reference to the features listed in Table 7.5. The neuropsychiatric consequences of a head injury are a result of the interaction of many of these factors and are listed in Table 7.6.

Lishman (1978) has described the common post-traumatic personality changes as a loss of refinement and a reduced vitality of behaviour. Such changes are sometimes transient and they represent the mild end of a spectrum of post-traumatic disorders that not only tend to show some correlation with the severity of neurological damage, but are also likely to be influenced by interaction with other aspects of the patient's environment, such as his work and family situation. Further along this hypothetical spectrum the changes of the Organic Personality syndrome (DSM III, 1980) may be seen.

The post-traumatic sequelae that may occur are shown in Table 7.6. Some of them may reflect damage to a specific area of the brain, particularly if there has been a penetrating injury. Any focal features resulting from blunt head trauma will usually be superimposed on other less specific consequences, resulting from more diffuse cerebral damage. Damage at the site of impact is called a "coup" injury, but movement of the brain in the skull may lead to cerebral damage on the opposite side ("contre coup"), or even in other areas. Levin *et al.* (1982) regarded the mechanical shearing and tearing of nerve fibres and blood vessels as the main cause of the primary diffuse brain damage that follows blunt head trauma.

Damage to the dominant (in contrast to the right) hemisphere, especially if there are sensorimotor deficits on the right side of the body or a right sided quadrantanopsia, have been found to be particularly associated with psychiatric problems (Lishman, 1968). Lishman found affective illnesses to be more common following damage to the non-dominant cerebral hemisphere. In the affective psychoses, predisposition in the patient's premorbid personality is often an important factor (Lishman, 1973). Other consequences of damage to this

Table 7.5 Factors influencing the sequelae of a head injury

PHYSICAL CONSEQUENCES OF THE TRAUMA	Open (displacement or penetration of the bones protecting the brain) or closed
	Dural penetration
	Intracranial haematoma and/or infection
	Duration of anterograde amnesia
	Occurrence of seizures (in the first post-traumatic week or later)
	Area(s) of brain damaged
	Amount of brain tissue damaged
OTHER ASPECTS OF THE TRAUMATIC EVENT	Who the patient perceives as responsible for the injury
	Other people injured (especially those emotionally close to the patient)
	Work related accident
PREMORBID DATA	Genetic predisposition to psychiatric illness
	Previous psychiatric illness (especially alcoholism)
	Personality, age, employment, socio-economic situation
POST-TRAUMATIC DATA	Litigation involved
	Effect of trauma on patient's employment and personal life

Table 7.6 The neuropsychiatric consequences of head injury

PERSONALITY CHANGE	Organic personality syndrome
	Frontal lobe type
	Temporal lobe type
	Aggressive behaviour
	Other
NEUROSES	Affective neurosis
	Post-traumatic neurosis
	Other
PSYCHOSES	Delirium
	Schizophrenic
	Affective
EPILEPSY	Simple partial seizures
	Complex partial seizures (TLE)
NEUROLOGICAL	Post-traumatic dementia
	Normal pressure hydrocephalus
	Subdural haematoma
	Other neurological deficits
OTHER	Employment
	Litigation
	Socio-economic

side, such as aprosody, may be identified, now that there is an increased awareness of the functions of the right cerebral hemisphere (Ross, 1981).

In the early stages of recovery, euphoria with lack of insight, or depression, may be present. Levin and Grossman (1978) found that the degree of affective disorder at this stage correlated with the severity of the injury. These affective changes tend to improve with time, but often leave an apathetic, socially withdrawn individual with limited insight into his problems. There is little evidence to support an organic basis for the chronic neurotic disorders that may develop after head injury, and the patient will usually be found to have had a pre-existing neurotic predisposition. However, careful evaluation is necessary in all these cases, as cognitive deficits may be present in the absence of the more obvious signs of brain damage. Subtle specific cognitive deficits have been demonstrated in children following head injuries (Chadwick *et al.*, 1981b), and neurological signs in children may disappear with time (Solomons *et al.*, 1963), obscuring the aetiology of such cognitive deficits.

The specific personality changes that can result from damage localised to certain areas have been described earlier in this chapter. In addition, Levin *et al.* (1979) found certain changes which they described as the "Post-traumatic Borderline personality", when evaluating a population of adult patients who had received closed head trauma about 6 months previously. These changes included disturbance of thinking (tangential fragmented speech with over-inclusive thinking) and motor retardation, as well as chronic socio-economic dependence. These features were particularly associated with a history of acute post-traumatic psychosis. They found that the anterograde amnesia (AGA) showed a strongly positive correlation with intellectual impairment, the patients having particular difficulty solving non-verbal problems, but with a relative preservation of verbal skills.

7.6 THE POST-TRAUMATIC SYNDROME

This is a constellation of symptoms that develop in a person usually following a relatively minor head injury. The syndrome can also be seen as a consequence of injury to other areas of the body, particularly the back. It can be grossly incapacitating for the patient and can develop a chronicity that makes it almost a change in personality. The commonest symptoms are headache and dizziness, but impairment of sleep, decreased concentration and libido, irritability, anxiety, depression, and sensitivity to noise, are also seen (Levin *et al.*, 1982). Impotence may develop.

The cause of the syndrome is a contentious issue and some regard it as having no basis in organic brain disease because: it can be produced by trauma to other parts of the body; the preceding head injury is usually relatively slight; there is commonly a relative absence of any significant post-traumatic cognitive or neurological disability; the frequent relationship between the development of the syndrome and litigation; and because, in some cases, there is a time delay between the occurrence of the trauma and the development of the symptoms (Field, 1981). Other authors (Kelly and Smith, 1981; Kelly, 1981) have proposed the opposite view on the basis of evidence such as the experimental demonstration that brain damage can be produced in animals by subjecting them to a minor head injury, and the fact that the resolution of the syndrome does not always follow the satisfactory completion of litigation, in those cases where litigation is involved. In addition, litigation is not always present. Some of these differences in opinion may reflect variations in the characteristics of the different populations studied, some physicians seeing more litigious cases than others (Levin *et al.*, 1982). It seems likely that the clinical features of many of these cases have a basis in the physical consequences of craniovertebral trauma, but that psychological factors then become superimposed and, with time, become the predominant cause of their continuing. This is more likely the milder the head injury and the longer the symptoms continue after the injury. The use of the term psychological should not be regarded as a synonym for malingering. It is not surprising that many patients who have sustained a head injury develop somatic preoccupation and anxiety when involved in litigation, particularly as the brain is an organ that possesses an immense personal significance to most people. However, it is important to look for other causes for the patient's symptoms, especially neck injury and labyrinthine damage (Guthkelch, 1981), as well as subclinical injury to the temporal lobe, cerebellum, and diencephalon/mesencephalon region of the CNS. Testing for postural vertigo may be helpful in some cases.

In Kelly and Smith's series (1981) a poor prognosis for recovery was associated with: a failure to return to work before the litigation was resolved, an attitude of resentment in the patient, and an age in excess of 60 years. *A poor prognosis was not significantly associated with prolonged litigation or psychiatric problems.* Patients in previously dangerous occupations usually did not return to their jobs. However, the majority of patients had returned to work before litigation was resolved. Clearly there is evidence for the presence of both organic and non-organic factors in this syndrome (Trimble, 1981b) and each cases should be considered on its individual merits.

CHAPTER 8

Neuropsychiatric Aspects of Aggression

8.1 INTRODUCTION

The term *aggression is used here to refer to hostile or destructive behaviour that is directed towards oneself or towards others*. The degree to which such activity is regarded as antisocial depends on factors such as the circumstances surrounding the aggressive act, the prevailing cultural norms, and the degree of aggression.

Table 8.1 shows the common causes of pathological aggression. One of the first steps in assessing the cause is to ascertain whether the aggressive behaviour is a long-standing behavioural trait. This is the most common cause of such behaviour, though there may be an interaction with psychosocial or organic events. If it is a consistent aspect of a personality disorder then, in most cases, there will be a past history suggestive of childhood conduct disorder. Careful questioning may be necessary to elicit such a history, as it may have been accepted as normal within the patient's childhood subculture, with other members of his peer group showing similar behaviour. In such cases it is common for there to be a history of aggressive behaviour in some of the patient's first degree relatives. He may make oblique reference to the latter, such as "he never put up with nonsense" and "he always stood up for his rights and would fight for them."

It is difficult to separate the genetic from the learned contribution in such cases and often both factors are probably operating. Studies of adopted children born to sociopathic parents suggest that the children have an increased incidence of antisocial behaviour that can only be adequately explained on the basis of some degree of genetic predisposition. The mean concordance for criminality is 58% in monozygotic twins and 21% in male dizygotic twins (Vassilopoulos, 1982).

The DSM III discriminates between four types of conduct disorder. They are divided according to whether socialisation is present or not, and whether aggression is present or not. Those diagnosed as having aggressive conduct disorders have shown consistently aggressive behaviour for over 6 months and vary in their ability to form bonds with their peers. Those with an *undersocialised aggressive conduct disorder* tend to show an absence of guilt when caught misbehaving, exhibit self-centredness, a lack of concern for their companions, and are unable to form peer friendships that last for any length of time (over 6 months). This disorder tends to start before puberty and has a poor prognosis, often progressing into the adult antisocial personality disorder. In contrast, the child with a *socialised aggressive conduct disorder* tends to develop his behaviour disturbance after puberty. This results in an adolescent who has some capacity for empathic and consistent relationships with his peers, and the prognosis is better in this group. Evidence of minimal brain dysfunction is frequently found in children with aggressive conduct disorders.

The adult *antisocial personality*, according to DSM III criteria, exhibits a behavioural disturbance starting before the age of 15 years. These adults frequently show immature EEG patterns and a high frequency of aggressive behaviour in their first degree relatives (Hill and Watterson, 1942). It has been suggested that these EEG patterns indicate dysfunction in the limbic system, possibly reflecting a delay in its neurological maturation. An interaction between such neurological dysmaturation and an adverse environment in childhood seems likely to be acting in many cases, in view of the proven importance of the environment in determining later psychological adjustment in children who have sustained brain damage (Rutter, 1981). It is emphasised, however, that the author is *not* equating the abnormal EEGs prevalent in this chronically aggressive population, with organic brain disease; he is merely emphasising the importance of the child's environment in the development of his personality.

The term *"episodic dyscontrol" is used here to refer to intermittent outbursts of aggression that occur out of proportion to any antecedent provoking event.* Authors differ as to whether such behaviour forms one aspect of a chronically aggressive personality (Mark and Ervin, 1980), or whether it is behaviour that is out of keeping with a well-adjusted premorbid personality. The DSM III adopts the latter view and uses the diagnosis *Intermittent Explosive disorder* to describe these cases, excluding anybody who has shown significant impulsive or aggressive behaviour between the outbursts. In these cases of isolated uncharacteristic aggression, the outburst may occur as a result of some persistent stress, such as chronic persecution by a nagging wife or boss. These patients often show obsessional traits and tend to over-control their aggressive impulses until they reach a stage where there is a sudden inappropriate and catastrophic explosion of aggression. In other cases the outburst is a sudden immediate response to some provocation, which the person is unable to control, despite the serious consequences such occurrences may have. When there is a single episode of aggression, the diagnosis of *Isolated Explosive disorder* is used in the DSM III.

Aggressive behaviour may form one aspect of almost any psychiatric disorder, particularly when interacting with a pre-existing predisposition to violence. Anxiety and depression may lead to irritability and a lowered threshold for aggression. The deluded, severely depressed patient sometimes will murder his family, and then commit suicide, to protect them from some terrible impending disaster that he imagines he has brought on them. The manic patient — full of energy, feelings of power and omnipotence — may become aggressive when obstructed from pursuing his grandiose and ill conceived aims. In milder forms of mania, particularly in the elderly, a dysphoric, irritable and paranoid picture may develop (Pitt, 1974).

Any acutely psychotic patient, whether or not there is an organic basis for the psychosis, who is bewildered and frightened by his delusions and hallucinations, may become aggressive. However, it is those psychotic patients, such as the older paranoid schizophrenic, with his well preserved personality and intact thought processes, who is particularly capable of carrying out a planned act of aggression. Mental illness in one of the latter group of patients may not be overtly apparent to others until he brings it to their attention when he acts to defend himself against his imagined persecutors. The rare condition of catatonic schizophrenia may produce aggressive outbursts, sometimes alternating with episodes of stupor, but these outbursts are usually unplanned and disorganised. Abnormal patterns on the EEG tracing are not uncommon in these patients and may cause some diagnostic confusion.

Morbid jealousy can be a manifestation of a psychotic or a neurotic illness or a personality disorder. Up to 25% of sane murderers commit their offences as a result of jealousy. A variety of organic disorders have been associated with morbid jealousy, but there does not appear to be a lesion in any particular area of the brain predisposing to its development (Cobb, 1979). Shepherd (1961) has drawn attention to a close association between this disorder, and addiction to amphetamine and cocaine. It is an interesting curiosity that he also described it as a transient post-ictal phenomenon in TLE. However, "alcoholism constitutes the most widely recognised physical association of morbid jealousy" (Shepherd, 1961) and this is probably a consequence of factors such as the patient's waning potency, his rejection by his spouse/girlfriend, his premorbid personality, etc.

8.2 BRAIN STRUCTURES
UNDERLYING AGGRESSIVE BEHAVIOUR

When aggressive behaviour develops after a closed head injury it is damage to the amygdala that is suspected of being the most important predisposing factor (Lishman, 1978). Electrical stimulation of the amygdala in animals produces behaviour that includes aggression, flight and defensive posturing. In man, aggression is more likely to be produced by such stimulation where there are pre-existing aggressive tendencies in his personality (Kim and Umbach, 1973). This underlines the influence of premorbid personality traits in determining the behavioural consequences of disturbed brain function. Many factors play a role in producing such behaviour and Hitchcock (1979) emphasised the close connection between the amygdala and the endocrine system (diencephalon), and suggested that there may well be an interaction between the two in the modulation of aggression.

Of the three most clearly defined limbic circuits the amygdala is part of two of them (it is not part of the third—the Papez circuit). The two circuits are the "Defense Reaction" and the "Basolateral" (Kelly, 1976). The *Basolateral circuit* is as follows:

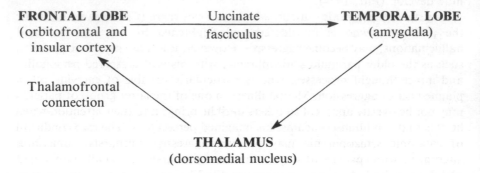

FRONTAL LOBE   Uncinate   **TEMPORAL LOBE**
(orbitofrontal and   fasciculus   (amygdala)
insular cortex)

Thalamofrontal
connection

THALAMUS
(dorsomedial nucleus)

The operation of partial temporal lobectomy, as carried out by Falconer at the Maudsley Hospital (Turner, 1969), involved removal of the uncus, amygdala and the anterior hippocampus, whilst leaving the superior temporal gyrus intact. In those cases where a unilateral temporal lobe epileptic focus is associated with aggressive behaviour, the successful control of the epilepsy by such a procedure is often also associated with a reduction in aggressive behaviour (Taylor, 1972).

The *Defence Reaction* circuit is as follows:

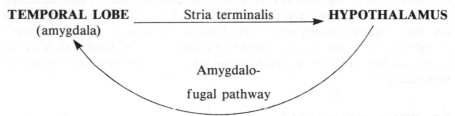

TEMPORAL LOBE   Stria terminalis   **HYPOTHALAMUS**
(amygdala)

Amygdalo-
fugal pathway

Stimulation of the rostral hypothalamus causes fear and autonomic arousal in man. Lesions in the postero-medial hypothalamus have been used to treat aggressive behaviour (Kim and Umbach, 1973). The stria terminalis has also been the site of psychosurgery for aggression, but the most effective site for such a lesion appears to be the amygdala. Heimburger *et al.* (1978) found that bilateral amygdalotomy reduced aggressive behaviour in 50% of patients with, and 33% without, seizure disorders.

Other operations have been used with varying success. Hemispherectomy has been found to be an effective treatment of behaviour disorder in patients with infantile hemiplegia. Anterior cingulectomy (the operative removal bilaterally of a section of the anterior part of the cingulate gyrus), which effectively interrupts the Papez circuit, has been found to benefit aggressive and obsessional behaviour. The operation of posterior cingulectomy appears to be less useful and has few advocates (Kelly, 1976).

Table 8.1   Differential diagnosis of recurrent aggressive behaviour

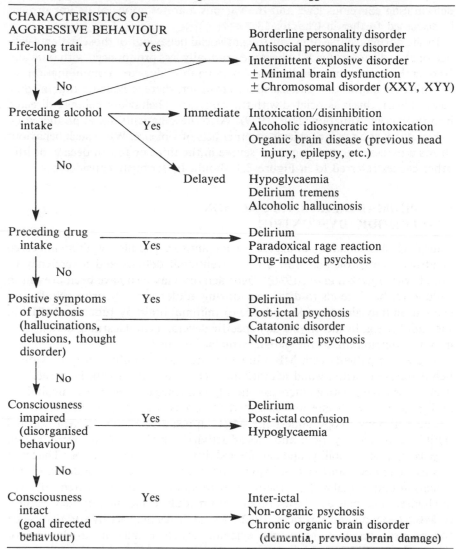

CHARACTERISTICS OF
AGGRESSIVE BEHAVIOUR

Life-long trait — Yes
Borderline personality disorder
Antisocial personality disorder
Intermittent explosive disorder
± Minimal brain dysfunction
± Chromosomal disorder (XXY, XYY)

No

Preceding alcohol — Immediate
intake   Yes
Intoxication/disinhibition
Alcoholic idiosyncratic intoxication
Organic brain disease (previous head
   injury, epilepsy, etc.)

No

Delayed
Hypoglycaemia
Delirium tremens
Alcoholic hallucinosis

Preceding drug — Yes
intake
Delirium
Paradoxical rage reaction
Drug-induced psychosis

No

Positive symptoms — Yes
of psychosis
(hallucinations,
delusions, thought
disorder)
Delirium
Post-ictal psychosis
Catatonic disorder
Non-organic psychosis

No

Consciousness — Yes
impaired
(disorganised
behaviour)
Delirium
Post-ictal confusion
Hypoglycaemia

No

Consciousness — Yes
intact
(goal directed
behaviour)
Inter-ictal
Non-organic psychosis
Chronic organic brain disorder
   (dementia, previous brain damage)

Table 8.1 shows one method of approach to the assessment of the patient exhibiting aggressive behaviour, emphasising some of the important areas to be enquired into.

It should be emphasised that a high level of emotional arousal can result in impairment of conscious awareness, albeit not in the organic sense. Impaired consciousness may be indicated by patients' descriptions such as "being confused", in a "dream-like" state, difficulty with thinking, or similar subjective experiences. Alternatively, if the patient exhibits disorganised aggressive behaviour that is inappropriate and not goal-directed, this would also imply the presence of a reduced level of conscious awareness. The difficulty of determining conscious level and the various manifestations of its impairment is discussed further in Chapter 13.

In the normal course of events the antisocial behaviour of those patients with personality disorders tends to become gradually less pronounced with time and frequently ceases by middle age, presumably due to a combination of neurological maturation and learning. However, there is evidence that in some cases at least, this is associated with their disturbed behaviour being re-directed into their home situation (Hill, 1979). Also these patients are at an increased risk of death as a result of suicide or other acts of violence. When such behaviour shows a tendency to become more severe in the third or fourth decade of life, other causes referred to in Figure 8.1 should be seriously considered.

8.3 MINIMAL BRAIN DYSFUNCTION AND EPISODIC DYSCONTROL

Neurological examination of aggressive and antisocial adults reveals an increased incidence of neurological soft signs, attentional deficits and a tendency to impulsivity (Quitkin *et al.*, 1976). Over-activity may also have been present in childhood, but it tends to disappear during adolescence. Neuropsychological evaluation may also provide evidence of minimal brain dysfunction (MBD) in such adults, e.g. by identifying any specific developmental learning deficits that may be contributing to the patient's maladjustment.

Aggressive patients with MBD have an increased family history of violent behaviour, over-activity and school failure (Huessy *et al.*, 1979). Hyperactivity itself is associated with an increased family incidence of sociopathy, alcoholism and Briquet's Syndrome, the so-called St. Louis triad (Cantwell, 1975).

The pathophysiology underlying MBD appears to be insufficient cortical inhibition of sensory input and motor activity, which results in over-activity, impulsivity, distractibility, and a limited ability to tolerate frustration. The latter can cause temper tantrums and aggressive behaviour. It is a condition that is usually found in males, and treatment with stimulant drugs is often effective in children, and may also be useful in certain adults exhibiting residual features of MBD (Amado and Lustman, 1982). These drugs may act by stimulation of the arousal reticular activating system, which results in a slowing or "normalisation" of nervous transmission in the brain of the hyperactive person (Perel and Dayton, 1977). The short action of methylphenidate makes it an ideal drug for a short trial, the dose being increased until a positive or negative response occurs. In the case of a positive response, controlled use of this or a similar drug may result in an increase in attention span and greater stability of mood. The tricyclic antidepressants may prove an effective substitute in some cases, if the potential for addiction to stimulants is considered too high. Alternatively, a trial of carbamazepine or lithium may be useful for stabilising mood swings and reducing aggressive behaviour (Oyewumi and Lapierre, 1981; Post *et al.*, 1982). Females with evidence of MBD may be particularly sensitive to fluid retention and so develop a dysphoric mood and aggressive behaviour in the premenstrual phase. In such cases a trial of treatment with diuretic medication, during the premenstrual period, is indicated (Huessy *et al.*, 1979).

Some patients who do not have clinical seizures may nevertheless exhibit episodic aggressive behaviour and in between outbursts they are found to have abnormal EEGs. They are also prone to perceptual experiences of a temporal lobe type. Monroe (1979) studied a population of criminals who exhibited episodic aggression and suggested that they fall into two main groups. The first group experienced episodes of dizziness, light-headedness, blurring of vision, headaches, perceptual distortions, such as "déjà vu" experiences, and outbursts of uncoordinated violence. These outbursts were preceded by prodromal autonomic symptoms, and were followed by a relief of tension, with remorse and partial amnesia for the preceding events. Their EEGs, in between their "attacks", were found to have a high theta (4–7 c/s) count on computer analysis. He labelled these outbursts "epileptoid". It was suggested that they represent a subgroup of patients with MBD, as they show a raised incidence of neurological soft signs and past neurological trauma, in comparison to the second group. Monroe recommended that a trial of stimulant or anticonvulsant medication should be considered for the members of this "epileptoid" group. Major tranquillisers, despite a tendency to lower the seizure threshold, have also been found to be effective in controlling disturbed behaviour in these type of patients (Johnson, 1979). In Monroe's second group the acts were equally explosive, but there was some degree of premeditation, and they were followed by complete amnesia for the outburst. This group were regarded as having a more "hysteroid" pattern of dyscontrol and the EEG was usually normal in between outbursts. These patients tend to respond poorly to medication and may require a more psychotherapeutic approach (Monroe, 1979).

Spitzer *et al.* (1979) described the characteristics of the patient with a *borderline personality disorder*. Such a patient is uncertain about some aspects of his personal identity; he experiences intense, but unstable, interpersonal relationships and mood states; he under-achieves in his academic work and occupations, and experiences anhedonia and an inability to tolerate being alone. Aggressive behaviour, which may involve self-injury, is also characteristic of these patients. It has been suggested that neurological trauma or genetic factors may interfere with the development of the limbic system in the child, resulting in a subgroup of patients with borderline personalities and also organic cerebral dysfunction (Andrulonis *et al.*, 1980). It was felt that such a combination might predispose to episodic dyscontrol. In support of this theory Andrulonis *et al.* (1980) looked at 91 borderline patients and found that 27% of them had a history suggestive of MBD and/or learning disability. In contrast to those without such a history, they were more often male, with an onset of psychiatric difficulties in the first decade, and a positive family history for alcohol and/or drug abuse. 62% of their total patients had no prior history of neurological insult, hyperactivity, attentional deficits, or learning disability. The latter group mainly consisted of female patients with an onset of psychiatric problems in adolescence, a predisposition to develop depressive illness, and a family history of affective disorder. It is highly arguable whether they are justified in equating MBD with organic brain dysfunction, but the different profiles of the MBD and the non-MBD groups may well have implications for treatment, prognosis and actiology of the dyscontrol disorder. It is notable that 11% of these 91 patients had a past history of neurological trauma, epilepsy or encephalitis.

8.4 EPILEPSY

Aggressive outbursts are rarely a manifestation of an epileptic seizure, though a history of episodic aggression raises the question of whether or not epilepsy is present. When dealing with epilepsy it is necessary to take into account the effects of numerous variables that can cause behavioural change, including the seizures, psychosocial factors, anticonvulsant drugs, brain damage, and genetic predisposition. Aggression is a personality trait commonly seen in a subgroup of patients with temporal lobe epilepsy (Betts *et al.*, 1976). This behaviour has been particularly related to young males of limited intellect and from poor social backgrounds, whose seizures had started at an early age (under 10 years). This suggests that there may be a critical period in male epileptics when limbic dysfunction, directly or indirectly, is particularly likely to predispose them to later behavioural disturbance (Serafetinides, 1965; Taylor, 1972). However, it seems more usual for inter-ictal aggression to be associated with EEG evidence of diffuse, bilateral cerebral disease, especially involving the baso-frontal area of the brain (Stevens and Herman, 1981).

A stereotyped pattern of complex purposeful behaviour is not seen in ictal aggression. This has been studied by means of videotelemetry. Delgado-Escueta *et al.* (1981) found it appears suddenly, without any evidence of planning, tends to last under a minute, is simple, unsustained and never involves a consecutive series of purposeful movements. Usually the fists or hands are used and no attempt is made to hide the act. It was usually a part of a TLE attack and was associated with or followed by the more typical features of such seizures, e.g. lip smacking, swallowing, etc. In two of their 13 cases the seizure was grand mal in type and the violence was the result of the patient being restrained during the period of post-ictal confusion. There was no attempt made to conceal the behaviour.

Aggression is a very real risk if an attempt is made to restrain a patient during the period of post-ictal confusion. This is particularly likely to be a problem in a patient who exhibits inter-ictal aggressive tendencies. In his confused state he will not have his normal level of cortical inhibition acting to restrain him. If he is interfered with he may well interpret this as a deliberate attack upon him and react accordingly.

Patients with epilepsy are prone to inter-ictal mood changes, especially prior to their seizures. When this involves marked irritability, given the appropriate circumstances, aggressive behaviour can result. In such cases better seizure control may improve, worsen or have no effect on the behaviour disorder. Each case must be evaluated individually, possibly with a trial of varying doses and types, of anticonvulsants.

Such destructive behaviour is not only directed externally, but an increase in the incidence of attempted suicide, compared with the general population rate, has been noted by several authors. Hawton *et al.* (1980) found that, compared to the general population, there was a five-fold excess of epileptic patients who had attempted suicide, 17% of attempts involving self-injury, in a series of 1291 parasuicides.

Though patients with episodic outbursts of violence are frequently referred for assessment and the question is often asked, "Does this patient have epilepsy?", *it is very unusual for epilepsy to present with episodes of aggressive behaviour*, unless one uses the term loosely so that it is synonymous with the term "epileptoid", as used by Monroe (1979).

8.5 CHROMOSOMAL DISORDERS

Certain chromosomal abnormalities have been particularly associated with aggressive behaviour. They involve the presence of an extra Y chromosome and, to a lesser extent, the presence of an extra X chromosome (Vassilopoulos, 1982). Before elaborating further it should be emphasised that *the majority of individuals with chromosomal disorders do not exhibit antisocial behaviour*.

Males with a sex chromosome complement of XYY (an extra Y chromosome), are found in 0.14% of the newborn, and in 0.52% of both a mentally ill population and a population of juvenile delinquents. However, the prevalence of this chromosomal abnormality is twice as commonly found (1.34%) among criminals (Jarvik, 1976). This antisocial XYY subgroup show compulsive aggressive behaviour, tallness (50% are over 183 cm in height), borderline intelligence and abnormal sexual development (usually involving undescended testes). They tend to be from relatively stable social backgrounds, but their disturbed behaviour is difficult to treat.

Males with a sex chromosome complement of XXY (an extra X chromosome) are described as having *Klinefelter's syndrome*. They are found in 0.14% of the newborn, 0.52% of a mentally ill population, and 0.22% of a population of juvenile delinquents. The quality of their upbringing appears to influence the severity of their psychopathology. The prevalence of the syndrome is 0.88% in a population of criminals. Aggressive behaviour is less frequent than in the XYY group, but these people also tend to be tall (the length of their lower body segment is greater than that of their upper body segment), of low normal intelligence (with delayed expressive language development and a low verbal IQ), and have abnormal sexual development (small testes, gynaecomastia, and an elevated level of follicle stimulating hormone in their blood). They occasionally develop neurological problems, such as extrapyramidal disease, and an atypical schizophrenia-like illness (Robinson, 1982).

8.6 ALCOHOL AND HYPOGLYCAEMIA

Alcohol can cause aggressive behaviour immediately after it has been consumed, and this is usually found in individuals who are already predisposed to such behaviour, the alochol acting by means of the mechanism of disinhibition. Occasionally it may have this effect in the absence of such predisposing factors and this has been called *Alcoholic Idiosyncratic Intoxication* (AII). AII (also called pathological drunkenness or *"Mania a Potu"*) is a term used to describe violent behaviour immediately following the intake of a relatively small quantity of alcohol, followed by sleep and some degree of amnesia for the preceding events (Coid, 1979). This term is usually used loosely, with little diagnostic specificity, and it can refer to a variety of alcohol-related conditions, some of which are listed in Table 8.2.

Alcohol may affect the nervous system in many ways. It may act as a direct toxin (dementia, Marchiafava–Bignami disease, central pontine myelinosis); by causing nutritional, especially thiamine, deficiency (Wernicke's encephalopathy); or by causing a withdrawal syndrome (delirium tremens). Any of these effects may contribute to or cause aggressive behaviour. Auditory hallucinosis can result from alcohol withdrawal and, if the voices assume a persecutory form, aggressive behaviour can result. This may result in murder when the alcoholic attempts to defend himself from his persecutors (Hamilton, 1974). In occasional cases alcohol may activate an epileptiform EEG abnormality (Marinacci, 1963), though this is rarely associated with a true seizure unless the patient has a preceding history of epilepsy.

AII is rare in its "pure" form, that is to say when drinking a minimal amount of alcohol results in violent behaviour that is totally out of keeping with the patient's premorbid personality.

Table 8.2   The neuropsychiatric effects of alcohol

Acute effects	*Simple intoxication
	Memory blackouts
	*Alcoholic idiosyncratic intoxication
	*EEG Abnormalities
Withdrawal effects	"Early morning" withdrawal syndrome
	*Hypoglycaemia
	*Delirium tremens
	*Hallucinosis—auditory or visual
	*Convulsions
Toxic effects	*Dementia
	Cerebellar degeneration
	Central pontine myelinosis
	*Marchiafava–Bignami disease
Vitamin deficiency	*Wernicke's encephalopathy
	Korsakoff's psychosis
	Peripheral neuropathy
	Amblyopia

*May predispose to aggression and/or delirium.

Alcohol-induced hypoglycaemia usually occurs 6 to 36 hours after a period of excessive alcohol intake. It can cause drowsiness, altered consciousness, depersonalisation, disinhibition, delirium, dysarthria, perioral paraesthesia and focal neurological signs. In addition there may be a feeling of hunger, sweating and palpitations. Aggressive behaviour may be marked. This is usually seen in chronic alcoholic patients who eat poorly. It is a *"fasting" hypoglycaemia* (in contrast to the "reactive" type), and results from inadequate glycogen reserves. Other causes of this type of hypoglycaemia (see Table 8.3) include severe liver disease, hypopituitarism, hypoadrenalism, and sarcomas (which are usually large and palpable in the abdomen, or visible on a chest radiograph).

Causes of particular importance to the psychiatrist are drugs and insulinomas (insulin-producing tumours of the pancreas). Malingering patients may self-administer insulin or hypoglycaemic drugs. The former can be identified by finding immunoreactive insulin, but no immunoreactive C-peptide, in the blood of a patient who should not be taking the drug. The latter is more difficult to diagnose and a high index of suspicion is required, combined with close observation of the patient (Turner *et al.*, 1981).

The *insulinoma* is a rare tumour that is benign in 90% of cases and can be found at any age. It produces a steady level of insulin, irrespective of the blood sugar level. Neurological symptoms predominate, but it can produce insidious intellectual deterioration and it can mimic most psychiatric disorders (including the psychoses). It characteristically produces drowsiness on waking in the morning, which is relieved by the intake of sugar. A low fasting glucose (less than 2 mmol/L) and a high plasma insulin (normal range 3–13 mIU/L) are virtually diagnostic. The tumours are usually palpable.

The *"reactive" hypoglycaemias* occur following meals and result from the inappropriately excessive release of insulin following food intake. It may be seen in the early stages of diabetes mellitus. It is also seen in alcoholic patients or following any gastrointestinal surgery (gastrectomy, or some other form of gastric resection) that results in rapid gastric emptying. Since alcoholics are prone to develop peptic ulceration requiring gastric surgery, both factors may be contributing to cause them to develop hypoglycaemia.

Table 8.3   The causes of hypoglycaemia

FASTING	Alcohol, insulin, hypoglycaemia drugs
	Insulinoma
	Severe liver disease
	Hypoadrenalism
	Hypopituitarism
	Sarcoma (large)
REACTIVE	"Essential reactive"
	Diabetes mellitus
	Alcoholism
	Gastric surgery

Essential "reactive" hypoglycaemia is the commonest "reactive" type. In many cases this diagnosis is probably made inappropriately in those anxious individuals whose symptoms are due to anxiety rather than hypoglycaemia. Following a glucose load it is normal for the blood sugar level to fall to about 2.5 mmol/L, but *pronounced symptoms of hypoglycaemia usually require a blood sugar level of less than 40 mg% (2.2 mmol/L)* (Marks and Rose, 1965). Less profound reductions of serum glucose may cause milder symptoms and it may be that the rate of the fall in the level of the serum glucose is a significant factor in producing symptoms in some of these patients. In cases of doubt a trial of frequent meals with a high protein and low carbohydrate content may produce symptomatic improvement.

It is important to note that *"reactive" hypoglycaemia is usually not due to organic disease, but it may be associated with "fasting" hypoglycaemia, which is often due to organic disorders.*

8.7 DRUGS

Drugs must always be suspected in cases where there is a behavioural disturbance of uncertain origin. Acute intoxication with cocaine, amphetamines, phencyclidine, and other structurally related drugs, can cause violent behaviour. In such cases the mood may be euphoric and the clinical pictures may resemble hypomania. These drugs can also cause paranoid ideation. The ingestion of such drugs may be suggested clinically by the presence of unusual exploratory behaviour, repetitive orofacial movements and hallucinations, usually in the visual modality. With cocaine and amphetamines, sympathomimetic overactivity is usually prominent and causes hypertension, tachycardia, perspiration and pupillary dilatation. However, to a certain degree, such features are only to be expected in any highly agitated patient. The symptoms usually settle in a couple of days, though certain drugs, notably phenyclidine, may cause more prolonged behavioural disturbance that can last up to 2 weeks. With this drug, which is often used in combination with other illicit drugs (intentionally or unintentionally), symptoms such as agitation, delirium or paranoid ideation, may result in disturbed behaviour. Other signs include hallucinations, catatonic phenomena, nystagmus, ataxia, hypertension, hypersalivation and intermittent apnoea. A profound amnesia for the period of psychosis is common, and it is not uncommon for the patient to remain alert during the period of the psychosis (Jacob *et al.*, 1981). Some of these signs should also suggest the possibility of alcohol or barbiturate ingestion, and the latter drug also has a tendency to induce dysphoric mood changes.

The recognition of the signs of minimal brain dysfunction is important as these patients may show bizarre or unusually sensitive responses to psychotropic medication. They may develop a paradoxical response to sedative drugs (Huessy *et al.*, 1979), with the attendant risk of precipitating a *paradoxical rage reaction* in certain patients (Gaind and Jacoby, 1978). DiMascio *et al.* (1969) found that minor tranquillisers were particularly likely to precipitate rage reactions in patients with poor impulse control.

Routine drugs prescribed by physicians may produce delirium and so may drugs which can be obtained legally, without a prescription being necessary. Care must be taken to look for any temporal relationship between mood change and a history of starting or altering the dosage of any particular medication. Such a history may indicate if a drug is causing, exacerbating, or is likely to be useful in the treatment of, aggressive behaviour.

8.8 OTHER CEREBRAL DISORDERS

Evidence for definite brain damage is present in the minority of chronically aggressive patients, but it is quite common to find evidence of minimal brain dysfunction.

Head trauma predisposes to aggressive behaviour in a variety of circumstances. Irritability following a head injury may lower the threshold for aggression, especially if alcohol is ingested. Such a predisposition to aggressive behaviour is well recognized in the immediate post-traumatic period. This may be a result of neuronal irritability or part of a post-traumatic confusional state. The temporal pole (wherein resides the amygdala) is particularly vulnerable to damage as a result of a closed head injury, and TLE or generalised epilepsy are the commonest types of late epilepsy, following such injuries (Marsden, 1976b). When a tendency to aggressive behaviour persists following a head injury it is likely that the crucial structure damaged is the amygdala (Lishman, 1978). Such trauma must be severe when this behaviour develops *de novo*, and it is more common for these patients to have been premorbidly predisposed to such behaviour.

The hypothalamus, septal nuclei and hippocampus have also been implicated as areas of the brain which, if damaged, can produce aggressive behaviour (Poeck, 1974). *Encephalitis lethargica* is an infection which tends to cause damage to the region of the diencephalon. It can result in episodes of compulsive aggressive behaviour involving violence towards others or self-mutilation, that may progressively worsen over the years, unlike the tendency to improvement seen in the aggressive personality disorders that are not the result of brain damage. The post-encephalitic patient tends to be remorseful about his antisocial behaviour, but nevertheless episodically feels a compulsion to behave this way. *Aggressive outbursts associated with a "loss of control" and "remorse" should raise the suspicion that organic factors are involved*, though such features are by no means diagnostic of "organicity".

Many of the causes of personality change discussed in the previous chapter, especially those disorders involving the temporo-limbic structures, can cause aggressive tendencies to develop or become exaggerated. This is also true of many of the brain disorders that cause acute or chronic organic brain syndromes.

CHAPTER 9

Delirium

9.1 INTRODUCTION

The term *delirium* is used in a variety of ways, and the third edition of the Diagnostic and Statistical Manual of Mental Disorders (DSM III, 1980) describes it as *"an acute organic disorder involving a reduced awareness of, and an inability to maintain appropriate sustained attention towards the environment"*. This attentional impairment is associated with disorientation, a diurnal fluctuation in symptoms, and impairment of memory. The DSM III also recommends that there be at least two of the following—perceptual disturbance, incoherent speech, disturbance of the sleep–wakefulness cycle, and a significant alteration in psychomotor activity (which may be increased or decreased). These criteria encompass most of the characteristic clinical features associated with this condition. However, other authors use the term in a less specific way, and Lishman (1978) describes it as *"a syndrome of impairment of consciousness along with intrusive abnormalities derived from the fields of perception and affect"*. It is understandably regarded as a disorder involving global cognitive impairment by authorities such as Lipowski, who has discussed the use of the term in some detail (Lipowski, 1980). He describes the essence of delirium as *"a defective ability to extract, process, retain, and retrieve information about oneself and one's environment"*.

A disorder of the mechanisms for maintaining attention is implicit in such definitions of delirium, and Geschwind (1982) has suggested that an attentional disorder underlies and explains the clinical features of confusional states. His view is helpful insofar as it alerts the physician to the more subtle clinical manifestations that may result from delirium. According to Geschwind *"confusional states are ones in which the normal coherence of thought or action is lost"*. Though this view is essentially similar to that of Lipowski's, Geschwind has extended the concept of confusion to include those disorders of attention which are part of normal everyday experience and can be found in those who have no organic brain disorder.

Geschwind's view also challenges the concept of a *"global cognitive impairment . . . due to widespread disturbance of cerebral metabolism"*

(Lipowski, 1980). He emphasises the close association between damage to the right parietal lobe and confusion (Mesulam *et al.*, 1976), a relationship he suggests is a consequence of disruption of the dominant function the right cerebral hemisphere plays in mediating attention. In contrast Plum and Posner (1980) view delirium as a stage between wakefulness and coma, and when unilateral lesions are present in the cerebral hemisphere, it is their size and remote effects which are the main determinant of the degree to which alertness is impaired.

These different views reflect differences in the attitudes towards the diagnostic criteria and the height of the threshold of suspicion required, for the diagnosis of delirium. The author is emphasising these different views since a too restricted view of what constitutes delirium can result in the diagnosis being missed, especially in those cases that involve relatively few clinical signs or that are in some other way atypical. Such errors in diagnosis can have serious implications for management, e.g. 16% of a series of 186 patients with Korsakoff's psychosis developed their memory impairment in the absence of any previous history suggestive of Wernicke's encephalopathy (Victor *et al.*, 1971), despite showing the neurological sequelae associated with it. This may well be due to the encephalopathy having been missed because clinically it varied from what was expected.

9.2 HISTORY OF ILLNESS

The onset of delirium is typically acute. If there is an underlying dementia, the delirium may be manifest as a sudden cognitive deterioration, superimposed on a more gradual decline. Such cases are often precipitated by the injudicious use of drugs or by an infection. A clear history may not be available in some cases and it may be the development of confusion that leads to the dementing patient being taken to the doctor for the first time. This is a frequent presentation of dementia in those patients aged over 65 years of age.

A more gradual onset may occur and the features may be difficult to separate from those of a neurotic affective disorder, which may be the diagnosis made when the symptoms remain persistent and subtle. Concentration becomes impaired, with the development of anxiety, restlessness and hypersensitivity to noise. The patient may complain of tiredness, an inability to think clearly, and experience vivid dreams, hypnagogic phenomena or "dream-like" experiences. The diurnal variation in clinical features is typically marked and the patient may be in clear consciousness during the morning, when he is able to describe the difficulty he has experienced in thinking clearly and concentrating during the previous evening. He may exhibit fear and trepidation as the night approaches and be frightened to go to bed because of the frightening experiences that occur at such times.

The history is usually of a short duration before the patient is seen by the doctor and the progression in the severity and quality of the symptoms can be variable. A profound disturbance of cognition may develop rapidly with illusions, hallucinations, delusions, distractability, and motor (including speech) over-activity. It is the patient who is exhibiting this *"hyperactive" delirium* (Lipowski, 1980) that is most likely to be brought to the doctor at an early stage because of the obvious abnormality of his behaviour, and the social disruption and management difficulties that he creates. Similarly, it is this type of delirium that attracts the attention of the medical staff when the patient is already in hospital, e.g. post-operatively.

Less obvious and more subtle are the manifestations of the *"hypoactive" delirium*. In this variant the patient is drowsy, quiet, out of contact with his surroundings and less liable to experience perceptual abnormalities. Such patients may show little abnormal behaviour and the diagnosis may be missed unless the patient is called upon, at such times, to carry out behaviour that requires fully intact higher cortical functions.

These two syndromes are not mutually exclusive and may alternate dramatically. Reversal of the sleep–wakefulness cycle is characteristic, with insomnia at night and drowsiness during the daytime. Relatives may say that they are able to hold a normal conversation with the patient during the day, when he behaves appropriately, but that he becomes irrational, irritable and behaves in an abnormal manner, in the evening or when he awakes from sleep during the night.

9.3 PREVIOUS DETAILS

Particular attention should be paid as to whether there is any history of similar episodes in the past, and if so, their duration, what was felt to be the cause, what treatments were used, and how the patient responded to them.

Previous and current physical or mental illnesses, current drug use (prescribed, illicit, and "across-the-counter" preparations), and any recent change in drug dosage, should be enquired about. Particular attention should be paid to the temporal relationship between any drug ingestion and the onset of the current illness. A careful note should be made of all medications brought in by the patient.

A specific request should be made for all the medications at the patient's home to be brought in by a relative or some other person. A home visit with this intention may reveal evidence of covert alcohol abuse or the use of multiple medications. This may be the first indication that the patient has been "shopping" around different doctors, or it may provide some other indication of the cause of the delirium. In such cases the family practitioner may be unaware of the patient's drug abuse.

Specific enquiry should be guided by the age of the patient and the causes listed in Table 9.1. Of particular importance in the older patient is whether there is any evidence of cognitive decline or cerebrovascular disease, antedating the onset of the delirium. A history of gradual cognitive decline may not be spontaneously volunteered, particularly if the illness involved a relatively abrupt change of behaviour, effectively overshadowing the more subtle preceding deterioration.

Table 9.1   The causes of delirium

Alcohol and other toxins	Heavy metals, organic solvents
Blood vessel disease	Cerebrovascular disease, hypertensive encephalopathy, cardiac disease
Collagen disorders	Polyarteritis nodosa, systemic lupus erythematosis
Drugs	Polypharmacy, major tranquillisers, antidepressants, lithium withdrawal, barbiturates and other anti-convulsants, psychotomimetic drugs, bromide, anti-inflammatory compounds (indomethacin), anti-histamines (especially in combination with*) cimetidine, L-dopa, anticholinergic drugs*, steroids, benzodiazepines, beta blockers
Endocrine, metabolic and vitamin disorders	Hypercalcaemia, hypoglycaemia, electrolyte imbalance, alkalosis, acidosis, porphyria, thyrotoxicosis, hypo-, hypercalcaemia, myxoedema and other endocrine disorders, renal and liver failure
Epilepsy	Petit mal status, temporal lobe status, post-ictal confusion, "spike-wave" stupor
Growth	Primary or secondary tumours, remote effect of tumour, e.g. limbic encephalitis, inappropriate antidiuretic hormone secretion, subdural haematoma and other space occupying lesions
Hypoxia	Cardiac, pulmonary disease
Infection	Encephalitis, meningitis, abscess
Injury	Post-operative, head injury, cerebral irradiation

9.4   MENTAL STATE EXAMINATION

Where appropriate, reference should be made to the chapters on catatonia and stupor (Chapter 14), and hypersomnia (Chapter 15). When the patient is admitted to hospital his delirium should become more obvious because he is in unfamiliar surroundings. The familiar environmental cues, that he will have been using at home to compensate for his tenuous contact with reality, will have been removed. He may respond to this change by becoming more paranoid and suspicious, by becoming aggressive or by withdrawing from contact with other people. He will tend to make excuses for his errors in areas such as memory and orientation. When the cause of his delirium is alcohol or some physically addictive drug, he may deteriorate further and show withdrawal phenomena. Usually, if he has been removed from some deleriogenic agent (and it is advisable to stop unessential medications on admission), he will show a fairly rapid improvement in behaviour, after a few days at the most. When disturbed behaviour remains and requires treatment, a drug such as haloperidol (which has little anticholinergic effect) is relatively safe and effective in most cases (Moore, 1977).

Motor behaviour may vary markedly and make the assessment of the patient difficult. Over-activity may be pronounced and there may even be dancing and singing behaviour. It may be more organised and the term "occupational delirium'' has been used to describe those confused patients who behave as they would if they were at their place of work, e.g. someone who has worked as a plumber in the past may repetitively inspect the pipes in the ward. In such cases the significance of any unusual behaviour of this type may become evident if enquiry is made about the patient's past occupations or interests. A variant of this type of behaviour is ''occupational jargon'', where the patient uses a style of speech which would have been appropriate in his place of work.

Other abnormalities of motor behaviour may be seen, especially *tremor and myoclonus*, which is found in toxic and metabolic disorders. The term ''jactitation'' was used in the past to refer to restless ''tossing about'' movements of the whole body. ''Carphology'' is a term used to describe the restless picking at the bedclothes seen in the apathetic delirious patient confined to his bed (Lipowski, 1980).

Dysphasic speech may be present and can vary from an incoherent ''jargon'' dysphasia, to speech characterised by the features of a sensory dysphasia, such as paraphasias and circumlocutions (Chedru and Geschwind, 1972a). Chedru and Geschwind (1972b) have noted that *dysgraphia* is an early sign of disturbance of language functions and is common in the early stages of delirium. Perseveration was one of the abnormalities of writing seen and may also be seen in non-verbal motor activity.

The predominant affect can vary, but fear and anxiety are frequent. Apathy is particularly common in the stuporose patient. The confused patient may show a lack of concern for his condition, even to the point of denial (Geschwind, 1982). In some cases playful or facetious behaviour may be present, but Geschwind felt that careful evaluation will usually reveal this to be a result of the patient's lack of concern and disordered thinking, producing chance associations in speech which are unintentionally humorous.

The characteristic features of *disordered attention* will be present, though not necessarily obvious on superficial examination. These features include distractability, an inability to follow a coherent line of thought or action, and an inability to grasp the essentials of a complex situation.

Disorientation, disorders of memory, confabulations and delusions, tend to show a degree of overlap with each other. Confabulations occur in about 15% of patients (Wolff and Curran, 1935) and are usually rather mundane and inconsistent. *Disorientation is usual* and initially involves the perception of time, though in milder forms of delirium orientation may appear to be unimpaired on examination (Romano and Engel, 1944). The pathological significance of errors of orientation are more obvious when the month or year are incorrectly stated, whereas incorrectly naming the day of the week may not be regarded as pathological by those who do not know the patient well. The patient may admit that he does not know where he is or who the people around him are. He may exhibit a degree of perplexity, but it is more common for him to produce confabulations or delusions. *Particularly characteristic of delirium is a tendency to misidentify the unfamiliar for the familiar*, e.g. a nurse may be identified as a relative.

Not only is paramnesia (memory distortion) present, but an anterograde and a persistent retrograde amnesia may be found. These *disorders of memory* cannot be explained solely on the basis of inattention. Defective retention and retrieval of memories is also found. When the patient looks back on his delirious period, partial amnesia and paramnesia for certain of the events is usual, and this may be helpful in making a retrospective diagnosis and evaluating the nature of past episodes of impaired consciousness. It contrasts with the more well defined and selective amnesia seen in dissociative disorders.

When asked a question, e.g. "Where are you?" The patient will tend to respond with incorrect responses that are based on past experience. At the same time he may produce correct answers, e.g. he says he is at home in his own flat, but that the flat is situated in the hospital, and then he gives the correct name and address of the hospital. This tendency to duplicate and distort memories is called *"reduplicative paramnesia"* (Weinstein and Kahn, 1955) and, if specifically sought, such responses are not uncommon in delirium. It has been suggested that reduplicative paramnesia is a result of an irresistible sense of familiarity, due to disturbed temporo-limbic function, which cannot be resolved with reality, possibly due to an associated impairment of frontal lobe function (Alexander *et al.*, 1979).

Another unusual clinical feature that can be seen is a tendency to attempt to justify errors, by misidentifying objects in the environment, sometimes in a dramatic way, in order to support false statements, e.g. one patient explained away his intravenous stand as a Christmas tree (Geschwind, 1982). This process of justification has been called *"propagation of error"*. Such responses cannot be understood as confabulations or delusions, and appear to be similar to the false explanations provided by anosognosic patients with right cerebral hemisphere lesions, when they attempt to explain away their inability to use the hemiparetic side of their body.

The incidence of hallucinations or illusions occurs in between 40 and 75% of patients with delirium, according to Lipowski (1980). These figures are significant insofar as they indicate that such disorders of perception are not always seen. *Visual and/or auditory hallucinations* are the modalities usually involved, but they can occur in any modality. It is notable that hallucinations of taste are uncommon though (Frieske and Wilson, 1966; Goodwin *et al.*, 1971). Abnormalities of perception are discussed further in Chapter 16.

Delusions that rapidly change over time, being subject to changing events in the patient's environment and his affective state (*unsystematised delusions*), are common. They can be difficult to differentiate from confabulations and hallucinations. They are most frequently delusions of persecution, but are liable to be affected by the patient's premorbid personality, previous experiences and the aetiology of this confusional state.

9.5 PHYSICAL EXAMINATION AND INVESTIGATIONS

Apart from the clinical features already described, physical examination may reveal evidence of specific disorders causing or predisposing the patient to delirium. Some of these features are shown in Figures 10.1 and 10.2 in the next Chapter. The causes listed in Table 9.1 should be considered in all cases and the patient's age may provide some indication of what disorders should be particularly looked for.

Causes particularly associated with the first two decades of life include the childhood infections (measles, mumps, scarlet fever, rheumatic fever, etc.), acute glomerulonephritis, migraine, hyponatraemia (water intoxication) and hypernatraemia (dehydration). In the third and fourth decade they include alcohol and drug use, infectious hepatitis, infectious mononucleosis, typhoid, multiple sclerosis and systemic lupus erythematosis. In the fifth and sixth decade they include alcohol and drugs, presenile dementia, the endocrinopathies and autoimmune diseases (Lipowski, 1980).

The three features that appear to be most potent in predisposing a person to delirium are an age of over 60 years (when senile dementia is the most frequent predisposing disorder), preceding cerebral damage, and the abuse of alcohol or drugs (Lipowski, 1967). An immature CNS is also important and the young are particularly at risk. If more than one of these features is present, then the predisposing risk will be greater.

The delirious patient who presents with evidence of current or past alcohol abuse can be a particular diagnostic problem. Alcohol can produce confusion due to its immediate depressant action on the nervous system, as a withdrawal effect, or (in the chronic abuser) by causing neurological damage (due to a toxic effect or by inducing a nutritional deficiency). Table 8.2 (see page 154) lists the effects of alcohol on the nervous system, most of which are capable of causing or predisposing the alcoholic to delirium.

Routine blood investigations, including a screen for drugs, should be carried out, but it is the EEG that is particularly important, not only for confirming the diagnosis, but also as a help in identifying the cause. *A generalised diffuse slowing of the background activity in the EEG tracing, is almost always present in delirium* (Lipowski, 1980). However, the "hyperactive" syndrome is associated with predominantly fast activity on the EEG, and it is commonly found in association with withdrawal from alcohol and minor tranquillisers, and as a result of intoxication with anticholinergic drugs.

The "hypo-active" syndrome is associated with diffuse slowing on the EEG. The degree of slowing correlates with the degree of drowsiness and the reduction of awareness, exhibited by the patient. It also correlates with the extent of reduction of cerebral metabolism (Ingvar *et al.*, 1976). Such an EEG pattern is particularly found in metabolic disorders (especially hepatic encephalopathy, when a characteristic triphasic pattern may be seen), infections and Wernicke's encephalopathy.

The EEG may appear to be normal in delirium. A normal EEG can be seen in association with steroid psychosis, pontomesencephalic lesions, and in Wernicke's encephalopathy (Victor *et al.*, 1971). The EEG may only appear to be "normal" due to the absence of baseline recordings and in the presence of a relatively mild delirium. In such cases the abnormality of the EEG may only be appreciated in retrospect, when a variation in the degree of cognitive impairment may be found to be accompanied by a change in the EEG pattern.

The use of intravenous barbiturates may be helpful in eliciting psychopathology in non-organic disorders and may even be therapeutic, e.g. by producing an abreaction. Relatively high doses of the drug may be needed. In organic conditions there will tend to be further cognitive deterioration which will occur when a relatively low dose of barbiturates is used (Ward *et al.*, 1978).

An alternative diagnostic procedure involves the use of physostigmine in suspected cases of the *Central Anticholingeric Syndrome* (CAS). CAS is a toxic state that usually results from the use of one or more drugs with anticholinergic effects. It is particularly prone to occur as a result of the types of drugs used in psychiatric practice. A substantial number of non-prescription drugs have this effect. The characteristic clinical features of CAS include some of the characteristic features of delirium, but particularly notable are the presence of dilated pupils that react poorly to light, disturbance of recent memory, facial flushing, a widened pulse pressure, tachycardia and hyperthermia. Certain of the features of the CAS can be better remembered by Cohen *et al.*'s (1944) description of the toxic patient as being *"hot as a hare, blind as a bat, dry as a bone, red as a beet and mad as a hen"*.

A careful history needs to be taken if the use of the anticholinesterase, physostigmine, is being considered, as there are many contra-indications (see Hall *et al.*, 1981a). Physostigmine injections are not purely cholinergic, but also have a sympathomimetic action due to preganglionic stimulation. As the drug inhibits anticholinesteras it will act to potentiate the effect of acetylcholine and thus functions as an antidote to the anticholinergic effect. 1 to 2 mg of physostigmine should be given by intramuscular injection and if the CAS is present a positive response should be seen within an hour. A positive response involves a significant improvement in mental status, a slowing of the tachycardia and a reduction in the dryness of the mouth. The dilated pupils may be more refractory to treatment.

If the drug induces toxicity this can be reversed by using 0.5 mg of intramuscular atropine sulphate for each 1 mg of physostigmine that has been given. If CAS is considered to be a possibility and the physician wishes to avoid the use of physostigmine, then one of the benzodiazepines can be used. This will avoid the potentiation of the CAS that may occur if drugs with an anticholinergic action, e.g. chlorpromazine, are used. In practice haloperidol is usually effective and safe.

9.6 DIFFERENTIATION OF DELIRIUM FROM OTHER DISORDERS

In many cases the delirious patient will present no diagnostic problem, but difficulties are particularly likely to arise with those patients who present to the doctor for the first time, often in an emergency setting, and with no one available to provide objective information about the preceding history.

Table 9.2 shows the features that may be found in delirium and will help in differentiating it from other disorders including dementia, organic amnesic disorders (particularly Korsakoff's psychosis), sensory dysphasia and non-organic disorders—acute or chronic schizophrenia, hysterical psychosis (the Ganser syndrome), hysterical dissociation, affective and brief reactive psychoses. In addition, *a fluctuating course with nocturnal deterioration, a tendency to misidentify the unfamiliar for the familiar, and a diffuse slowing of the EEG, are features that are commonly found only in delirium.*

Only in dementia and delirium is it possible to see a truly global impairment of cognition, and in Table 9.2 dementia primarily refers to the earlier stages of the Alzheimer's type, when attention is usually preserved, as it is in the other disorders listed. Other types of dementia may show some of the features seen in delirium, including an acute onset (post-traumatic dementia), a short course (Creutzfeldt–Jacob dementia), and involuntary movements (Huntington's chorea). Delirium may clear to reveal a dementia (Multi-Infarct dementia), a memory deficit (Korsakoff's psychosis) or an aphasia, but focal neurological or cognitive deficits should then be found on examination.

Any of the non-organic disorders can result in altered attention, but organic features such as aphasia, perseveration and dysgraphia are not found. Memory disturbance will not involve confabulation and retrograde amnesia, and in hysteria there may be the characteristic selective loss of memory, possibly with a loss of personal identity. Hysterical psychoses may take the form of the Ganser syndrome or involve a different picture with psychotic features developing in response to stress, often in a person with premorbid hysterical personality traits (Merskey, 1979). Lipowski (1980) grouped together the schizophreniform disorders, brief reactive psychoses and atypical psychoses, and feels that, in some cases, on the basis of symptomatology, such diagnosis may have to be made by excluding an organic cause.

The delirious patient may talk incomprehensible nonsense. The differential diagnosis in such cases involves a sensory aphasia, hypomania and schizophrenia. Denial of disability (anosognosia) and, in some cases, euphoria are often seen in association with sensory aphasia. There may be no neurological signs and the patient may produce excessive speech made incoherent with numerous paraphasic substitutions (jargon aphasia). These patients usually do not exhibit abnormalities of motor activity, unlike the delirious patient who may show a similar affect and speech pattern but should not show the same degree of comprehension or repetition difficulties. Both of these disorders will have an acute onset, but if the EEG is abnormal in the aphasic it should show a predominantly left-sided abnormality, whereas the delirious patient is more likely

Table 9.2 Differential diagnosis of delirium

COMMON FEATURES OF DELIRIUM	Dementia of Alzheimer's type	Organic amnesia	Sensory dysphasia	Hysterical psychosis	Hysterical dissociation	Affective psychosis	Chronic schizophrenia	Acute non-organic psychosis
Acute onset		+	+	+	+	+		+
Short history		+	+	+	+	+		+
Variable motor activity					+	+		+
Involuntary movements								
Incoherent speech			+	+		+	+	+
Dysgraphia	+		+					
Perceptual disorders				+		+	+	+
Unsystematised delusions						+	+	+
Impaired attention	+			+		+		+
Retrograde amnesia and confabulation		+						
Cognitive deterioration with IV amytal	+	+	+					

+ = commonly present.

to have a diffusely abnormal tracing. However, delirium may be present in the acute phase of a cerebrovascular accident, subsequently resulting in aphasia.

The EEG will usually be normal in the non-organic psychoses. In hypomania, the onset of the disorder will be more gradual and, apart from the other features of hypomania, the speech will tend to show bizarre, though often understandable, connections between the words or phrases. The hypomanic patient connects his words using methods such as rhyming, assonance (words sounding alike) and conceptual linkage (e.g. "red, blue"). Schizophrenic patients may produce profuse nonsensical speech, which has been described as a word salad. This is usually seen in patients with established chronic schizophrenia, and other features should be expected including a deterioration in social behaviour, loss of affect, delusions and auditory hallucinations. Gerson *et al.* (1977) compared schizophrenic and sensory aphasic speech and found the diagnostically significant features in the aphasic were the presence of paraphasias, circumlocutions, the awareness of the patient that he was having difficulty communicating, and his attempt to enlist the help of others. In contrast the schizophrenic patient exhibited circumstantiality and expressed bizarre ideas in his speech. In conclusion it can be said that *the acute onset of incoherent speech is usually organic in origin*.

The ability to write normally is usually impaired in the aphasias, dementia and delirium, but not in the non-organic disorders. In chronic schizophrenia (also in TLE) "hypergraphia" — a tendency towards extensive, and sometimes compulsive writing — may be seen (Critchley, 1970).

In chronic schizophrenia, involuntary movements (usually orofacial dyskinesia) may be seen, hallucinations are usually auditory and the delusions, if present, systematised. The first rank symptoms of schizophrenia are not usually seen in the organic psychoses. A dominant and persistent disturbance of mood is more suggestive of an affective disorder. A comparison of the clinical features of the non-organic psychoses and dementia is discussed further in Chapter 10.

If doubt remains, recourse may need to be made to the EEG or even the patient's response to intravenous amytal. The course of the disorder may help to confirm the diagnosis in retrospect. Most cases of delirium do not last more than 3 months, though Geschwind (1982) has described occasional chronic confusion as a sequel to right hemisphere infarction.

CHAPTER 10

Dementia

10.1 INTRODUCTION

For practical purposes the term dementia can be regarded as being synonomous with the term chronic organic brain syndrome. An *organic brain syndrome can be described as a group of symptoms and/or signs that are found in association with an acute or chronic impairment of brain function.* On the basis of DSM III criteria, the term does not imply that there is any organic aetiological factor, unlike the organic mental disorders which require at least the assumption of some organic cause. Primary degenerative dementia (Alzheimer's dementia, senile dementia and Pick's dementia) is one of the diagnoses included in the latter group, despite there being no conclusive evidence for any specific cause for these dementias. Primary degenerative dementia and Multi-Infarct dementia (MID) are further subdivided in the DSM III according to whether or not delusions, delirium or depression are present.

Delirium and dementia tend to be grouped together on the basis that it is only in these two disorders that there is commonly a global cognitive impairment. However, in the early stages of dementia there may be localized areas of cognitive impairment, the clinical features of which depend on the area of the brain involved, unlike delirium where impairment has a tendency to be global from the onset. *A diagnosis of dementia should not be made for the first time when delirium is present* and the patient should be re-evaluated for cognitive impairment when the delirium has cleared. In the ICD-9 dementia, like delirium, is one of the organic psychoses, but it is described as being a progressive disorder which, if not treated, is irreversible and terminal, unlike the reversible confusional state seen in delirium. The DSM-III criteria for diagnosing dementia requires the presence of all of the following—clear consciousness, memory impairment, and cognitive impairment of a degree sufficient to interfere with social or occupational functioning. Also, at least one of the following is required—impairment of abstract thinking, impaired judgment, alteration in personality, or evidence of cerebral cortical disease (agnosia, aphasia or apraxia). An organic aetiology is assumed providing the clinical picture and investigations are consistent with a diagnosis of primary degenerative dementia and functional psychiatric conditions have been excluded as a cause for the findings.

Too rigid adherence to the DSM III criteria will result in diagnostic problems in the early stages of some disorders. For example, in the patient with early Pick's dementia a change in personality may be the predominant clinical feature, or the patient with early Alzheimer's dementia may only exhibit memory impairment. In this book the term dementia of the Alzheimer's type (DAT) will be used to refer to the two conditions that were formerly referred to separately as Alzheimer's dementia and senile dementia. There is little evidence to justify separating these two disorders (Schneck *et al.*, 1982), but some of the clinical differences that have been found are shown in Table 10.1. *The main evidence for Alzheimer's and senile dementia being separate entities is genetic.* Larson *et al.* (1963) found no evidence of presenile dementia in over 2000 first degree relatives of a series of patients with senile dementia, but this separation has not been confirmed by other authors (Lauter and Meyer, 1968). Many of the other differences that have been found between the two disorders are inconsistent and understandable as the result of a variability in clinical severity and rate of progress of the disorder, rather than their being two fundamentally different conditions.

Using the inclusive concept of DAT and pathological confirmation of the diagnosis, Heston *et al.* (1981) found evidence that supported the view that the more severe the dementia, i.e. the shorter the survival time, the greater was the risk to the proband's relatives of acquiring the disease, and the younger the age of onset in those who were affected. The risk to the siblings of probands who had an onset of dementia before the age of 70 years and had an affected parent, was that of an autosomal dominant trait. Evidence supporting this form of inheritance was also found by Sjögren *et al.* (1952).

However, not all the data support this view, and Heston *et al.* (1981) found that the risk of DAT developing in the siblings of probands whose illness began after the age of 70 years was no different from the random population risk. This raises the question—what is the difference between an acceleration of the normal aging process and DAT in these older patients? One of the main clinical differences is in the pattern of cognitive deficits found in the two conditions (Miller, 1974). Albert (1978) has found marked similarities between the psychological features of subcortical dementia and aging. The latter type of cognitive deficits may be the result of slowing in nervous transmission in certain crucial subcortical brain pathways, similar to the decrease in peripheral nerve conduction that has been found in demented patients (Levy, 1969).

The combining of DAT and Pick's dementia in one group (the primary degenerative dementias), in the DSM III, has been justified on the basis that it is not possible to differentiate between these two disorders on clinical or radiological grounds, and the diagnosis depends on postmortem examination of the brain (Merritt, 1979). In DAT the gross findings consist of generalised cerebral atrophy involving the cortex and the ventricular system, with senile plaques and neurofibrillary tangles being found histopathologically, in

Table 10.1 Clinical differences between Alzheimer's and senile dementia

	ALZHEIMER'S DEMENTIA	SENILE DEMENTIA
AGE OF ONSET (YEARS)	45–60	Over 65
ILLNESS	More severe and rapidly progressive	Less severe and progressive
	(Currier *et al.*, 1982; Heston *et al.*, 1981)	
EXTRAPYRAMIDAL SIGNS, SEIZURES AND OTHER FOCAL FEATURES	Occasionally (Trimble, 1981a)	
APHASIA, APRAXIA AND AGNOSIA	Common	Uncommon (McDonald, 1969)
PHYSICAL WASTING	Terminal feature only	Progressive with cognitive deterioration
KLÜVER–BUCY SYNDROME	Common late feature	Uncommon
	(Sourander and Sjögren, 1970)	

Table 10.2 Clinical differences between Pick's and Alzheimer's dementia

	PICK'S	ALZHEIMER'S
EARLY FEATURES	Change in personality of the frontal lobe type	Memory loss
	Speech affected with dysphasia and stereotyped phrases	Speech affected late
	Facile hilarity	Depressed/anxious
	Aspontaneity	Overactive
	(Stengel, 1943)	
	Incontinence	No
	Features of the Klüver–Bucy syndrome	No
	(Cummings and Duchen, 1981)	
LATE FEATURES	*Seizures infrequent	Common
	(Sourander and Sjögren, 1970)	
EARLY PHYSICAL SIGNS	*Not a feature	*"Direct forward staring"
	*Not a feature	*Extrapyramidal rigidity
	*(Sjögren *et al.*, 1952)	

numbers proportionate to the degree of cognitive impairment. In Pick's dementia, circumscribed "knife blade" atrophy is found in the frontal and temporal lobes, and "balloon" (Pick) cells are found histopathologically, though they are not essential for the diagnosis.

Unfortunately such a view does not do justice to the fact that failure to be aware of the characteristic features of Pick's disease can cause particular clinical problems to the psychiatrist. The clinical differences between the two disorders differ in different studies, but the main ones are listed in Table 10.2.

The dementias will now be divided into the cortical and subcortical types, depending on where in the brain are the main pathological changes.

10.2 THE CORTICAL DEMENTIAS

The category of "cortical" dementia includes those disorders commonly considered as dementias, such as Multi-Infarct dementia, which are typically associated with the impairment of the "instrumental" functions of the cortical association areas. These "instrumental" functions involve language, perception and skilled motor activity. Disruption of these higher cortical functions results in aphasia, apraxia and agnosia, which are not present in the subcortical dementias. In the latter it is the "fundamental" functions, e.g. attention and arousal, which facilitate the higher cortical functions, that are affected (Albert, 1978). The clinical features of the subcortical dementias are the result of interference with neuronal conduction at the subcortical level.

At postmortem examination the majority of cases of dementia are found to be of the Alzheimer's type, which constitutes the cause in 75-90% of demented patients over the age of 65 years. Cerebrovascular disease is the second most common cause, and evidence for it being present is found in up to 50% of cases of Alzheimer's dementia (Tomlinson, 1977). However, it is probably much less frequently of clinical significance. In many elderly dements cerebrovascular disease will be the sole cause. The prevalence of these common causes of dementia appear to be less frequent in presenile cases (under 65 years of age). Marsden and Harrison (1972) reviewed 106 patients who had previously been diagnosed as having presenile dementia, and the cause was felt to be arteriosclerosis in eight, a cerebral tumour in eight, alcohol in six, and normal pressure hydrocephalus in five. *Cerebral atrophy of unknown cause was found in 48 patients* and some of these cases were probably due to Alzheimer's disease, though this large figure indicates the limitations of our knowledge concerning the causes of dementia in clinical practice. Other causes of dementia in this series were less frequent, being found in three or less cases, each.

Alcoholic dementia has probably been underdiagnosed in the past due to the clinician's preoccupation with the Wernicke–Korsakoff syndrome (Cutting, 1978a). Current studies using the CAT head scanner have revealed a high incidence of cerebral atrophy, the severity of which shows some correlation with cognitive impairment, in chronic alcohol abusers (Lishman, 1981). Another problem in identifying how many patients develop dementia as a result of alcohol abuse, is what are the criteria that indicate alcohol has been abused to a sufficient degreee to cause neurological damage. Different studies of patients with dementia have used different criteria and so it is not surprising that there is a marked variation in the prevalence of patients found with "alcoholic dementia."

Marsden and Harrison (1972) were unable to confirm the presence of dementia in 22 of their cases, ten of whom had psychiatric disorders (eight with depression, one with hysteria and one with mania). They concluded that 15% of the demented patients had a condition amenable to treatment. The degree of reversibility may depend on how early the correct diagnosis is made. Hence, an awareness of the early clinical features of these conditions is important. Atypical age of onset and mode of presentation may mislead the clinician. In normal pressure hydrocephalus (NPH) resulting from a head injury, there may be a delay of several years between the responsible traumatic event and the onset of NPH. Huntington's Chorea may present atypically in the young. When a neurodegenerative disorder, such as Wilson's disease, arises in childhood or adolescence, the presence of concurrent environmental stresses may mislead the physician into considering the initial symptoms as being those of a neurotic disorder or a disorder of personality. In addition, a diagnosis may have important implications for other members of the patient's family when the condition is an inherited one.

The physician is advised to be careful before attaching too much significance to psychiatric symptoms, at the expense of other symptoms and signs. Almost any psychiatric illness can be associated with disorders such as Huntington's chorea, and some of the previous studies relating the "non-organic" to the associated "organic" diagnoses in such conditions may have been unreliable due to factors such as a lack of consistency in the diagnostic criteria used by different physicians and the absence of sophisticated investigatory tools that are now readily available, e.g. the CAT scanner. Also the method of cognitive evaluation and the type of control groups used, vary in different studies. The findings of such studies need to be re-evaluated in the light of new concepts such as "subcortical dementia".

Primary Degenerative and Multi-Infarct dementias

A prolonged and insidious course of cognitive deterioration, of uncertain duration, is most typical of the *Primary Degenerative dementias*. Early deterioration of memory is usual in DAT and the early phase has been referred to as the "forgetfulness phase". The signs at this stage may be very subtle, though compensatory behaviour, such as keeping notes or avoiding changes in routine, may come to the notice of those who know the patient well. In the early stages this dysmnesia may not be separable from the memory difficulties that accompany normal aging, the so-called "benign senescent forgetfulness" (Kral, 1962), where only relatively minor, unimportant details are forgotten. Gradually a more "malignant forgetfulness" will become apparent, with important data and whole sections of experience being forgotten. This gradual process may take many months and, in the interim, the only other signs may be affective changes (typically anxiety or depression), clumsiness of gait, and topographical disorientation. For a brief, but comprehensive, review of this illness, the reader is referred to Schneck *et al.* (1982).

There is usually a preponderance of frontal lobe features in the early stages of Pick's dementia. In such cases the organic nature of the change may not be obvious. When a frontal lobe change in personality is seen other causes should be considered including tumours, Wilson's disease and hepatic insufficiency (see Table 7.1, page 127). Urinary incontinence may occur early in such "frontal lobe" disorders and is characteristically, though not invariably, associated with a relative indifference on the part of the patient.

For the diagnosis of *Multi-Infarct dementia* (MID) the DSM III requires the diagnostic criteria already mentioned for dementia, and also a stepwise downhill course, a variable distribution of cognitive deficits, focal neurological features, and evidence of cerebrovascular disease that is sufficient to be, at least in part, responsible for the dementia. Table 10.3 shows the clinical features which differentiate DAT from MID.

Table 10.3 Clinical differences between dementia of the Alzheimer's type and Multi-Infarct dementia

	ALZHEIMER'S	MULTI-INFARCT
Age of onset (years)	Over 45	60–80
Sex ratio	Marked female preponderance	M = F
Family history	Dementia, Down's syndrome, lympho-reticuloses, auto-immune disorders	Cerebrovascular disease, hypertension
Course	Insidious	Acute onset and stepwise progression
EARLY FEATURES		
Clinical	Memory deterioration, may be topographical disorientation	Patchy cognitive deficits, memory often preserved. Episodes of delirium
Physical	Normal	Hypertension, cardio- or cerebrovascular disease, focal neurological signs, pseudobulbar palsy
EEG	Normal or reduction in alpha activity	Alpha activity preserved, may be focal slow activity
Neuropsychology	Memory impairment, constructional apraxia	Patchy deficits

Disease of the small vessels of the brain may cause a more insidious development of neurological deficits to occur, whilst producing a subcortical dementia or Binswanger's disease (Caplan and Schoene, 1978; Janota, 1981). There is usually a past history of episodes of cerebrovascular insufficiency, when cognitive impairment is secondary to cerebrovascular disease (Caplan and Schoene, 1978). However, Jacoby *et al.* (1980b) found cerebral infarcts in the CAT brain scans of 25% of their 40 patients with senile dementia and no previous history of cerebrovascular disease. This scan finding correlated with the presence of a relatively elevated diastolic blood pressure, when they were compared with a group of age-matched demented patients without evidence of infarction on their scans. These findings support the validity of the concept of "silent infarcts" occurring in patients with dementia and hypertension. Corsellis (1969) found that a previous history of a blood pressure exceeding 210/110 mm Hg was usually found in patients with dementia and multiple infarcts in their brains at postmortem.

Alcoholic dementia

With the advent of CAT brain scanning it is now becoming clear that alcoholic patients tend to have an increased incidence of cortical atrophy and ventricular enlargement. The severity of this atrophy shows a degree of correlation with the cognitive deterioration (Lishman, 1981). These changes can be found in young alcoholics under the age of 30, who have only been drinking for a few years (Bergman et al., 1980). It is possible that in some of these cases the brain changes antedate and may in some way predispose the patient to alcohol abuse. There is evidence that the brunt of this damage is on the frontal areas of the brain (Cutting, 1978b; Lishman, 1981; Tarter, 1980) which may well partly explain the antisocial personality change that develops in chronic alcoholic patients. It is not necessary for there to be correlation between the severity of neurological impairments that follow alcohol abuse and the cognitive impairments (Grant and Mohns, 1976), so a relative absence of the former need not rule out alcohol as a cause for dementia, and the appropriate enquiries about alcohol intake should be made in all cases of dementia. There is also evidence that this secondary cerebral damage may be, at least partially, reversible with abstinence from alcohol (Lishman, 1981).

10.3   THE SUBCORTICAL DEMENTIAS

Impaired cerebral cortical function can result from subcortical lesions in various sites, but they tend to produce a particular pattern of deficits which consist of the following:-

1.   Change in personality.
2.   Memory impairment.
3.   Impairment of the processing of incoming information.
4.   Impairment of the ability to manipulate acquired knowledge.

This syndrome has been called subcortical dementia and one of the first papers describing this disorder was by Albert et al. (1974), who described it in association with progressive supranuclear palsy. Subcortical gray or white matter, or both can be involved. Figures 10.1 and 10.2 show some of the subcortical gray matter structures that have been associated with this syndrome.

They include the caudate and putamen (Huntington's chorea), the thalamus and mamillary bodies (Korsakoff's psychosis), and the substantia nigra, globus pallidus and caudate nucleus (Parkinson's disease). It can also be found in association with diffuse cerebrovascular disease involving the small vessels of the brain (Caplan and Schoene, 1978).

These patients exhibit a defect in retrieval of memories, producing characteristic "I don't know" responses to questions but, unlike depressed patients, they will tend to produce the correct answer provided the question is persisted with. The characteristic features of this disorder suggest that the primary problem is an impairment of the fundamental functions, involving learning, flexibility of sets and the processing of incoming information, due to interference with the connections between the frontal lobe and the thalamus and other subcortical structures. Hence, the term "fronto-limbic dementia" has been used to describe it. The syndrome includes "frontal lobe" disorders of emotion and personality, such as apathy, irritability and loss of initiative. They also typically have difficulty in manipulating acquired knowledge (Albert, 1978).

Due to their lack of initiative these patients may respond surprisingly well to a structured environment and can perform complex tasks provided they are taken through each stage step by step and are allowed sufficient time. They are slow to process information and so instructions and other material should be given slowly. Though they may appear to be depressed, antidepressants, particularly those with a significant anti-cholinergic effect, should be avoided as they may cause further cognitive impairment (Ghoneim and Mewaldt, 1977; Glen, 1979; Granacher and Baldessarini, 1976).

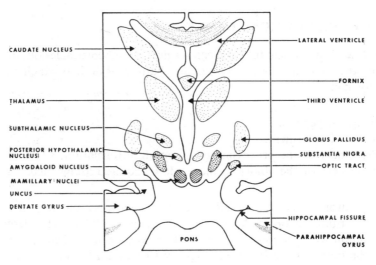

Figure 10.1   Coronal section of the brain to show subcortical gray matter

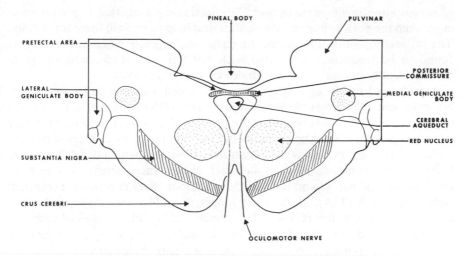

Figure 10.2 Transverse section of the brain stem at the level of the upper mid-brain

10.4 HISTORY OF ILLNESS

History taking will be facilitated if different aspects of the illness are evaluated systematically. The author suggests that they can be divided into the following five categories:-

1. Onset and course.
2. Memory and related functions.
3. Personality and emotional behaviour.
4. Speech.
5. Other features suggestive of focal neurological dysfunction.

The onset of mental disturbance in patients who are in their sixth decade of life or older, often creates a degree of suspicion (in the mind of the physician) that the patient may be dementing. In such cases *the clinical features expected with the common three dementias—Alzheimer's type, Multi-Infarct, and alcoholic dementia—should be looked for, and the significance of any variations from what is expected, evaluated carefully.* The other major illness that commonly starts in this age group is depression, and depressive pseudodementia is discussed in the next chapter.

The demented patient is often accompanied by relatives and it is characteristic that he denies having any problems. He may appear surprised that he has been brought to the doctor. Such a presentation in an elderly patient is highly suggestive of dementia, and Wells (1977) has described three other suggestive modes of presentation. One presentation is where the patient complains of neurotic symptoms which do not fit into any clear diagnostic category. In another he complains of multiple physical complaints that defy diagnosis. The third mode of presentation involves vague and ill-defined complaints that remain obtuse, even when the patient is given ample time and help to explain them more fully. The vague complaints of headache, forgetfulness, depression and insomnia, were found to be frequently associated with NPH in one study, whereas gross neurological abnormalities were absent (Botez *et al.*, 1977).

A prolonged course of a year or more, without a clearly delineated onset, is usually seen in dementia of the Alzheimer's type (DAT) and alcoholic dementia (AD) but when associated with an acute onset or acute exacerbations, the nature of these episodes should be considered. Did they result from alcohol or drug withdrawal? Did they follow the initiation of treatment with a drug? Were they followed by focal neurological deficits? When such deficits result from cerebrovascular disease and last less than 24 hours they constitute a transient ischaemic attack (TIA). If they last longer than 24 hours they constitute a cerebrovascular accident (CVA) (McCormick, 1983). Other causes of enduring sequelae should be considered, e.g. a short-term memory impairment (Korsakoff's psychosis), following Wernicke's encephalopathy.

In the common dementias there is usually some event(s) that precipitates the patient's referral. This may be the death or illness of a spouse or some other person who has been helping the patient to cope with his cognitive deficits; a change in behaviour which makes him more difficult to manage, often involving urinary incontinence, aggression, or other antisocial behaviour, which has brought the patient into conflict with the law, e.g. shoplifting or sexually indiscreet behaviour; the development of depression; or the onset of delirium, usually precipitated by drugs or infection. A short course suggests one of the less common and potentially reversible causes of dementia, particularly when the patient is under 50 years of age.

A history of *memory impairment is particularly characteristic of DAT*, but it is usually described by secondary informants. In fact it is so unusual for the ''demented'' patient to complain spontaneously of this that, when he does, it suggests a diagnosis of depressive pseudodementia (Wells, 1977). Denial of memory impairment is also charactcristic of chronic alcoholic patients with Korsakoff's psychosis. Denial of illness in general is particularly likely to occur when the cerebral impairment involves the posterior part of the right cerebral hemisphere, such as may result from a parietal lobe tumour. Such denial is more likely to be a transient phenomenon when the cause is a CVA. A tendency to get lost in familiar surroundings may be regarded as another sign of a failing memory. However, careful questioning may reveal other causes for such difficulties, such as inattention to visual cues in the left side of the visual field.

Changes in personality may be the prominent feature of dementias where the accent of the pathology is on the frontal lobes. Changes in personality with organic brain disease can vary from a subtle alteration in premorbid personality traits, to a dramatic change in behaviour. Such a dramatic change can be seen following herpes simplex encephalitis, when the behavioural features of the Klüver–Bucy syndrome may occur (Greenwood *et al.*, 1983). Features of this syndrome may also be seen in the early stages of Pick's dementia (Cummings and Duchen, 1981). It is occasionally seen in dementia of the Alzheimer's type, but then it usually occurs late in the course of the disease.

In the elderly dement there may be an exacerbation of those personality traits associated with ageing, notably a narrowing of interests, a tendency to be intolerant of change and a "turning in to oneself" (Roth and Myers, 1969). It tends to be those patients who had premorbidly maladjusted personalities who are admitted to psychiatric units, as they are more likely to present behavioural difficulties (Post, 1965).

When subject to stress, e.g. during psychological testing, the demented patient will use certain ploys to try and cope with the situation. Katz *et al.* (1961) investigated these responses and classified them into those where the patient tries to delay the examiner (time buying), those where he assumes control of the interview (warding off), those where he responds inappropriately to the situation, e.g. assumes the role of interviewer (anxiety binding), and other responses, such as confabulations. These methods indicate that the patient has some awareness of his limitations, and if they fail a catastrophic reaction may result.

Apathy is a common emotional concomitant of dementia, but depression, and occasionally mania, are not uncommon in the early stages (especially in Multi-Infarct dementia). These mood changes tend to fluctuate in intensity over time, and if delusions are present they tend to be excessively bizarre. Depression and elation may alternate, and serious suicidal attempts are a particular risk when consciousness is impaired (Roth and Myers, 1969). There may be a marked failure to modulate affective responses, with a slowness to respond to a particular event, an excessive response, and then a delayed return to a euthymic state.

10.5 FAMILY AND PERSONAL HISTORY

A history of death occurring in a first degree relative in the fifth or sixth decade, associated with dementia, a choreiform movement disorder and psychiatric problems, is suggestive of *Huntington's chorea* (HC). In patients with this condition such a history is usual, but not invariable. It was found in 80% of patients in Heathfield's series (1967). In younger patients a rigid form of this disorder, with seizures and cerebellar signs, may rarely occur. This variant has a poorer prognosis and may be selectively inherited. The Westphal variant is the name given to a rigid form of this disorder occurring in adults (Trimble, 1981a).

Dementia of Alzheimer's type also tends to have a more rapid course the earlier the age of onset (Currier *et al.*, 1982). There is evidence that the severe cases tend to have an autosomal dominant pattern of inheritance and a genetic association with Down's syndrome, lymphoma (Hodgkin's disease, lymphosarcoma and reticulum cell sarcoma) and autoimmune disorders, notably insulin dependent diabetes mellitus and rheumatic heart disease (Heston *et al.*, 1981). The female preponderance is lost and sex incidence tends to be equal in these familial cases, and atypical clinical features, such as spastic paraplegia, may be present (Lishman, 1978).

Neurofibromatosis and *tuberous sclerosis (epiloia)* are both inherited as autosomal dominant disorders and are often associated with intracranial tumours. A family history of epilepsy, mental retardation and a nodular "butterfly" rash on the face, are characteristic of epiloia. There are wide variations in the clinical features of this disorder, and it may be clinically "silent", being found only at postmortem, or it may only become manifest by causing epilepsy in later life. It can cause not only mental retardation, but also progressive mental deterioration, and even a "secondary" cognitive impairment as a result of other complications, such as cardiac failure (Cytryn and Lourie, 1980). Like HC and DAT it tends to have a poorer prognosis the earlier the age of onset. Neurofibromatosis and epiloia characteristically involve skin nodules and abnormalities of skin pigmentation, but mental subnormality is less common in the former. Mental subnormality or dementia may also be found in pseudohypoparathyroidism and dystrophia myotonica. Some of the physical signs of these autosomal inherited disorders have been shown in Figure 1.1 (see page 8).

Dominant inheritance may be seen in Pick's dementia and rarely in Creutzfeldt — Jacob disease. The porphyrias (the acute intermittent and variegata types), though rare, are inherited in this way. Clinically they usually cause episodic neuropsychiatric disorders, rather than a dementiform illness, though the occurrence of hypertension, seizures and neurological deficits, may suggest a vascular disorder.

The family history may also reveal a predisposition to alcoholism or hypertension. Consanguinity in the parents may alert the physician to an increased risk of the patient developing an autosomal recessively inherited disorder, such as Wilson's disease, though sometimes several members of a single family may develop this disease (Lishman, 1978).

Occasionally factors in early life may have diagnostic significance in relation to later dementia. Evidence of mental retardation may be elicited and can be the result of Down's syndrome or other disorders mentioned in the previous section, some of which can cause a progressive intellectual impairment in later life. In some of these cases recurrent epileptic seizures may play a role in causing intellectual deterioration (Gomez *et al.*, 1982).

Delay in menarche may indicate impaired function of the hypothalamo–pituitary axis, e.g. in one study an adult patient who had developed progressive obstructive hydrocephalus, due to aqueduct stenosis, gave a history of delayed menarche (at age 19 years) and was found to have an enlargement of the head circumference to greater than the 95th percentile. These findings were felt to indicate that subclinical hydrocephalus had been present since infancy, probably with the enlarged third ventricle causing the endocrine disorder (Roberts *et al.*, 1983). A history in a female patient of amenorrhoea following excessive bleeding postpartum suggests that pituitary necrosis, with resulting hypopituitarism (Sheehan's syndrome), might have developed.

Indiscriminate sexual activity or homosexuality will indicate an increased risk of syphilis. This may not be admitted to in the medical history, or infection may have been subclinical. Syphilis is also suggested by a history of repeated miscarriages in a female patient.

The past or current occupation of the patient may involve a particular risk of exposure to certain toxins, e.g. alcoholism in a bartender. A history of travel to foreign places carries the risk of exposure to potentially chronic neurological infections, e.g. cysticercosis in Mexico. The country of origin may indicate an increased risk of an acquired or an inherited neurological disorder.

10.6 PAST MEDICAL HISTORY

A previous history of neurological insult should be looked for. The commonest causes of *normal pressure hydrocephalus* (NPH) are meningitis, subarachnoid haemorrhage, head injury or neurosurgery, though no cause may be found in many cases. Such events may antedate clinical presentation of NPH by several years (McHugh, 1964). After any severe head injury the usual course is for the post-traumatic cognitive impairment to show some degree of gradual recovery, though this may take several years. Head injury may, in some cases, reveal an underlying dementia that was present before the accident, and there is some evidence that head trauma may precipitate presenile dementia (Strich, 1956). If there has been a period of post-traumatic intellectual improvement and then deterioration develops, this is most likely to be caused by complications such as NPH, intracranial infection, depression or a subdural haematoma.

Minor head injuries may cause a *chronic subdural haematoma*. Occasionally there is no history of any preceding CNS trauma. This condition often has an insidious course and a variable clinical picture with little in the way of neurological signs. It should be particularly suspected when a headache, which may be relatively mild in intensity, is associated with a cognitive impairment that fluctuates from day to day (Mertens and Schimrigk, 1974). It is particularly likely to occur in chronic alcoholic or elderly patients. These two groups, and other patients with pre-existing brain damage, have nervous systems that are particularly vulnerable to damage or dysfunction as a result of trauma, toxins, drugs, hypoxia or a reduction in cerebral circulation, for whatever reason. In such cases the cause of any cognitive impairment may be obscured by the multiple factors involved and the presence of other physical disorders that are particularly likely to be found in the alcoholic (delirium tremens) and the elderly (recurrent falls).

Any history of long-standing or recent onset non-neurological organic disorders, should be noted. Respiratory, renal, cardiovascular or hepatic disorders, can cause a reversible dementia. They may also contribute a superimposed reversible element to an underlying irreversible dementia. Cummings *et al.* (1980) described a 48-year-old patient whose precarious cognitive adjustment depended on his pulmonary function and, when anoxic, he showed myoclonic jerking and cognitive impairment, such that initially a diagnosis of Creutzfeldt–Jacob disease was considered. Cerebral atrophy of uncertain origin was present on his pneumoencephalogram and was probably responsible for the sensitivity of his cognitive functions to minor variations in his cerebral oxygen level.

Such predisposed patients may become impaired by drugs taken in normal doses, particularly when combinations of drugs are used. Cummings *et al.* (1980) classified the main predisposing drugs into four groups—psychotropic, anticonvulsant, anticholinergic and antihypertensive drugs. Drugs can greatly complicate the clinical picture, e.g. hypertension can cause cerebrovascular disease, but the drugs used to treat it can cause intellectual impairment and depression in their own right (Kurland, 1979). Any or all of these three factors may be acting in any case and the role of a particular drug may be revealed by taking a careful history of when it was started or its dose was increased, and the temporal relationship of such events to the patients level of cognitive functioning. Deliberate or accidental overuse of such drugs may be occurring, but an atypical response to a drug taken at normal doses, even in the absence of predisposing factors, should also be considered.

Disorders of gastrointestinal function may cause vitamin deficiency which may be manifest clinically months or years later, when the body stores of the vitamin are exhausted, e.g. vitamin B_{12} deficiency as a result of a total gastrectomy. Other factors may act to provoke an abrupt increase in the severity of a vitamin deficiency, e.g. nutritional deficiency in alcoholics may be facilitated by a partial gastrectomy for treatment of a peptic ulcer. Severe nutritional deficiency itself has been implicated as a cause of dementia (Willanger *et al.*, 1968).

The question that must always be considered is—could a particular event in the patient's medical history have any bearing on his current state? If so, how do we confirm or disprove this relationship?

10.7 PREVIOUS PSYCHIATRIC HISTORY

The relationship between psychiatric disorders and dementia is discussed in Chapter 11. In this chapter such a history is of importance in relation to those disorders which can cause both dementia and psychiatric disturbance concurrently. This relationship may be indirect in so far as a psychiatric disorder may result in exposure to drugs (legally or illegally), electroconvulsive treatment, psychosurgery, or other events which can cause cognitive impairment. A more direct relationship may be seen in alcoholism, epilepsy, Huntington's chorea, multiple sclerosis, Wilson's disease, systemic lupus erythematosis, and the endocrinopathies.

Transient or chronic psychoses may be seen in association with epilepsy, particularly temporal lobe epilepsy (TLE), and may or may not be related to the seizures. Also, a dementing process is recognised as occurring in epileptic patients and involves deterioration in personality and cognition (Trimble, 1981a). The patients referred to here are not those who have developed seizures secondary to an encephalopathy which is also causing progressive cognitive deterioration. *Epileptic dementia* may be due to anticonvulsant drugs or subclinical seizure activity, but many cases appear to be of uncertain origin. Such a dementia is particularly associated with TLE, the presence of a specific brain lesion, a long history of epilepsy involving grand mal seizures (Lishman, 1978), and an associated chronic psychosis (Slater *et al.*, 1963). A gradual dementing process was found in over 50% of Slater *et al.*'s epileptic patients who had developed a chronic schizophrenia-like psychosis.

In *multiple sclerosis* a variety of neurological symptoms and signs are found. Because they tend to be transient, varied and leave no residual signs in the early stages of the illness; because the onset is usually in the third decade of life; and because euphoria, emotional lability and depression are often found; other diagnoses, especially hysteria, are frequently considered. Intellectual impairment of varying degrees of severity is present in the majority of cases (Surridge, 1969), and should be suspected in patients exhibiting euphoria or denial of disability. Rarely the disorder presents as a progressive dementia (Bergin, 1957; Koenig, 1968). Schizophrenia-like psychoses do not occur in this condition more often than would be expected from chance, but when they do occur they often appear to have a close temporal relationship to the onset of the neurological features (Davison and Bagley, 1969).

In *Huntington's chorea* dementia is a common mode of presentation, but psychiatric disorder may antedate this and did so in 50% of Dewhurst *et al.*'s (1969) series. Oliver (1970) found schizophrenia in 12% and depression in 35% of his patients. In one case psychiatric illness preceded the onset of the chorea by 20 years. Psychiatric disorder is to be expected in families where a parent is affected by this disorder and is exhibiting disturbed behaviour; and depression is an understandable reaction in a person who is aware that he is at risk of developing HC. In view of these factors the presence of a psychiatric disorder need not indicate that Huntington's chorea is present or is going to develop, even if the person is genetically at risk. When schizophrenia antedates the movement disorder it may be difficult to tell whether the latter is drug-induced or not. A family history, a progressive dementia, choreiform movements involving the limbs, an abnormal EEG and caudate atrophy on the CAT scan, are features which would suggest a diagnosis of Huntington's chorea (see Table 3.3, see page 47).

Hepatolenticular degeneration (Wilson's disease) presents with psychiatric symptoms in about 20% of patients (Bearn, 1972). Like multiple sclerosis, Wilson's disease presents in the young (usually the first two decades). It may involve transient neurological symptoms and they may be exacerbated by emotional events in the patient's life. All types of psychosis and behavioural disturbance may occur and a chronic schizophrenia-like illness has been described in association with the neurological deterioration (Davison and Bagley, 1969). Some of the features of Wilson's disease that will help to differentiate it from a purely psychiatric disorder are an onset before the age of 20 years, abnormal movements involving the upper limbs, and an abnormal EEG and CAT head scan (which may show atrophy of the lentiform nuclei). The diagnosis can be confirmed by a low serum caeruloplasmin and a corneal Kayser–Fleischer ring (see Table 3.3).

Systemic lupus erythematosus is a disorder of the connective tissue, most commonly occurring in young adult women. It involves many body systems, and the nervous system in about 60% of cases. It is not an uncommon disorder and it may present with any type of psychiatric disorder. 44% of patients had psychiatric features before or at the time of diagnosis in one study (Hall *et al.*, 1981b). These psychiatric phenomena varied at different stages of the disease, but tended to be accompanied by involvement of other systems, particularly involving skin lesions, arthritis and muscle pains.

The *porphyrias* are rare. They usually present in the second or third decades, and characteristically involve an episodic course. The attacks are precipitated or exacerbated by organic factors, especially infections, alcohol and drugs (barbiturates, dichloralphenazone, methyldopa). Any type of psychiatric disorder may be seen and a histrionic emotionality is particularly common, sometimes with an apparent psychological elaboration of the organic features. Suggestive features include a family history, episodic course, and severe pain, which is usually abdominal and may lead to surgical intervention. Neurological features such as a motor neuropathy and epilepsy are often seen. Enquiry should be made for a history of passing dark brown urine. Photosensitive skin lesions are seen in the South African variegata type.

10.8 MENTAL STATE AND PHYSICAL EXAMINATION

The examination of the patient's mental state has been discussed in Chapter 2. Particular care should be taken to look for attentional deficits and other evidence of delirium which, if present, will require evaluation and treatment before the diagnosis of dementia can be confirmed or disproved. Also evidence for an affective disorder and any psychotic symptoms should be looked for. Some of the important physical signs found in disorders that can cause potentially reversible dementia-like pictures, are shown in Figures 10.3 and 10.4, and the causes are listed in Table 10.4.

The primary degenerative dementias are not associated with focal neurological localising signs, if one excludes aphasia, apraxia and agnosia, the presence of the latter indicating cerebral cortical disease. *Constructional apraxia is an early sign of dementia of the Alzheimer's type* (Sim, 1979).

Focal signs are found in Multi-Infarct dementia. Pseudobulbar palsy is characteristic of, but not always present in, MID. It has been found to be particularly associated with cognitive impairment, presumably because it indicates bilateral disease of the cerebral hemispheres (Paulson, 1977). The features of pseudobulbar palsy are emotional lability, defective conjugate gaze upwards, a brisk jaw jerk, dysarthria and dysphagia.

Paulson (1977) described several physical changes that occur with ageing, but do not necessarily indicate dementia. These include a bent posture, muscle hypertonicity, tremors and akinesia. There appears to be a reduction in the ability

TREATABLE CAUSES OF DEMENTIA: PHYSICAL SIGNS (1) HEAD AND NECK

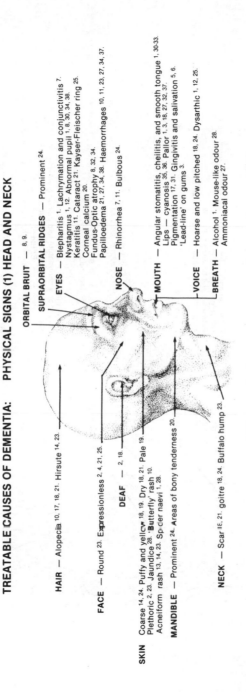

ORBITAL BRUIT — 8, 9.

SUPRAORBITAL RIDGES — Prominent [24].

EYES — Blepharitis [1]. Lachrymation and conjunctivitis [7].
Nystagmus [1, 12]. Abnormal pupil [1, 8, 30, 34, 38].
Keratitis [11]. Cataract [21]. Kayser-Fleischer ring [25].
Corneal calcium [20].
Fundus-Optic atrophy [8, 32, 34].
Papilloedema [21, 27, 34, 38]. Haemorrhages [10, 11, 23, 27, 34, 37].

NOSE — Rhinorrhea [7, 11]. Bulbous [24].

MOUTH — Angular stomatitis, cheilitis, and smooth tongue [1, 30, 33].
Lips — cyanosis [35, 36]. Pallor [1, 3, 18, 27, 32, 37].
Pigmentation [17, 31]. Gingivitis and salivation [5, 6].
'Lead-line' on gums [3].

VOICE — Hoarse and low pitched [18, 24]. Dysarthric [1, 12, 25].

BREATH — Alcohol [1]. Mouse-like odour [28].
Ammoniacal odour [27].

HAIR — Alopecia [10, 17, 18, 21]. Hirsute [14, 23].

FACE — Round [23]. Expressionless [2, 4, 21, 25].

DEAF — 2, 18.

SKIN   Coarse [14, 24]. Puffy and yellow [18, 19]. Dry [18, 21]. Pale [19].
Plethoric [2, 23]. Jaundice [28]. 'Butterfly' rash [10].
Acneiform rash [13, 14, 23]. Spider naevi [1, 28].

MANDIBLE — Prominent [24]. Areas of bony tenderness [20].

NECK — Scar [16, 21]. goitre [18, 24]. Buffalo hump [23].

Figure 10.3   Treatable causes of dementia: physical signs (1): Head and neck. Refer to Table 10.4 for key

186

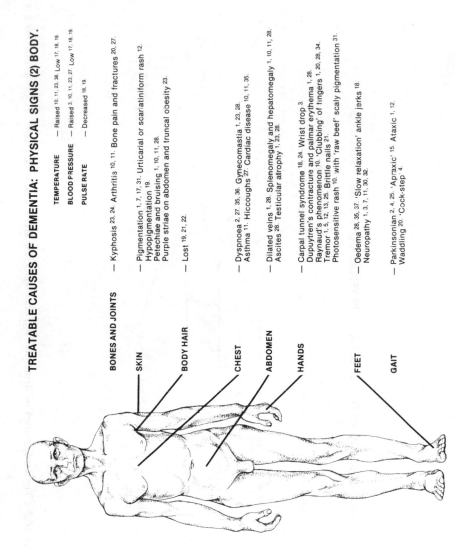

TREATABLE CAUSES OF DEMENTIA: PHYSICAL SIGNS (2) BODY.

TEMPERATURE — Raised 10, 11, 23, 38. Low 17, 18, 19

BLOOD PRESSURE — Raised 3, 10, 11, 23, 27. Low 17, 18, 19

PULSE RATE — Decreased 18, 19.

BONES AND JOINTS — Kyphosis 23, 24. Arthritis 10, 11. Bone pain and fractures 20, 27.

SKIN — Pigmentation 1, 7, 17, 31. Urticarial or scar/atiniform rash 12. Hypopigmentation 19. Petechiae and bruising 1, 10, 11, 28. Purple striae on abdomen and truncal obesity 23.

BODY HAIR — Lost 19, 21, 22.

CHEST — Dyspnoea 2, 27, 35, 36. Gynecomastia 1, 23, 28. Asthma 11. Hiccoughs 27. Cardiac disease 10, 11, 35.

ABDOMEN — Dilated veins 1, 28. Splenomegaly and hepatomegaly 1, 10, 11, 28. Ascites 28. Testicular atrophy 1, 23, 28.

HANDS — Carpal tunnel syndrome 18, 24. Wrist drop 3. Dupuytren's contracture and palmar erythema 1, 28. Raynaud's phenomenon 10. 'Clubbing' of fingers 1, 20, 28, 34. Tremor 1, 5, 12, 13, 25. Brittle nails 21. Photosensitive rash 10: with 'raw beef' scaly pigmentation 31.

FEET — Oedema 28, 35, 37. 'Slow relaxation' ankle jerks 18. Neuropathy 1, 3, 7, 11, 30, 32.

GAIT — Parkinsonian 2, 4, 25. 'Apraxic' 15. Ataxic 1, 12. Waddling 20. 'Cock-step' 4.

Figure 10.4 Treatable causes of dementia: physical signs (2): Body. Refer to Table 10.4 for key

Table 10.4 Potentially treatable causes of dementia

Alcohol	1.
Other toxins	2. Carbon monoxide
	3. Lead
	4. Manganese
	5. Mercury
	6. Organic mercury
	7. Arsenic
Blood vessel disease	8. Aneurysm
	9. Angioma
Collagen disorders	10. Systemic lupus erythematosus
	11. Polyarteritis nodosa
Drugs	12. Barbiturates
	13. Bromism
	14. Phenytoin
Degenerative	15. Normal pressure hydrocephalus
	16. Creutzfeldt–Jacob disease
Endocrine	17. Hypoadrenalism
	18. Hypothyroidism
	19. Hypopituitarism
	20. Hyperparathyroidism
	21. Hypoparathyroidism
	22. Pseudohypoparathyroidism
	23. Cushing's Syndrome
	24. Acromegaly
Metabolic	25. Wilson's disease (also see 28)
	26. Hypoglycaemia
	27. Renal failure
	28. Hepatic failure
	29. Electrolyte imbalance
Vitamin deficiency	30. Thiamine
	31. Nicotinic acid
	32. B_{12}
	33. Folate
Growth	34. Cerebral abscess, subdural haematoma, cerebral neoplasia (primary, secondary, or remote effect)
Hypoxia	35. Cardiac disease
	36. Respiratory disease
	37. Anaemia
Infection	38. Cerebral tuberculosis, syphilis, yeasts, parasites; progressive multifocal leukoencephalopathy

to converge the eyes and in conjugate gaze upwards. The pupils tend to be constricted and respond poorly to light. The ankle jerks are often absent and there is a reduction in the threshhold of peripheral sensory perception, e.g. reduced vibration sense at the ankles. Levy (1969) found that this reduction in nerve condition rate correlated with cognitive impairment in demented patients.

Frontal lobe disorders may be relatively silent and may be indicated by relatively few signs on examination, such as primitive reflexes (Pick's dementia), anosmia, facial weakness of the upper motor neurone type and papilloedema (mass lesions), and incontinence of urine or gait apraxia (normal pressure hydrocephalus). Botez *et al.* (1977) found that NPH was characterised by a normal neurological examination, except for a tonic foot response and a grasp reflex of the foot. Abnormal extraocular movements may be present, such as nystagmus (alcohol and barbiturate abuse) and pupillary abnormalities (syphilis, the sequelae of Wernicke's encephalopathy).

The commonest *cerebral tumour* causing dementia is the meningioma. It has a predilection for the region of the olfactory groove, where it can grow slowly to a large size, producing minimal neurological signs and a progressive dementia (Hunter *et al.*, 1968). More rapidly growing tumours tend to produce focal neurological signs or raised intracranial pressure, at an earlier stage. This is true of metastases, which are most commonly from carcinoma of the bronchus. Other common sites for primaries are the prostate, pancreas, breast and gastrointestinal tracts (Lishman, 1978). Remote effects of carcinoma may less commonly cause dementia, most notable being the development of limbic encephalitis, usually as a consequence of carcinoma of the bronchus (Corsellis *et al.*, 1968).

Patients with psychiatric disorders associated with brain tumours may respond to psychotropic medication in such a manner as to confuse the diagnosis. Binder (1983) described a 40-year-old woman who had been manic for 3 months and had a right intraventricular meningioma, and a 32-year-old man who had a 15 year history of episodic violence, inappropriate affect and visual hallucinations, associated with a large bilateral occipital falx meningioma. The first case had shown no neurological or cognitive abnormalities and the second had bilateral papilloedema only. Both had responded clinically in the past to neuroleptics, but underwent a more permanent improvement following surgery. A temporary post-operative exacerbation of symptoms, requiring neuroleptics, was seen in both. A clinical response may be seen to other psychiatric drugs, and Oyewumi and Lapierre (1981) have described the use of lithium to control mood swings secondary to brain stem damage.

Abnormal movements may be seen in many disorders (see Table 3.2), most notably Huntington's chorea, Wilson's disease, Creutzfeldt–Jacob disease, metabolic disorders and chronic schizophrenia (tardive dyskinesia). Focal neurological signs usually appear early in the first three of these disorders. The differential diagnosis of abnormal movements has already been discussed in section 3.3.

10.9 INVESTIGATIONS

The investigations will need to be tailored to the findings in the history and on examination of the dementing patient. The following investigations are recommended (Cummings *et al.*, 1980; Kaufman, 1981):

Full blood count, erythrocyte sedimentation rate, electrolytes, urea, calcium, phosphorus, thyroid function tests, liver function tests, vitamin B_{12} and red cell folate. Serology for syphilis. Electrocardiogram, urine analysis, skull and chest radiography, electroencephalogram.

CAT brain scanning, and evaluation of the extra-cerebral vasculature using the technique of ultrasound.

A lumbar puncture should be considered provided there is no evidence of raised intracranial pressure. The cerebrospinal fluid obtained should be examined (and cultured where appropriate) for cells, protein, glucose, oligoclonal banding and infectious agents.

More specialised tests that should be considered including serum caeruloplasmin, screening for heavy metal poisoning, urinary examination for porphyrins and metachromatic granules, cerebral angiography, air encephalography and RIHSA cisternography.

In the early stages of dementia a normal EEG almost rules out a metabolic, toxic, focal or infectious cause. In DAT and Huntington's chorea, the EEG is relatively normal in the early stages (Harner, 1975). However, focal changes in the EEG occur in about 10% of the primary degenerative dementias. Potential pitfalls are hypothermia, hypothyroidism, vitamin B_{12} deficiency and a subdural haematoma, where little abnormality may be seen on the EEG.

With ageing the alpha rhythm slows in frequency and quantity. Focal theta activity tends to develop, becoming more frequent with increasing age, and usually being found in the left anterior temporal region. There is also a tendency for symmetrical anterior slowing to develop, and there is a decrease in the response to hyperventilation. In DAT in the elderly the EEG changes are an exaggeration of the normal ageing changes, but in the younger age groups a loss of alpha activity is a frequent and early sign (Gordon and Sim, 1967).

An exaggeration of the ageing process is also seen in the EEG in MID, but the changes are more severe and focal abnormalities, which may be paroxysmal, may be seen. The alpha activity is relatively preserved (Lishman, 1978).

Care must be taken in the evaluation of the significance of the CAT head scan findings in the elderly patient. *Cerebral atrophy can occur without cognitive impairment and is more likely to be found the older the patient.* However, statistically only a limited relationship has been demonstrated between cognitive impairment and cerebral atrophy in some studies of the elderly (Jacoby and Levy, 1980a). From this it can be seen that in assessing the significance of cerebral atrophy on the CAT head scan, the age of the patient, and other evidence for dementia, must be taken into account.

A population of patients with primary degenerative dementia will have a greater degree of cerebral atrophy than an age-matched non-demented population, but dementia can occur in the absence of cerebral atrophy, and vice versa. However, the absence of "major atrophy" in a demented patient should make the physician particularly suspicious that a treatable illness is present (Huckman *et al.*, 1975). The CAT head scanner is of little use in discriminating

Pick's from DAT. The scan may help in the diagnosis of MID, and evidence of infarction was found unexpectedly in 25% of 40 demented patients, in one study (Jacoby *et al.*, 1980b).

Normal pressure hydrocephalus produces a characteristic picture with gross enlargement of the cerebral ventricles, which are even visible on the highest scan slices. The cortical mantle is so reduced in size as to make visualisation of the cortical sulci difficult. Cortical atrophy is not present.

The presence of a focal lesion (a tumour or an infarct), or the presence of cerebral atrophy in a young or middle-aged patient, are of more significance in indicating the presence of structural brain disease. However, problems may arise with a subdural haematoma which may be difficult to visualise on a scan, as they can be isodense with brain tissue, and in about 40% of cases they are bilateral. In such cases distortion, by compression, of the ventricular system, may be the main indication of the presence of the haematoma. When it is unilateral, lateralised distortion of the brain structures will be seen and is easier to recognise.

Other neuroradiological procedures may be necessary and the insertion of radioiodinated human serum albumen (RIHSA) into the CSF, will demonstrate the CSF dynamics and can be used to confirm a diagnosis of normal pressure hydrocephalus. Cerebral angiography may be necessary to demonstrate the cerebral vasculature in more detail, and air encephalography to demonstrate the ventricles and subarachnoid spaces.

10.10 PROGNOSIS

Except in rapidly progressive dementias, such as Creutzfeldt–Jacob disease, where the vast majority of patients die within 2 years, the prognosis tends to be influenced by numerous factors as well as the nature of the disorder, including genetic loading, age of onset, duration of illness before the correct diagnosis is made and the appropriate treatment instituted, and the occurrence of complicating disorders that can prematurely shorten the survival time, e.g. bronchopneumonia.

Dementia of the Alzheimer's type has a survival time that varies markedly, but is about 5 years on average (Lishman, 1978). Heston *et al.* (1981) found that the mean survival time varied between 4 and 25 years, but was of a fairly consistent duration of about 8 years, when the onset was between 55 and 75 years of age. In this limited series the duration was shorter with an earlier age of onset. Pick's dementia has a duration of from 2 to 10 years, and Multi-Infarct dementia about 5 years. Admission to hospital is a poor prognostic sign in MID and DAT in the elderly, with the majority of patients subsequently dying within 2 years (Roth, 1955).

Small vessel cerebrovascular disease may become more frequently diagnosed now that CAT brain scanning is available, and Binswanger's disease (subcortical arteriosclerotic encephalopathy) tends to last over 10 years (Wells, 1977). It may be possible to slow down or even arrest the progression of a dementing disorder resulting from hypertensive cerebrovascular disease, by controlling the blood pressure, irrespective of whether it is the small or large vessels of the brain that are affected. Over-vigorous antihypertensive treatment should be avoided due to the risk of precipitating cerebral ischaemia, with further deterioration in cognition.

Huntington's chorea has a variable duration, with an average of about 15 years in adults, but 8 years when the onset is in childhood. Untreated Wilson's disease has a duration of less than 4 years in children, but longer in adults. The earlier the treatment is started the better is the prognosis, but liver damage, which is the dominant feature in children, is less responsive to treatment. In contrast, treatment can lead to marked recovery of the neurological and psychiatric complications of this disorder (Lishman, 1978).

In idiopathic Parkinson's disease and progressive supranuclear palsy, survival time is less than 10 years. However, there are always exceptions, and apparently successful treatment of two cases of Creutzfeldt–Jacob dementia, using amantidine, has been documented (Braham, 1971; Sanders and Dunn, 1973). In another of Sanders and Dunn's cases the drug produced a remission in symptoms.

CHAPTER 11

Pseudodementia, Pseudodepression and Related Problems

11.1 INTRODUCTION

Pseudodementia has been defined as a "syndrome in which dementia is mimicked or caricatured by functional psychiatric illness" (Wells, 1979). Such a definition has the advantage that it does not restrict the use of the term to those cases of depression, usually in the elderly, where cognitive impairment has become so pronounced as to cause diagnostic problems. However, depression is probably the commonest cause of pseudodementia (Nott and Fleminger, 1975), though even this conclusion was questioned by Wells (1979). Pseudodementia has also been seen as a manifestation of post-traumatic neurosis (Lishman, 1968), somatisation disorder, hysterical conversion, the Ganser syndrome, chronic schizophrenia, hypomania, schizo-affective disorder, personality disorder, and mental subnormality (Caine, 1981). An element of malingering may be found in cases of hysterical conversion, but the deliberate simulation of dementia is almost impossible to maintain for any length of time (Anderson *et al.*, 1959). Lishman (1968) has suggested that diagnostic difficulties may arise in occasional cases of obsessional neurosis, and neurotic affective illness.

Pseudodementia was found in 10% of one series of 106 patients who had been routinely diagnosed as demented prior to their evaluation at a neurological hospital (Marsden and Harrison, 1972). Careful assessment of these patients found no evidence for *any* neuropsychiatric abnormality in a further 2%. This latter 2% indicate that the diagnosis in difficult cases of suspected dementia may become clearer if a period of observation is employed, rather than premature diagnosis and discharge. This made the diagnosis of dementia incorrect in 12% of the total number of patients. 12% represents a particularly significant proportion for the psychiatrist, who is particularly likely to encounter patients with the kind of disorders that will produce pseudodementia.

The relationship between "non-organic" and "organic" disorders can be complex and varied. The diagnostic problem may require more than just separating dementia from pseudodementia. It may involve identifying the

Table 11.1   The possible relationships between organic and non-organic brain disorders

1. OBD (organic brain disease) *mimicked by* functional psychiatric illness (FPI)
   e.g. depressive pseudodementia
2. OBD *mimicking* FPI
   e.g. Pick's dementia and pseudodepression
3. OBD *masking* concurrent FPI
   e.g. right hemisphere damage and depression
4. OBD *superimposed on* FPI
   e.g. dementia and personality disorder
5. OBD *coexisting with* FPI
   e.g. cerebral ventricular enlargement and chronic schizophrenia
6. OBD *with superimposed* FPI
   e.g. aphasia and affective disorders
7. OBD of the *focal type mimicking diffuse OBD*
   e.g. angular gyrus syndrome and dementia

relationship between, and relative contributions of, "organic" and "functional" factors, in a particular illness. Table 11.1 shows the different ways in which these elements may be related.

In addition to the classical depressive pseudodementia, the converse may be seen and depression may be mimicked by an organic disorder. For example, a patient with a slowly progressive disorder involving the frontal lobes, such as Pick's dementia, often exhibits prominent features of apathy and motor retardation, without any pronounced neurological or cognitive abnormalities being present in the early stages (Robertson *et al.*, 1958). Particularly disorders affecting the dorsolateral region of the frontal lobe produce this "pseudodepressed" clinical picture (Blumer and Benson, 1975).

Brain damage, particularly when it involves the non-dominant cerebral hemisphere, may effectively mask a concurrent depressive illness. These patients may develop aprosody and a loss of the ability to communicate emotion by non-verbal behaviour, such as facial expression. In some cases they may even deny depressive symptoms (Ross and Rush, 1981). In such cases the diagnosis of depression may have to be substantially based on objective data, including sleep disturbance, loss of libido and anorexia. Other behavioural changes may occur, such as suddenly becoming "uncooperative" or "difficult", during rehabilitation from the original acute neurological illness. In some cases brain damaged patients, who become impaired in their ability to express emotion, may have their emotional "flatness" incorrectly diagnosed as a manifestation of depression, particularly when certain other features of organic brain disease, notably emotional incontinence, are present.

In a random population of people over 65 years of age, dementia is a frequent finding and is present in about 10% (Kay *et al.*, 1964). In view of this it is reasonable to expect dementia to develop in a substantial number of patients with pre-existing psychiatric disorders, simply on the basis of coincidence. Such a presentation of dementia may be affected, and in some cases can be masked by, pre-existing factors, such as the patient's premorbid personality (Post, 1968).

Lishman (1978) used the term "pseudo-pseudodementia" to describe those cases where a patient who is developing dementia reacts in such a way as to mislead the clinician into suspecting that he has a pseudodementia. However, it should be borne in mind that affective disorders, such as anxiety and depression, are commonly seen in the early stages of Alzheimer's dementia and Multi-Infarct dementia.

In other disorders, though organic and functional factors appear to be present, the significance of the association is not clear. Using the CAT scanner, Jacoby and Levy (1980b) studied patients with depression of late onset. They found a subgroup of patients who had cerebral ventricles that were significantly larger in size than those found in an age-matched group of patients who had depressive illnesses which had started at an earlier age. Whether or not this finding indicates that organic brain disease is playing an aetiological role in the development of depression in the former group, remains to be seen, though patients in this group were found to have a significantly higher mortality, on follow up 2 years later (Jacoby, 1981).

A functional psychiatric disorder may develop on a pre-existing neurological disorder. This is seen in the aphasias when a depression (motor aphasia), euphoria or paranoid psychosis (sensory aphasia) may develop (Benson, 1979).

Finally, there is a group of patients who have definite organic brain disease and who are diagnosed as demented, but have a pseudodementia, in the sense that there is no global impairment of cognitive functions. This mistake may be made when the patient has a focal brain lesion. It has been described in association with a relatively focal lesion in the angular gyrus region, which caused an apparent global cognitive impairment (Benson et al., 1982). Similar errors can be made with Parkinson's syndrome, severe organic memory impairment, and delirium. Dementia may never develop in many of these cases and by making the wrong diagnosis the physician places the patient at risk of receiving incorrect management and an inappropriately poor prognosis.

Whether the syndrome of subcortical dementia can be regarded as a true dementia or a pseudodementia, depends on the criteria adopted for the diagnosis of dementia. However, subcortical dementia is an important concept to be aware of because of its potential reversibility, the atypical cognitive deficits associated with it (Albert, 1978), and because of the similarities between this syndrome and pseudodementia (Caine, 1981).

Pseudodementia versus dementia

Dementia of uncertain origin is a common diagnosis after neurological evaluation of a patient has been completed and has revealed evidence consistent with a dementing process. By adding together all the demented patients in three series, 47% of a total of 233 patients had no clear cause for their dementia (Freemon, 1976; Marsden and Harrison, 1972; Smith et al., 1976). When a population of patients with this diagnosis have been followed up, 57% in one series (Nott and Fleminger, 1975), and 31% in another series (Ron et al., 1979),

Table 11.2 The major clinical features differentiating pseudementia from dementia

PSEUDODEMENTIA	DEMENTIA
Clinical course and history	
Family always aware of dysfunction and its severity	Family often unaware of dysfunction and its severity
Onset can be dated with some precision	Onset can be dated only within broad limits
Symptoms of short duration before medical help is sought	Symptoms usually of long duration before medical help is sought
Rapid progression of symptoms after onset	Slow progression of symptoms throughout course
History of previous psychiatric dysfunction common	History of previous psychiatric dysfunction unusual
Complaints and clinical behaviour	
Patients usually complain much of cognitive loss	Patients usually complain little of cognitive loss
Patients' complaints of cognitive dysfunction usually detailed	Patients' complaints of cognitive dysfunction usually vague
Patients emphasize disability	Patients conceal disability
Patients highlight failures	Patients delight in accomplishments, however trivial
Patients make little effort to perform even simple tasks	Patients struggle to perform tasks
	Patients rely on notes, calendars, etc., to keep up
Patients usually communicate strong sense of distress	Patients often appear unconcerned
Affective change often pervasive	Affect labile and shallow
Loss of social skills often early and prominent	Social skills often retained
Behaviour often incongruent with severity of cognitive dysfunction	Behaviour usually compatible with severity of cognitive dysfunction
Nocturnal accentuation of dysfunction uncommon	Nocturnal accentuation of dysfunction common
Clinical features related to memory, cognitive, and intellectual dysfunction	
Attention and concentration often well preserved	Attention and concentration usually faulty
"Don't know" answers typical	Near-miss answers frequent
On tests of orientation, patients often give "don't know" answers	On tests of orientation, patients often mistake unusual for usual
Memory loss for recent and remote events usually severe	Memory loss for recent events usually more severe than for remote events
Memory gaps for specific periods or events common	Memory gaps for specific periods unusual*
Marked variability in performance on tasks of similar difficulty	Consistently poor performance on tasks of similar difficulty

*Except when due to delirium, trauma, seizures, etc.
From C. E. Wells (1979) *The American Journal of Psychiatry*, vol. **136**, p.898.
© 1979 The American Psychiatric Association. Reprinted by permission.

had shown no evidence of intellectual deterioration, and some of these patients had improved. These figures emphasise the importance of being aware of the various ways in which a progressive dementing disorder may be mimicked by other non-progressive cerebral conditions.

The rest of this chapter will be concerned with the differentiation of dementia from pseudodementia. Some of the important features separating the two disorders are summarised in Table 11.2.

11.2 HISTORY OF ILLNESS

Dementia and depressive pseudodementia are primarily diseases of those aged over 50 years. Young patients presenting with pseudodementia will present fewer diagnostic problems, as they lack many of the features that complicate its differential diagnosis in the older patients. Such features include age-related cerebral atrophy (seen on the CAT head scan) and EEG changes. Functional disorders other than depression, as a cause of pseudodementia, are more frequently found in patients under the age of 50 years.

Certain aspects of the initial contact with the patient and the associated circumstances, may suggest that pseudodementia is present. These patients usually need little persuasion to see the doctor and may arrive at the clinic unaccompanied. They may have travelled a long distance and navigated a complex route with an ease that contrasts with the severity of the cognitive impairment they claim. Though the onset of the illness is relatively acute, a depressive illness may involve an initial stage during which there is only a general loss of interest and a disturbance of biological functions, before the more florid picture develops (F. Post, 1975).

The patient's adjustment during the period apparently preceding his intellectual deterioration must be evaluated. Someone who appears to be dementing may come to the physician's attention when he (the patient) has just retired from his work. Careful assessment of the circumstances surrounding the patient's retirement may reveal that he was managing to cope normally with his work immediately prior to his retirement. This is in contrast to the dementing patient who, because of his deteriorating ability to manage, may have been encouraged to leave by his employers. Depression may be precipitated by life changes, such as retirement or the death of a spouse. However, if the patient was already cognitively impaired any change in his daily routine will probably lead to further difficulties in coping and an apparent worsening in his cognitive abilities. The dementia may then be revealed as he struggles to adjust to the lack of structure and support in his day-to-day life. Only by obtaining the details and context of such life-events is it possible to assess their aetiological significance.

The pseudodemented patient makes little secret of his disability and complains bitterly of his poor memory, impaired concentration, loss of interest in everything, and he may have many somatic complaints (Post, 1975). Because of these complaints and an early deterioration in personal care and social behaviour, those close to the patient will be in little doubt as to when the illness began. The duration of the illness is usually a matter of months at the most. The rapid progression and the patient's awareness of his difficulties, results in early contact with the physician.

When there is an acute onset, precipitating events should be enquired about, such as any emotionally or physically traumatic event that may have precipitated a psychiatric disorder (hysterical conversion reaction, Ganser syndrome, post-traumatic neurosis, or some other neurotic reaction). Similarly any primary or secondary gain should be looked for.

A short history suggestive of cognitive impairment may be seen in hypomania, with poor judgement and distractability occurring. This is uncommon as a first episode of affective illness in patients over the age of 50 years, and if it should occur, then a neurological disorder (particularly a tumour) or drug intake (especially alcohol, stimulant drugs or steroids), should be suspected (Klerman, 1978). Moreover, the features of hypomania are often atypical in older patients and mixed affective states are particularly common (Post, 1965) and may give the impression that an organic emotional lability is present. There may be a history of disinhibited behaviour, sexual or otherwise, and such uncharacteristic behaviour may also be seen in depressed, as well as dementing, patients.

Dementing patients are usually brought by relatives or friends. They will have difficulty defining the onset of the patient's illness and will usually underestimate its duration, which will be found to have been a matter of years, on closer enquiry, as they recall more distant events that in retrospect were indicative of cognitive deterioration. These patients usually come with some reluctance or an attitude of apathetic disinterest. They have few complaints, and may deny any problems at all. However, some patients may have multiple somatic complaints which may be inseparable from those found in neurotic patients (F. Post, 1975). The history may be dominated by some new development that has made the demented patient more difficult to manage and precipitated his referral, e.g. the onset of delirium. Attention to personal care and social behaviour usually remain intact in the early stages of dementia.

11.3 PREVIOUS HISTORY

A family history may suggest some predisposition to dementia or psychiatric illness. 10–25% of patients with manic/depressive illness have first degree relatives who have had a similar illness (Klerman, 1978). A previous history of affective illness, particularly when a family history is also present, is an important finding in pointing to the possibility of a depressive pseudodementia (Post, 1965; Ron et al., 1979).

There may be a past history of depression with a similar clinical picture, as a pseudodementia-like picture has a tendency to recur with further depressive episodes (Lishman, 1978). Though Wells (1979) found a previous psychiatric history uncommon in his demented patients, Post (1968) found that an abnormal premorbid personality predisposed a dementing patient to show clinical features suggesting a functional disorder, usually involving paranoid or depressive tendencies. These different findings probably reflect the different patient populations encountered by these two authors. Post dealt mainly with elderly depressed patients, and Wells with patients as young as 33 years of age, whose diagnoses included conversion hysteria and post-traumatic neurosis.

There may be a previous history suggestive of conversion phenomena, such as aphonia or limb weakness, or other disorders where the diagnosis was never satisfactorily established. The similarity between the clinical picture now and that seen in previous admissions to other hospitals may only be apparent on reviewing the discharge summary from the other hospitals. Such information may also be helpful in indicating the most appropriate treatment to be used, e.g. antidepressant drugs, ECT, etc., as well as the diagnosis and prognosis.

Evidence of maladjustments in the patient's premorbid personality should be looked for. Elderly patients who present for the first time with a psychiatric illness, frequently show evidence of a predisposing premorbid maladjustment (Post, 1965). The personality may have been antisocial (indicating a predisposition to malingering or somatisation disorder), histrionic or passive-immature-dependent (hysterical conversion), or schizoid (schizophrenia). The history may suggest an inadequate personality type, that is to say, one unable to cope with the stresses of normal living, unable to learn from experience and establish mature, long-lasting interpersonal relationships. Such a premorbid personality may be found in patients with mental subnormality, and a history of academic and social failure during the school years may support this impression. It is the intellectually limited and other people who have limited mechanisms for coping with emotionally stressful events, who are prone to develop hysterical conversion symptoms. Wells (1979) has demonstrated that *dependency traits are frequently present in the premorbid personality of the patient with pseudodementia.*

11.4 NURSING OBSERVATIONS

A rapid improvement within a few days of admission would suggest a situationally dependent condition (a brief reactive psychosis or a hysterical conversion disorder) or a transient organic disorder (drug or alcohol induced). An initial deterioration would be expected in the dementing patient.

Nursing observations will provide further information about the patient's pattern and consistency of behaviour, social and otherwise, and his degree of attention to personal care and hygiene. The depressed patient will tend to make little attempt to take part in the ward activities and will either remain withdrawn and apathetic, or agitated and restless, constantly requesting reassurance from the nursing staff. He will communicate a sense of distress, though this may alternate with periods of hypomania, if a mixed affective psychosis is present. Often he will be able to function normally when persuaded to do so, though negativism and other catatonic features, may be present. Marked variations in motor activity are a feature of the Ganser syndrome, over-activity is usual in hypomania and agitated depression, and is also seen in "hyperactive" delirium.

Hysteria can be associated with a histrionic emotional display and this may involve regressive behaviour, such as baby talk, bed wetting and thumb sucking. This type of behaviour has been described as "hysterical puerilism" (Lishman, 1968). However, in hysteria, attention to personal care is preserved and there may even be an excessive concern about personal appearance. Hysterical features are also seen in the Ganser syndrome.

In dementia the patient will usually cooperate in the ward tasks and attempt to either hide, deny or compensate for his cognitive difficulties. He may use environmental cues to attempt to cope with his impaired memory and orientation. Excuses will be made up to explain his failures, and a catastrophic reaction may develop when he is confronted with a task he cannot cope with. He may actively try and avoid situations that he has failed in before. Usually he will continue blindly on, apparently oblivious to his errors. There may a worsening in his cognition during the evening and frank delirium may develop.

Reversal of the sleep–wake cycle is common in dementia, but insomnia is also common in functional disorders, both neurotic and psychotic. Severely depressed patients often wake in the early hours of the morning and lie in bed preoccupied with morbid thoughts. This contrasts with the manic patient who will sleep little and get out of bed full of energy and start a variety of different tasks, usually failing to complete one before becoming distracted and moving on to another. When the demented patient wanders at night, cognitive impairment will be evident and he will exhibit disorientation and uncoordinated, purposeless behaviour.

11.5 MENTAL STATE AND PHYSICAL EXAMINATION

This will complement the nursing observations, but will not have the advantage of providing information about the patient's behaviour when he is unaware of being observed. When the patient functions at an improved level when unaware that he is being observed, malingering and/or hysteria is suggested. However, deliberate simulation of dementia is uncommon as a pure phenomenon and, in such cases, some gain will usually become obvious with time. Anderson *et al.* (1959) compared patients with true dementia, hysterical pseudodementia and simulated dementia. They came to the conclusion that it is almost impossible to simulate dementia, certainly for any length of time. Such patients will tend to be defensive, angry or otherwise uncooperative in their behaviour, when examined. This contrasts with the behaviour of the demented patient, who will usually cooperate and appear unconcerned at his failures. Any marked change in behaviour in a demented patient, when he is on his own, would be in the direction of a deterioration, as he would not try to hide his deficits and so his performance would be at a lower level.

In practice there is an element of malingering present in many patients with hysterical conversion phenomena and it is a moot point whether the Ganser syndrome is a hysterical, organic, or simulated phenomenon, or a combination of all three (Lishman, 1978). The author believes it is primarily a hysterical phenomenon. Hysterical patients may exhibit la belle indifférence, and other diagnoses may be suggested by observing the quality of the affect shown by the patient. Patients with affective disorders will communicate their predominant affect, in contrast to the shallow or labile affect of the demented patient. A flattened affect is commonly found in chronic schizophrenic patients, the physician feeling "as if there is a glass wall" between himself and the patient. Chronic schizophrenic patients may also show an incongruous affect, laughing or crying inappropriately, and this should not be confused with the emotional incontinence or lability, of the patient with organic brain disease. "Silly" behaviour may be seen in schizophrenic patients, as well as in those with hypomania, hysterical conversion, frontal lobe disease and delirium (Geschwind, 1982). A combination of hysterical and schizophrenic features has been described by Bleuler (1950) as the Buffoonery syndrome. In the rare Ganser syndrome, apathy or anxiety are more common.

"Don't-know" verbal responses are typical of patients with depressive pseudodementia and are one manifestation of resistance to the physician (negativism). Such a response may also result from abulia or a limited intellect. It is seen in schizophrenia, mental retardation and subcortical dementia. When such responses are overcome the depressed patient is found to be relatively orientated. His immediate memory may be impaired but his short-term memory is relatively intact in contrast to his apparent cognitive impairment. It is difficult to overcome the attentional deficits found in these patients (Caine, 1981) and this has contributed to the failure of clinical tests of orientation and memory to discriminate between true and pseudodementia (Nott and Fleminger, 1975; Ron *et al.*, 1979).

However, memory impairment in pseudodementia may only involve certain specific periods, in contrast to the diffuse recent memory impairment of dementia. Dense amnesia for a discrete period of time, during which an event of emotional or other personal significance to the patient occurred, or loss of memory for all (or most) of the events of his previous life, is particularly suggestive of psychogenic (hysterical) amnesia. It may be associated with a history of the patient wandering off (fugue) and losing his identity. Loss of one's personal identity as a result of dementia is only seen in the terminal stages. However, organic brain disease frequently coexists with, and may act to precipitate, hysterical conversion phenomena (Merskey, 1979). Inconsistency in memory deficits, often with a convenient quality, will be seen in the malingerer.

"Near miss" answers are common in demented patients, according to Wells (1979), but Anderson *et al.* (1959) found they were used more frequently in hysterical pseudodementia. He also found "confabulation" common in this population. Perseveration is more suggestive of dementia (Benton and Spreen, 1961), though it can occur in other disorders, as a catatonic symptom. "Near miss" answers should be differentiated from *"answering past the point"*

(vorbeireden) which is the "false response of a patient to the examiner's question where the answer, although wrong, is never far wrong and bears a definite and obvious relation to the question, indicating clearly that the question has been grasped by the patient" (Anderson and Mallinson, 1941). For example, to the question "What colour is the sky?" a typical response would be "Green". Though vorbeireden is particularly associated with the Ganser syndrome, it is more common in other organic or functional disorders, when it is referred to as the Ganser response. Vorbeireden should not be confused with the use of word substitutions (verbal paraphasias) found in sensory dysphasia.

In the *Ganser syndrome* the patient develops an acute illness, usually with impairment of consciousness, altered motor activity and hysterical conversion phenomena, including pseudohallucinations. It is an uncommon syndrome and has been associated with prisoners awaiting trial, but it can occur under other circumstances. An organic precipitant may be involved, often a minor head injury. There is some disagreement over the type of illness it represents but it seems to be understandable as a hysterical conversion disorder which is often "released" by an "organic" event. As a consequence of the latter, "organic" features may be present in the clinical picture (Lishman, 1978).

The patient with *chronic schizophrenia* may appear to be demented, exhibiting paucity of thought content, loss of abstract reasoning and loss of social behaviour. The term "aphanisis" (McGlashan, 1982) has been used to describe the picture of emotional flattening and social withdrawal that these patients present. This is particularly likely to be a diagnostic problem when the patient appears to the physician for the first time, with no previous history available. In fact it is arguable whether they have a pseudodementia or a true dementia, as they often show a combination of cerebral ventricular enlargement and neuropsychological impairment (Luchins, 1982). If the patient does not give an adequate history, certain features will suggest the diagnosis, such as residual psychotic symptoms (hallucinations, delusions, thought disorder) or neuroleptic-induced orofacial dyskinesia.

Premorbid limitation of intellect may interfere with the assessment of the patient, who will be slow to respond to questions. He will interpret proverbs and other test situations requiring abstract thinking, in a concrete manner. He will have difficulty grasping the complexities of a test situation. Circumstantiality of speech may be pronounced, giving an impression of vagueness. Such patients, particularly if depressed, may exhibit a profound lack of awareness of events that are not of immediate concern to them. Their long-standing cognitive limitations may be misinterpreted as an indication of recent cognitive decline.

If the patient exhibits inconsistencies in his performance it is worthwhile drawing his attention to them and then observing his response to this. Patients who are malingering will tend to be defensive and attempt to explain away any inconsistencies in their behaviour, in contrast to the apathy or the catastrophic response, seen in the demented patient. In depression and other disorders, the patient will be relatively unaffected by having his attention drawn to his variable responses.

Observation should be made of the rate of speech production, its semantic and syntactic structure, its content and the degree of logical connection between the ideas expressed. Apraxia, agnosia, aphasia and memory impairment should be looked for. Nott and Fleminger (1975) found that language functions and apraxia were confined to their patients with dementia and differentiated them from the pseudodemented.

Delusions, hallucinations or thought disorder, may be present and suggest the presence of a functional psychosis. Whether or not the phenomenology of these symptoms is consistent with the patient's mood, suggesting an affective psychosis, should be assessed, as should the degree to which they dominate the clinical picture. Hallucinations are a feature of the Ganser syndrome and may be seen in hysterical pseudodementia, though they are then more typically pseudohallucinations. Obsessional ruminations and other neurotic disorders may preoccupy the patient and lead to self-neglect or regressed behaviour that can mimic a dementia (Lishman, 1968).

Physical examination

Physical and neurological examination should be carried out looking for any "hard" neurological signs, and for evidence of primitive reflexes and other signs that may indicate the presence of an otherwise "silent" organic brain disorder, particularly in the frontal lobe region. Ron *et al.* (1979) found the combination of depression and Parkinsonism was particularly associated with an incorrect diagnosis of dementia, so patients showing extrapyramidal signs must be evaluated with particular care. However, there is evidence of dementia in about 30% of patients with Parkinson's disease (Grimes, 1983). The elderly depressed patient often gives an appearance of Parkinsonism, exhibiting a shuffling gait, and this has been called "pseudoparkinsonism" (Post, 1965).

11.6 INVESTIGATIONS

These should be aimed at identifying possible causes of dementia or functional illness. Blood tests may point to an abnormality known to be aetiologically related to dementia. Neuropsychological testing, like the EEG tracing, is frequently unhelpful when the clinical picture is unclear (Caine, 1981), though a marked variability and inconsistency in responses is particularly suggestive of pseudodementia. Such testing will also be useful as a baseline against which later test results can be compared. Pseudodementia patients can produce test results virtually indistinguishable from those produced by demented patients and this is most likely to occur in elderly patients with severe depression (Post, 1966). Caine (1981) found a similarity between the neuropsychological profile of the patient with pseudodementia and the patient with subcortical dementia, with defects in those cognitive functions dependent on preservation of attention, arousal and concentration. This resulted clinically in a lack of spontaneous speech and an inability to solve complex problems.

Useful investigations include CAT head scanning, though it should be borne in mind that in the older patients the presence or absence of cerebral atrophy can be difficult to interpret. In some cases the scan may produce a highly significant result, e.g. a cerebral tumour or normal pressure hydrocephalus, but such findings need not exclude an associated depression.

Other investigations that may help are the dexamethasone suppression test, hypnosis, and the use of intravenous barbiturates.

Trial of treatment

If a patient is admitted on medication, a trial off all unessential medication, for a period of assessment, may result in clinical improvement. If depression is missed and inappropriate medication is used, e.g. minor tranquillisers, this may result in the diagnosis being obscured and if depression is present, it may be made worse. In patients with organic brain disease injudicious use of psychotropic drugs, especially those with a marked anticholinergic action, may induce, or worsen, cognitive impairment (Ghoneim and Mewaldt, 1977; Glen, 1979; Granacher and Baldessarini, 1976).

If there is any reasonable evidence that depression exists, judicious use of antidepressants may prove worthwhile, providing an adequate dosage is used over a reasonable period of time (3 to 4 weeks). In those frequent cases where OBD and depression coexist, the choice of antidepressant treatment must be made carefully. In selected cases a trial of ECT may clarify the diagnosis, and unilateral ECT, applied to the non-dominant hemisphere, may be preferable to minimise cognitive impairment.

11.7 PROGNOSIS

Ron et al.'s (1979) study looked retrospectively at patients previously diagnosed as suffering from presenile dementia, and found a high incidence of incorrect diagnoses. These incorrect diagnoses constituted 33% of their cases, which were taken from a psychiatric hospital. Though these patients had improved cognitively when reassessed at a later date, they still demonstrated a high incidence of psychiatric disability. When compared to those patients who had undergone a progressive dementing course, the pseudodementia patients were more frequently found to have had a previous history of affective illness, evidence of depression during their initial assessment, a verbal/performance WAIS IQ discrepancy which failed to reach the 5% level of significance, normal EEG's, and no radiological evidence of cortical atrophy. They had also shown a greater incidence of abnormal premorbid personalities.

The clinical progress in pseudodementia will depend on the underlying illness and whether or not concurrent OBD is present. In some cases observation of the course of the illness may be necessary to clarify the diagnosis. Any of the following three courses may be followed:

1. Full recovery can occur in the affective psychoses, hysteria, the Ganser syndrome, and malingering.

2. Deterioration may occur when irreversible dementia is also present. The prognosis should be guarded in certain cases, e.g. following head injury, when cognitive recovery may continue for a year or more; or when a potentially reversible cause of dementia is present.

3. In some cases where brain damage of uncertain cause is also present, progression may not occur (Ron *et al.*, 1979).

Chronic schizophrenic patients tend to show their maximum deterioration during the initial 5 years of their illness, after which they will continue to show a defect state (Bleuler, 1974). Some depressed patients may continue to exhibit depressive symptomatology of varying degrees and in others a similar pseudodementia picture may recur with later depressive episodes. There is also evidence that in late-onset depression, enlarged cerebral ventricles visible on the CAT head scan are statistically associated with an increased mortality at follow-up (Jacoby, 1981).

Where there is an underlying disturbance of personality, it will of course remain. There is a tendency for many patients with pseudodementia to have a dependent premorbid personality, and they will continue to exhibit features of dependency (Wells, 1979). Malingering tends to be short-lived as it is extremely difficult to simulate dementia and puts considerable demands on the patient, but there is usually an underlying maladjusted personality.

The short-term prognosis is good for the rare Ganser syndrome and rapid recovery usually occurs, but in many patients who show Ganser responses, there is underlying organic brain disease or a nonorganic psychosis, which may only become apparent after recovery from the acute illness or on later follow-up (Lishman, 1978). In hysterical pseudodementia the disorder may become chronic if the underlying conflicts are not identified and resolved.

CHAPTER 12

Recurrent "Falling" Attacks

12.1 INTRODUCTION

In order to simplify the diagnostic process involved in evaluating the patient subject to recurrent episodes of altered consciousness, the author has divided such cases into those which involve loss of postural muscle tone ("falling") and those which do not. In this chapter disorders associated with the former (both with and without impairment of consciousness) will be considered. For the purpose of this discussion the phrase "impairment of conscious level" excludes sleep attacks, which will be discussed in Chapter 15. *Sleep attacks are usually gradual in onset and the patient will be rousable.*

Table 12.1 lists the main causes of recurrent "falling" and, in those cases where this symptom forms one part of a complex clinical picture, identifying the cause may shed light on the aetiology of other aspects of the patient's condition. This table breaks down the causes of "falling" according to whether or not there is impairment of the conscious level, and the patient's age. Table 12.2 is a flow diagram demonstrating one approach to the differential diagnosis of falling attacks. This diagram should be considered in the light of the text, which will elaborate on the important causes of loss of postural muscle tone. Examination of the patient who is unresponsive after falling is discussed further in Chapter 14.

The basic mechanisms underlying such "falling" attacks are cerebral hypoxia, hypoglycaemia, ischaemia, aberrant neuronal activity which is excessive for the maintenance of normal consciousness or inadequate for the maintenance of muscle tone and posture, neuromuscular, and psychogenic disorders (hysteria and/or malingering). The latter cause is certainly not the least and the brunt of this chapter will be concerned with epileptic seizures and pseudoseizures (episodes which resemble epileptic seizures, but are not the result of a seizure discharge in the brain, and are usually psychogenic). After considering these two disorders, the hysterical faint and syncope will be discussed. Those conditions where postural muscle tone is lost, but conscious level unaffected, will be mentioned at the end of the chapter.

Table 12.1 Causes of recurrent "falling" due to loss of postural muscle tone

| | CONSCIOUSNESS | |
MAIN AGE GROUP	Impaired	Preserved
Under 40 years of age	Vasovagal syncope Vertebrobasilar migraine Hyperventilation syndrome Pregnancy ("Supine Hypotensive" syndrome)	Hysteria/malingering (pseudoseizures) Cataplexy Myotonia—Familial Periodic Paralysis Myasthenia gravis
Over 50 years of age	Micturition syncope Cough syncope Carotid sinus syncope Stokes–Adams attacks or other cardiac disease	Vertebrobasilar insufficiency ("drop attacks") Normal pressure hydrocephalus
Any age	Epilepsy Orthostatic hypotension Aortic stenosis, patent ductus arteriosus, pulmonary hypertension, "subclavian steal" syndrome	Symptomatic cataplexy

12.2 EPILEPSY

Hughlings Jackson described an *epileptic fit* as *"an occasional, an excessive and a disorderly discharge of nerve tissue"* (quoted in Marsden, 1976b), but it should be emphasised that whereas about 5% of the general population will have one such fit during their life, less than 1% will have recurrent fits, and the term epilepsy should only be applied to the latter group (Marsden, 1976b). Therefore a person who has had a single fit does not automatically require anticonvulsant treatment, but evidence indicating that he is predisposed to further attacks should be sought.

The International league against Epilepsy have proposed a classification of the epilepsies (Gastaut, 1969). The two main categories in this system are Partial seizures (which are focal in origin) and Generalised seizures (which are generalised in origin). In this section the following generalised seizures will be referred to:

> Absences (petit mal)
> Myoclonic
> Tonic and/or clonic
> Atonic
> Akinetic

Partial seizures are divided into simple or complex (in which there is an associated impairment of consciousness). Simple partial seizures may involve motor, sensory and/or autonomic phenomena, but *consciousness remains intact*.

Complex partial seizures are, in effect, what has been referred to in the past, as temporal lobe epilepsy, involving a variety of behaviour and experiences, e.g. hallucinations, illusions, etc., which are listed in more detail in Table 16.1.

Epilepsy is a common cause of recurrent falling. *The commonest type of epileptic seizure associated with falling is the grand mal (tonic/clonic) seizure.* Less common are "atonic", "akinetic", petit mal variant and, occasionally, petit mal epilepsy. If there is a focal site of discharge in the brain, the falling may be preceded by symptoms or signs (the aura) which will depend on the area of brain involved, and may be sensory (e.g. paraesthesia), motor (e.g. clonic movements), autonomic (e.g. salivation), or complex (associated with impaired consciousness). The aura usually lasts for less than a minute, has an intrusive quality, and may be forgotten after the seizure, due to a retrograde amnesia.

When the seizure generalises it becomes grand mal in type and the clinical features are the same at this stage, irrespective of whether it was generalised or focal in origin. Typically the muscles of the body go into tonic spasm, the patient falls and then there are clonic jerking movements of the whole body. The jerking gradually slows in frequency until the patient enters the post-ictal state of drowsiness, confusion, and headache. The motor component involves the muscles of the body symmetrically, lasts under 2 minutes, and tends to cause tongue biting and urinary incontinence.

The *"atonic" seizure* involves a sudden and complete loss of consciousness and muscle tone, and there are no convulsive movements. In the *"akinetic" seizure*, posture is maintained and consciousness less severely impaired, but the patient is unable to move. The people affected by these disorders can be divided into two groups, children and adults. In children the seizure usually occurs as a febrile event and has a good prognosis. In adults it is the result of focal brain disease, usually involving the frontal lobes, and is associated with grand mal seizures (Gastaut *et al.*, 1974). A third group of patients with such seizures starting in late life, but with no evidence of OBD, may be present (Fisher, 1979). A trial of anticonvulsants has been recommended by Fisher for those cases of loss of consciousness of uncertain origin, which do not appear to be the result of vasovagal or orthostatic hypotensive attacks, even if the EEG is normal.

A *petit mal seizure* involves a transient loss of consciousness sometimes with a reduction of muscle tone. The latter involves the legs and is usually insufficient to cause falling. In the typical petit mal attack the loss of consciousness has an acute onset and cessation, lasts a matter of seconds, and is usually only manifest as a brief "absence", followed by immediate recovery without falling. There is no confusion after, in contrast to TLE, which can produce "absence-like" episodes, which clincally resemble petit mal. The patient is often unaware that he has had an attack. A characteristic EEG pattern of 3 c/s spike and wave activity, is seen, and this EEG abnormality is inherited as an autosomal dominant disorder (Metrakos and Metrakos, 1961). Clinical petit mal stops before adulthood is reached, in 80% of cases. The presence of grand mal seizures is

Table 12.2   Differential diagnosis of recurrent "falling"

PRECEDING EVENT

Exercise	Yes →	Orthostatic hypotension, aortic stenosis, "subclavian steal" syndrome, patent ductus arteriosus, pulmonary hypertension
No ↓		
Emotional Stress	Yes →	Vasovagal syncope, cataplexy, hyperventilation syndrome, hysteria/malingering
No ↓		
Neck Movement	Yes →	Vertebrobasilar ischaemia, "carotid sinus" syncope
No ↓		
Coughing, micturition, defaecation, eating, swallowing	Yes →	Reflex syncope
No ↓		
Following rising from bed	Yes →	Ostostatic hypotension, "micturition" syncope

CLINICAL FEATURES

No loss of consciousness (LOC)	Yes →	Hysteria/malingering, vertebrobasilar insufficiency, cataplexy, myotonia—familial periodic paralysis, myasthenia gravis, NPH
No ↓		
Acute LOC while sitting/lying	Yes →	Epilepsy, cardiac disease
No ↓		
Gradual LOC while sitting/lying	Yes →	Migraine, pregnancy, reflex syncope

a poor prognostic sign and is seen in 45% of cases of petit mal, of whom a third will continue to have seizures in adulthood (Marsden, 1976b).

Petit mal variant or the *Lennox–Gastaut syndrome*, involves petit mal-like attacks, but with a more gradual onset and cessation, and a briefer duration of about 5 seconds. The EEG is abnormal, but does not show 3 c/s spike and wave activity. The disorder is usually associated with significant organic brain disease. The attacks may be accompanied by myoclonus and akinetic seizures, the combination being called the Petit Mal Triad.

Unusual epileptic seizures may be seen which involve laughing (gelastic), running (cursive) or autonomic phenomena (diencephalic epilepsy). The presence of focal neurological signs, e.g. dysphasia, as an aura or post-ictally (Todd's paralysis), is important and indicates the presence of a focal cerebral lesion, and may help to identify its site in the brain.

12.3 PSEUDOSEIZURES

A pseudoseizure is any experience or behaviour that mimics an epileptic seizure, but is not the result of an abnormal discharge of cerebral neurones. The term is usually applied to pseudoseizures that are the result of psychological factors, involving dissociation and/or malingering. This is the way the term will be used in this section. *Pseudoseizures commonly occur in patients who are also subject to true seizures.* In one series, 20% of patients with "intractable seizures" were found to have *both* true seizures and pseudoseizures (Ramani *et al.*, 1980). Moreover, emotional stress, which is a frequent precipitant of pseudoseizures, can also commonly precede true seizures and was found to be present in 21% of Currie *et al.*'s (1971) series of 666 patients with TLE. It may be very difficult to disentangle the contributions of each type of attack to the overall clinical picture, in such cases, and specialist techniques, particularly videotelemetry, are often helpful.

Table 12.3 shows the features in the patients' history and on examination which tend to be associated with pseudoseizures. Their presence or absence in any particular patient will vary, because the pseudoseizure is not a diagnosis in itself, but a sign found in association with many different neuropsychiatric disorders. The psychopathology in these patients varies along a continuum of severity. At the mild end of this continuum there is the patient who has relatively minor psychopathology and presents with a history of a recent onset of pseudoseizures, usually following some major psychological precipitant(s). In these patients the pseudoseizure represents a true hysterical conversion phenomenon. They have a good prognosis and often respond to measures such as reassurance and an explanation of the cause of their attacks. Other interventions are made where appropriate, according to the patient's problems (Guberman, 1982).

At the other extreme is the patient who has a gross disturbance of his personality and a history of multiple previous psychiatric admissions. This type of patient may show the features of Briquet's hysteria, with a history of multiple physical and psychiatric illnesses, involving repeated hospitalisations. Patients with severe disturbances of personality and pseudoseizures, often have a long history of attacks, which may even exceed 20 years duration, and clear psychological precipitants for their pseudoseizures are often not found. They respond poorly to explanation and reassurance, are non-compliant with psychiatric treatment and will often attempt to obtain anticonvulsants from other doctors after discharge.

Table 12.3 **Important factors in the history and on examination of the patient with pseudoseizures**

Family history of psychiatric disorder.
No previous history of neurological trauma (birth complications, head injury, febrile convulsions, encephalitis or meningitis).
Previous history of psychiatric illness (including suicide attempts).
Previous history of unexplained neurological deficits.
Previous history suggestive of sexual maladjustment.
Hysterical or passive–immature–dependent personality type.
Attacks preceded by psychological factors.
Audience usually present during attacks.
Failure of attacks to respond to adequate anticonvulsant treatment.
Current affective illness.

A family history of epilepsy may be found in association with pure pseudoseizures (Guberman, 1982), and this may indicate that the patient has been influenced as a result of observing seizures in relatives or, alternatively, that he has actually had true seizures in the past.

Table 12.3 emphasises the significance of previous and current psychiatric problems in relation to pseudoseizures, but it must be remembered that there is evidence that patients with temporal lobe epilepsy have a raised psychiatric morbidity (Shaffer, 1973), though not all studies support this association (Currie *et al.*, 1971).

Table 12.4 shows the clinical signs associated with pseudoseizures, compared to those found in epileptic seizures. This table refers to true grand mal seizures, and pseudoseizures *with* a motor component. Particular attention should be paid to the characteristics of any observable motor activity as pseudoseizures involving a motor component (in contrast to just psychic phenomena) are easier to differentiate from true seizures (Gulick *et al.*, 1982; King *et al.*, 1982). Pseudoseizures are often found in patients in whom they are not suspected and the motor component may be remarkably similar in appearance to that seen in epileptic seizures, e.g. there may be licking of the lips, rapid blinking of the eyelids, chewing movements, or focal motor disturbances. The patient may also complain of unusual focal sensory symptoms.

A true seizure has an acute onset. If an aura is present, it only lasts a minute or two, though it may be preceded by vague premonitory feelings. Some patients experience alterations of mood, with a build-up of tension and irritability for several days beforehand. The seizure may be beneficial, in such cases, by relieving this dysphoric mood. Motor activity in pseudoseizures usually does not have the quality of that seen in grand mal seizures, nor the stereotyped sequence of events that can be understood as the logical behavioural consequence of a spreading epileptic discharge in a particular area of the brain.

A brief cry, due to expiration through the larynx in spasm, may herald the onset of the true seizure, but persistent moaning and crying, and

Table 12.4 Features differentiating between true seizures and pseudoseizures

	PSEUDOSEIZURE	TRUE GRAND MAL SEIZURE
SEIZURE ONSET		
	Gradual	*Sudden
Aura duration	Over 5 mins.	Under 5 mins.
Cyanosis	—	+
Motor activity	Intermittent with "rest spells"	Orderly sequence
	Trembling, thrashing, opisthotonus, coordinated movements may be seen	Tonic and/or clonic phases
Vocalisation	May moan and scream	Brief cry at onset only
Breathing	May hyperventilate	Initial arrest of breathing
DURING SEIZURE		
Loss of consciousness	—	* +
Self-injury	—	+
Tongue biting	—	+
Urinary incontinence	—	+
Abnormal EEG	—	* +
FOLLOWING SEIZURE		
Confusion	—	* +
Dilated, unresponsive pupils	—	* +
Extensor plantar responses	—	* +
Abnormal EEG	—	* +
Serum prolactin	Normal	*Elevated
Henry and Woodruff's sign	May be present	—

+ Usually present.
— Usually absent.
*Invariably present.

other evidence of distress, are unusual during a true seizure. Respiratory arrest during the tonic phase of the seizure and post-ictal stertorous breathing may be seen, but hyperventilation or other abnormalities of respiration, are not usual. However, it should be remembered that hyperventilation, for whatever reason, may precipitate a seizure discharge in predisposed patients.

In pseudoseizures the movements tend to involve flailing, tremulousness, are sometimes purposeful, and may involve behaviour that is complex, coordinated and purposeful, e.g. a deliberate attack on another person. The movements may be episodic with periods of relaxation in between. These features are not seen in true seizures, where cerebral dysfunction prevents coordinated, goal-directed behaviour. In status epilepticus, repeated seizures may occur, but the same tendency to an orderly progression of clinical features is seen during each seizure and the patient rapidly becomes exhausted and in obvious distress. Occasionally repeated pseudoseizures may convincingly mimic status epilepticus (Guberman, 1982; Toone and Roberts, 1979).

Though pseudoseizures are often unusual in quality, Gulick *et al.* (1982) found that they can be associated with subsequent amnesia for the events of the attack, though recall may be produced by hypnosis (Peterson *et al.*, 1950). It is commonly thought that pseudoseizures are not associated with self-injury, but this is not always true, and in cases where a severe disturbance of personality is present, self-injury may be severe, e.g. in one case of confirmed pseudoseizures, the patient would repeatedly fall face down to the ground, with no attempt to protect himself from injury (Toone and Roberts, 1979).

A grand mal convulsion is incompatible with preservation of consciousness. A meaningful interaction with the patient during a generalised motor seizure, with his responding appropriately to commands such as "elevate your right hand", is incompatible with a true epileptic seizure. However, during the stage of post-ictal confusion the patient will gradually regain contact with his surroundings and be capable of simple but increasingly appropriate interaction with others, as his confusion gradually subsides.

Following a grand mal seizure, confusion, extensor plantar responses and dilated unreactive pupils are the rule. Urinary incontinence and tongue biting often occur during the seizure. The plantar responses and unreactive pupils are not seen in pseudoseizures, though it is possible that malingering patients with some medical knowledge may instill mydriatic drops, such as atropine, in their eyes. The absence of confusion immediately following a grand mal convulsion is unusual. However, if the seizure merges into a state of sleep, confusion may not be present on waking. Patients with pseudoseizures may complain of confusion, but, on careful questioning, the nature of the confusion will usually be found to differ from that found post-ictally.

A useful sign, that will be referred to as *Henry and Woodruff's sign*, will now be described. If following a "seizure" the patient remains immobile and apparently unresponsive, he should be turned onto his side. If his eyes then deviate conjugately towards the ground, he should be turned on his other side. If his eyes deviate towards the ground again, then it indicates that he is feigning unresponsiveness (Henry and Woodruff, 1978). In true seizures, if there is conjugate deviation of the eyes to one side, the side will remain constant irrespective of the patient's position.

Trimble (1978) demonstrated in a series of nine patients that *a true generalised seizure was associated with an elevation of the serum prolactin* to over 1000 μU/ml (normal range: 240–650 μU/ml), in all but one case. The prolactin was at its maximum level about 15 to 25 minutes post-ictally. This is believed to be due to the neuronal discharge spreading to involve the hypothalamus, and so causing a release of prolactin. Trimble did not find this elevation of prolactin following pseudoseizures, nor after some cases of temporal lobe seizures. Presumably this elevation is not seen in some focal seizure discharges, because they remain relatively localised to one area of the brain.

The increase in prolactin is unlikely to be due to muscle activity or cerebral anoxia, because it is seen following ECT, which involves the use of muscle relaxants, anaesthesia and oxygen. It is necessary to obtain a baseline level of prolactin before or after the attack, as a substantial elevation can be caused by other factors, such as the use of psychotropic drugs. This value of prolactin as a means of differentiating true seizures from pseudoseizures, has since been confirmed by Collins *et al.* (1983).

A grand mal seizure is incompatible with a normal EEG recording taken at the same time. However, when a seizure occurs the recording may be difficult to interpret, due to patient movement and muscle artefact. Obviously this procedure requires that there be an attack while the EEG is being recorded. Often this does not occur, especially if the patient's seizure rate prior to admission was less than one per week (King *et al.*, 1982). In such cases some form of provocation can be used to provoke pseudoseizures, in suggestible patients. Guberman (1982) used the method of placing a tuning fork on the patient's head, preferably in front of an audience, after explaining to him that the vibration was going to induce a seizure. The subsequent attack should then be evaluated as to what degree it resembles the patient's usual "seizure". If it is the same and all the attacks are of this one kind, then it is reasonable to conclude that they are all pseudoseizures.

It is important to correctly diagnose pseudoseizures because the psychological and other factors predisposing the patient to this disorder, require identification and treatment. The use of anticonvulsants in patients without epilepsy not only puts the patient at risk of developing side effects, but may also cause iatrogenic seizures, as such patients often take their drugs erratically and put themselves at risk of withdrawal seizures. This risk is made worse if they also abuse alcohol, minor tranquillisers or barbiturates. Pseudoseizures will not respond properly to anticonvulsant drug treatment, and this may lead to the use of increasing doses and, possibly, combinations of two or more anticonvulsants. Some transient symptomatic improvement may occur initially though, for reasons such as placebo effect and the beneficial effects these drugs may have on mood (Reynolds, 1983).

Other consequences of incorrectly labelling a patient epileptic include restrictions on his driving and obtaining certain types of employment, social ostracism and loss of self-esteem; any or all of which may cause psychological disturbance and so add on to the pre-existing psychological problems.

12.4 THE HYSTERICAL "FAINT"

Stressful circumstances may cause a hysterical "faint". In this the patient, typically, falls gracefully to the ground. This is usually found in young female patients. In its uncomplicated form it is less commonly seen nowadays, though it was a more socially acceptable form of behaviour in the past. During such attacks self-injury is uncommon, there is a dramatic quality to the fall, and it only occurs in the presence of others. More importantly, there is clinically no change in skin colour, no bradycardia, and no hypotension. There may be unusual movements and postures, in which case the clinical picture may resemble a pseudoseizure. If the patient remains supine and unresponsive, examination will reveal normal pupillary responses to light, and flexor plantar responses. Other behaviour such as blepharospasm, with resistance to eye opening, and Henry and Woodruff's sign, may be present. The EEG should be normal during and after the attack.

Hysterical "fainting" is a prominent feature in several recorded outbreaks of epidemic hysteria (Merskey, 1979). In view of this, enquiry should be made, particularly in younger patients, if anyone else at their school or place of work is similarly afflicted. Such a history may indicate an infective cause for the illness, but a hysterical cause should be considered, particularly if suggestive features, such as hyperventilation or a dramatic quality to the "faint", are present.

12.5 SYNCOPE

The term *syncope refers to a transient loss of consciousness due to the temporary failure of the cerebral circulation* (Bannister, 1973), usually occurring while the patient is standing. The normal cerebral blood flow is about 50 ml/100 g/min., and if this falls below 30 ml/100 g/min., symptoms of cerebral hypoxia will develop. Syncope can be caused by orthostatic hypotension, when there is a failure of the physiological mechanisms that maintain the level of the blood pressure when posture is changed, or as the result of a vasovagal attack, anaemia, cardiac disease, vascular disease, cerebrovascular disease or the valsalva manoeuvre. In many cases two or more causes may be interacting.

Clinically syncope has a gradual onset, with nausea, weakness, dizziness, tinnitus, yawning, blurred vision, epigastric discomfort and sweating. Pallor and hyperpnoea are usually seen. Bradycardia, pupillary dilatation and hypotension, are found on examination. Some muscle twitching and, occasionally, two or three tonic–clonic movements and urinary incontinence, may occur, but a true grand mal convulsion is rare. After falling, recovery is rapid, occurring in less than a minute, but it may be followed by some generalised weakness, nausea, headache, nervousness and minimal confusion. Reflex flushing will be seen and bradycardia may remain for a short while. An EEG carried out during unconsciousness will show high voltage delta activity, which rapidly becomes normal after recovery (Heyman, 1971).

The crucial features of syncope which help to differentiate it from epilepsy, are the erect posture of the patient at the onset, the mode of onset and cessation, the pallor, bradycardia and hypotension, and the rapid recovery without significant confusion, when the patient is horizontal.

Reflex syncope is produced by the valsalva manoeuvre (forced expiration against a closed glottis). This decreases the cerebral blood flow, either by raising the cerebrospinal fluid pressure and thus "squeezing" the blood out of the brain;

by decreasing venous return to the heart and thus reducing cardiac output; by stimulating the baroreceptors causing a reflex fall in the blood pressure; or by a combination of these. This technique is sometimes used by schoolboys to produce fainting and may also be used by malingerers. A similar mechanism is probably operating in patients with chronic respiratory disorders who lose consciousness while coughing (cough syncope), and in patients who get out of a bed at night and faint while passing urine (micturition syncope). In the latter, there may also be a contribution from reflex peripheral vasodilation, resulting from deflation of the bladder. In some cases, syncope may occur simply on arising from the bed at night, and may be due to the baroreceptors becoming "hyporeactive" during sleep. This mechanism may play a role in causing syncope when the patient gets out of bed in the morning (Fisher, 1979). These mechanisms probably contribute to the development of vasovagal syncope.

Vasovagal syncope (vasodepressor syncope or the "common faint") is commonly seen in the young and is due to widespread vascular dilatation in the limbs, causing hypotension, without a compensatory increase in heart rate that is adequate to maintain cerebral perfusion. The resulting cerebral ischaemia can cause loss of consciousness if the patient is standing. This is usually precipitated by pain or some other emotional shock, such as fear.

Occasionally, vasovagal syncope is found in association with abdominal pain, eating ("prandial" syncope) or defaecation (Fisher, 1979). Dilatation of the upper gastrointestinal tract, pleura or bronchi, can cause reflex cardiac arrest, due to stimulation of the vagus, causing bradycardia, and resulting in a transient loss of consciousness, or death.

Orthostatic hypotension occurs when there is an excessive drop in blood pressure when the patient stands. This is particularly likely to occur in psychiatric patients who are receiving drug treatment with the phenothiazines, barbiturates, monoamine oxidase inhibitors or tricyclic antidepressants. Other predisposing factors include hypoadrenalism (Addison's disease), hypovolaemia, sodium or potassium deficiency, physical debility, or an autonomic neuropathy. The latter may be found in many disorders, notably in chronic alcoholism, parkinsonism, diabetes mellitus and, rarely, tabes dorsalis. Parkinsonism may also cause falling because of the shuffling gait and postural instability found in this disorder.

Postural hypotension is often most marked on arising in the morning and it may be facilitated by the ingestion of alcohol the previous evening. Sudden episodes of hypotension can also be caused by ingestion of small quantities of alcohol, especially when taken on an empty stomach (Fisher, 1979).

Autonomic neuropathy may be indicated by the patient's history or the findings on physical examination. The features will vary depending on whether the sympathetic or the parasympathetic parts of the autonomic nervous system, are predominantly involved. Sympathetic failure can cause orthostatic hypotension, urinary urgency, and failure of ejaculation. On physical examination, the pupils may fail to dilate on painful stimulation to the back of the neck (ciliospinal reflex). Bradycardia and a marked fall in the blood pressure on standing, without a compensatory increase in the pulse rate, will be seen. Parasympathetic failure can cause a dry mouth, dry eyes, heat intolerance with anhidrosis, constipation, retention of urine and impotence. On examination, the pupils may fail to constrict in response to light, and the heart rate may fail to change with posture. The latter was suggested as a test for autonomic neuropathy by Ewing *et al.* (1978), who found that there is a rapid increase in the heart rate in the first 10 to 15 seconds following standing up from the lying down position, in normal controls. In diabetics with autonomic neuropathy, there was little alteration in the pulse rate following this change in posture. For references to more sophisticated tests of autonomic nervous system function, the reader is referred to Ewing *et al.* (1978) and Khurana *et al.* (1980).

Orthostatic hypotension is seen in the Shy–Drager syndrome, an uncommon disorder occurring in middle-aged men. It involves degeneration in multiple neurological systems, including progressive autonomic failure (primarily involving the parasympathetic nervous system), and parkinsonism (Shy and Drager, 1960). There are other uncommon disorders of the autonomic nervous system, which can cause orthostatic hypotension, but they are relatively unassociated with involvement of the parasympathetic nervous system or other system in the body (Demanet, 1976; Kontos *et al.*, 1975).

Cardiac disease may cause syncope, and any alteration in cardiac rhythm producing an excessively rapid or an excessively slow heart rate, may compromise cerebral perfusion. If cerebrovascular disease is present, a relatively mild reduction in heart rate, such as may be produced by a beta blocker drug, may reduce the cerebral circulation to a profound degree.

Cardiac dysrhythmias can cause altered consciousness, dementia, automatic behaviour, syncope and episodes resembling TIA's. The diagnosis should be suspected if the patient is found to have an unexplained tachycardia, an irregular pulse, or a bradycardia (less than 50 beats/minute). A family history may be present. However, prolonged ECG monitoring may be necessary, and even then arrhythmias are not uncommon on monitoring asymptomatic individuals, and so all the clinical data and results must be evaluated, before coming to any firm conclusions (Schott *et al.*, 1977). In some cases it is necessary to use an artificial cardiac pacemaker for a trial period (Fisher, 1979).

Syncopal attacks are particularly characteristic of complete heart block (Stokes-Adams attacks). In this condition the heart rate is about 40 beats/minute. Loss of consciousness is abrupt and unassociated with any particular activity or posture. The syncope is due to an abrupt change in heart rate and if it is short lived, recovery without confusion occurs. In one series of 100 cases, 41% experienced the symptoms of cerebral ischaemia, without loss of consciousness (Fisher, 1979).

If *cerebrovascular disease* is suspected, focal neurological signs and symptoms should be enquired for. However, *focal cerebral ischaemia is rarely the cause of recurrent loss of consciousness* (Hachinski, 1981). Attacks of transient ischaemia (TIA) of the brain may last a few minutes or several hours, and diagnostic errors are more likely with the brief episodes.

If ischaemia involves the area of the brain perfused by the vertebrobasilar vessels, certain neurological phenomena will usually, though not always, be present. They include vertigo, tinnitus, dysphagia, dysphonia, diplopia, ataxia, dysarthria, blurred vision, scintillation scotomata, homonymous hemianopia, and lateralised sensory or motor signs. In the older patient this may be due to the vertebrobasilar arteries being compressed by osteophytes, when the neck is turned or extended. It is uncommon for "drop attacks" due to vertebrobasilar insufficiency, to result in loss of consciousness (Hachinski, 1981). In adolescent girls such phenomena may be seen at the onset of an attack of *vertebrobasilar migraine*. This condition involves a gradual loss of consciousness, resembling sleep. It is followed by a severe headache.

Ischaemia involving the internal carotid artery and its branches usually results in weakness or sensory abnormality (paraesthesia) on the contralateral side of the body, dysphasia, contralateral hemianopia or ipsilateral visual impairment, which may be total.

Other cardiovascular causes include aortic stenosis, which is characterised by exertional dyspnoea and angina pectoris; syncope on exercise occurs in 10% of cases (Heyman, 1971). A characteristic "plateau" pulse, an aortic systolic ejection murmur and a low pulse pressure, should be looked for during the examination. Syncope may also be seen with pulmonary hypertension and patent ductus arteriosus.

Other uncommon causes of fainting may be found. In the elderly, it may result from pressure on a *hypersensitive carotid sinus*, due to a tight collar or turning the head. Cautious massage of each carotid sinus in turn, while monitoring the patient's ECG, may demonstrate the sensitivity. The *"Subclavian Steal"* syndrome is a rare cause and may cause falling without loss of consciousness. It results from a stenosis of the subclavian artery, proximal to the origin of the vertebral artery. Exercise of the arm on the side of the stenosis causes vasodilation and a reversal of the blood flow down the vertebral artery in order to supply the muscles of the arm, at the cost of vertebrobasilar ischaemia and ischaemia of the arm (Toole, 1964). A lower blood pressure and diminished pulse in the affected arm and an audible bruit heard over the area of the stenosis (supra- or infraclavicular fossa) should be looked for.

Overbreathing may reduce cerebral blood flow substantially and is particularly effective at facilitating valsalva-induced syncope. Hyperventilation can cause a variety of symptoms, such as depersonalisation and dizziness, but loss of consciousness is uncommon.

When the pregnant woman is in the supine position, especially during the second trimester, the uterus compresses the vena cava and decreases venous return to the heart. This causes a reduced cardiac output and can result in marked arterial hypotension and fainting, which can be stopped by adopting the prone posture. This is called the *"Supine Hypotensive" syndrome* (Pritchard and ·MacDonald, 1980).

12.7 "FALLING" WITH PRESERVED CONSCIOUSNESS

This category does not include persistent weakness, but refers to transient and recurrent episodes of muscles weakness involving the legs. It is often due to *hysteria and/or malingering* in the young. Such cases should be approached in a similar way to pseudoseizures, with full assessment of the past history and current mental state, looking closely at the circumstances surrounding the episodes, and their clinical features.

Transient ischaemic attacks involving the distribution of the vertebrobasilar artery may cause "drop attacks" in the elderly and they usually do not involve loss of consciousness. Recovery of muscle tone is almost immediate following the fall. A history of the neurological features of vertebrobasilar insufficiency should be enquired for, though it is not always present. 30% of patients with TIA's develop strokes within 5 years. Those patients whose TIA's are increasing in frequency are particularly at risk of developing a CVA and should be regarded as a medical emergency (McCormick, 1983). Compression due to cervical osteophytes or the "Subclavian Steal" syndrome may account for some of these cases (Botez, 1982).

Cataplexy involves loss of muscle tone and may be either focal, e.g. the jaw dropping open, or generalised, resulting in falling. It is precipitated by emotion, surprise or sudden muscular exertion. The attacks last under 2 minutes and are followed by full recovery. This condition is found in 70% of patients with the Narcoleptic syndrome (sleep attacks, hypnagogic hallucinations, sleep paralysis). The sleep attacks will usually dominate the clinical picture and precede the development of the cataplexy.

Symptomatic cataplexy has been described in association with tumours of the brain, especially in the frontal lobe region, and as a post-encephalitic phenomenon. Other lesions in this region and in the area of the third and fourth ventricle may cause it. If there is an accompanying transient increase in intracranial pressure, the fall may be accompanied by a severe headache. A transient loss of consciousness may occur in some cases (Botez, 1982).

A disturbance of gait, which can involve falling, can be an important early sign of *normal pressure hydrocephalus* (Botez *et al.*, 1977). Fisher (1982c) found that 34% of 50 elderly patients with this combination, responded to a reduction in cerebrospinal fluid pressure.

Falling may occur in *myotonia*, which involves a failure of muscle relaxation (myotonia dystrophica, myotonia congenita, or paramyotonia congenita), or as a result of transient alteration (an increase or decrease) in the serum potassium (*familial periodic paralysis*). Any of these disorders may be precipitated as an acute episode, by emotion or cold temperatures. They are all dominantly inherited and so a family history should be enquired for. In myotonia the failure of muscle relaxation may be evident on shaking hands with the patient, who will have difficulty in relaxing his grip, and may also show the other features of frontal baldness, cataracts and a characteristic facial appearance. Patients with *myasthenia gravis* may occasionally develop acute weakness of the legs after exertion, but ptosis, diplopia, dysarthria, and difficulty chewing, are more common symptoms. A response to intravenous edrophonium chloride within 2 minutes should confirm the diagnosis (Wolf, 1980). A placebo injection can be used to help to rule out a psychogenic cause.

Cataplexy, the myotonias, familial periodic paralysis and myasthenia gravis all usually present before the age of 30 years, though exceptions occur.

CHAPTER 13

Altered States of Consciousness

13.1 INTRODUCTION

This section deals with the diagnosis in those patients who have experienced one or more episodes of altered consciousness during which they have experienced some degree of loss of contact with their surroundings. Those disorders commonly associated with "falling" due to a loss of postural muscle tone have been discussed in the preceding chapter. Pathological altered consciousness may be the results of cerebral dysfunction (delirium); of a period of subclinical sleep (hypersomnia); of normal awareness being altered by intense emotion (episodic dyscontrol, phobic anxiety); or it may be due to a "narrowing" of consciousness (psychogenic fugue). In some cases this may be an incidental finding in patients being evaluated for other reasons, but the patient will usually complain about these episodes, because of his concern over what has caused them and what he might have done during the periods for which he is amnesic.

A full history is necessary, paying particular attention to the events immediately preceding the attack, the setting in which it took place, the time of day, duration, the quality of its onset and cessation (acute or gradual), and how the patient felt after (relieved, alert, confused, focal neurological deficit). If consciousness is not totally lost how did the patient feel during the attack (dreamy, frightened)? Did he have any abnormal experiences (hallucinations, illusions)? Those features that are repeated, in different attacks, should be looked for.

The diagnosis will be made more easily if there is an informant available who can provide an objective account of the patient's behaviour before, during and after his attack(s). Particular attention should be paid to any motor behaviour exhibited during the attack. This may involve involuntary facial movements (TLE, amphetamines or other stimulant drugs); aggressive behaviour (post-ictal, inter-ictal, pathological or simple intoxication with alcohol, paradoxical rage reaction, episodic dyscontrol); "escape" behaviour (phobic anxiety, psychogenic fugue); and the degree to which the behaviour is coordinated, complex and purposeful (suggesting relatively intact higher cortical functions), in contrast

220

to the random, purposeless behaviour, seen in the patient with an organic disturbance of brain function.

Where objective information about the patient's behaviour is unavailable, his subjective experiences during the attack assume particular importance. He may experience only a "blank" period for which he has no memory (epilepsy); unusual subjective experiences, such as hallucinations or illusions, which may involve the primary senses, the body image or memories (TLE, phobic anxiety); the experience of fear and/or autonomic symptoms, such as palpitations, shortness of breath or "butterfly-like" epigastric sensations (TLE, phobic anxiety, hyperventilation); feelings of anger and tension (episodic dyscontrol); the need to get away from his surroundings (psychogenic fugue); or the intense experience of being unable to initiate any appropriate behaviour (obsessional indecision).

Table 13.1 lists most of the important causes of altered consciousness, and some of these disorders are particularly associated with certain age groups, such as childhood (petit mal, the parasomnias, delirium), 10 to 30 years of age (hysterical dissociation, hyperventilation, phobic anxiety, depersonalisation, psychotomimetic drugs, narcolepsy, Kleine–Levin syndrome), and over 40 years (transient global amnesia, cerebrovascular disease, delirium).

Table 13.1 Causes of altered states of consciousness

Alcohol	Simple intoxication, idiosyncratic intoxication, hypolycaemia, withdrawal convulsions, delirium tremens
Blood vessel disease	Transient global amnesia, transient ischaemic attack, vertebrobasilar migraine
Drugs	Minor tranquillisers (paradoxical rage reaction), psychotomimetic, psychotropic drugs, clioquinol, digitalis, etc.
Metabolic	Hypoglycaemia, hypocapnia
Epilepsy	Ictal (petit mal status, temporal lobe status), post-ictal, twilight or fugue states
Functional	Episodic dyscontrol, hysterical/malingering/depressive fugue states, phobic anxiety, depersonalisation/ derealisation, hyperventilation
Vestibulocerebellar	Menière's disease, etc.
Sleep disorders	Narcolepsy, the hypersomnias, the parasomnias
Catatonic syndrome	
Causes of delirium	

Table 13.2 demonstrates a number of questions that will help in clarifying the cause(s) of the altered consciousness. Coordinated goal-directed behaviour indicates that the patient's higher cortical functions are relatively intact. This makes an organic impairment of consciousness unlikely. However, automatic behaviour of a limited level of complexity can occur in organic disorders, and other features of the attack should be taken into account before coming to any conclusions about its nature. When the patient has had several attacks of varying severity it is preferable to get an account of the most severe and most recent

222

Table 13.2 Differential diagnosis of altered consciousness

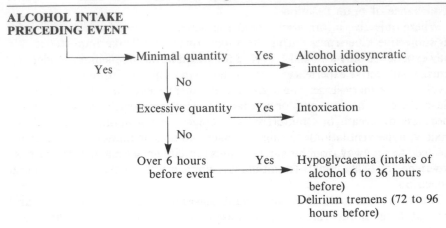

ALCOHOL INTAKE PRECEDING EVENT

Minimal quantity — Yes → Alcohol idiosyncratic intoxication

No

Excessive quantity — Yes → Intoxication

No

Over 6 hours before event — Yes → Hypoglycaemia (intake of alcohol 6 to 36 hours before)
Delirium tremens (72 to 96 hours before)

CLINICAL FEATURES

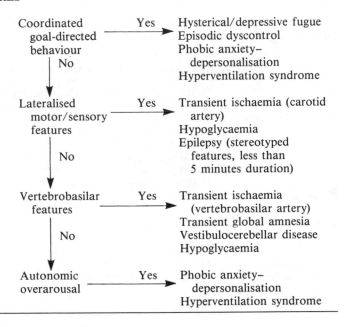

Coordinated goal-directed behaviour — Yes → Hysterical/depressive fugue
Episodic dyscontrol
Phobic anxiety–depersonalisation
Hyperventilation syndrome

No

Lateralised motor/sensory features — Yes → Transient ischaemia (carotid artery)
Hypoglycaemia
Epilepsy (stereotyped features, less than 5 minutes duration)

No

Vertebrobasilar features — Yes → Transient ischaemia (vertebrobasilar artery)
Transient global amnesia
Vestibulocerebellar disease
Hypoglycaemia

No

Autonomic overarousal — Yes → Phobic anxiety–depersonalisation
Hyperventilation syndrome

ones as they will be most clearly remembered, are more likely to involve features of diagnostic significance, and are more likely to be remembered by other observers, who may be able to provide further valuable details.

If the patient exhibits features that include aggressive behaviour (Chapter 8), delirium (Chapter 9), falling attacks (Chapter 12), catatonic phenomena (Chapter 14), or hypersomnia (Chapter 15), then further discussion will be found in the appropriate chapters in this book.

13.2 EPILEPSY

Epilepsy can cause recurrent episodes of altered consciousness, without necessarily involving loss of postural muscle tone, and enquiry should be made for a family history or a previous personal history, suggestive of epilepsy (including febrile convulsions) or any other neurological disorder. It is particularly helpful if the patient has "hard" evidence for epilepsy, e.g. a history of a well documented grand mal convulsion, especially if this is temporally associated with one of his episodes of altered consciousness.

A common cause of diagnostic confusion is the epileptic automatism, and Table 13.3 shows some of its features. Fenton (1972) has defined an *epileptic automatism* as *"a state of clouding of consciousness which occurs during or immediately after a seizure and during which the individual retains control of posture and muscle tone, but performs simple or complex movements without being aware of what is happening"*. Automatic behaviour has been divided into three stages, and loss of contact with the surroundings is most profound in the first stage, which involves an arrest of behaviour, often with staring, an alteration in body posture and facial pallor; in the second stage there are repetitive movements, such as lip smacking, chewing, or fumbling movements of the arms, possibly with the production of muttering or mumbling sounds; and in the final stage motor activity gradually becomes more integrated with events going on around the patient and involves behaviour, such as wandering or more coherent (but not entirely appropriate) speech.

All the three stages need not be present. The first two are a result of ongoing epileptic activity (ictal), i.e. they are directly caused by an abnormal neuronal discharge in the brain, in the same way that the tonic–clonic movements of a grand mal seizure are. Because focal neuronal discharges tend to follow certain specific pathways, these two stages are relatively stereotyped from one attack to the next, and they usually originate in the temporo-limbic structures.

The third stage occurs in the period following the seizure discharge and may or may not be preceded by the first two stages. The seizures may be focal (usually temporo-limbic) or generalised in origin, and the automatism is probably the result of post-ictal inactivity in neurones which are transiently refractory to any further nervous transmission, as a result of being involved in the preceding seizure. This third stage (or post-ictal automatism) is therefore liable to vary in quality from one episode to another, and is liable to be influenced by environmental events. Post-ictal aggression is particularly a problem in people with inter-ictal aggressive personality traits, who may become aggressive as a result of post-ictal impairment of function in those areas of the brain which normally modulate their aggressive behaviour. Aggression is particularly likely to occur if attempts are made to restrain the patient or if he is subject to other forms of physical interference during the post-ictal period.

If an EEG is carried out it will almost always be abnormal, showing either a focal or a generalised abnormality which will be epileptiform during the seizure and will show slowing of activity post-ictally.

Epileptic automatisms usually last a few minutes at the longest, but occasionally they can continue for hours. Such prolonged periods of automatic behaviour can be seen in petit mal status, sometimes called "spike–wave" stupor because of the EEG picture of multiple spike and wave foci on a background of disorganised activity. The aberrant neuronal discharge is non-focal in nature in these two uncommon disorders, and the automatic behaviour is less stereotyped and often gives the appearance of a stupor. Moreover, petit mal attacks may occasionally start for the first time in adults and present as petit mal status (Lishman, 1978).

Prolonged *"fugue-like"* states may occur and involve the patient wandering away. These episodes can last days and some probably represent dissociative fugues, in which case the patient may lose his personal identity and assume a new one. Presumably the neuronal processes underlying the epileptic seizure in these patients acts in some way to facilitate their developing a state of dissociation. Such a predisposition is supported by recent evidence that hysterical dissociation is probably more frequent than was previously realised in epileptic patients (Schenk and Bear, 1981). This facilitating process may be similar to that which occurs when a head injury precipitates a hysterical fugue, in non-epileptic patients (Berrington *et al.*, 1956). Epileptic patients sometimes develop episodes of altered consciousness which though "fugue-like", appear to be intermediate in type between hysterical dissociation and an epileptic automatism. In these an underlying ictal discharge probably plays an aetiological role and

Table 13.3 Comparative features of four important causes of altered consciousness

	EPILEPTIC AUTOMATISM	TRANSIENT GLOBAL AMNESIA	PHOBIC ANXIETY	PSYCHO-GENIC FUGUE
Age	All ages	Over 50 yrs.	20–40 yrs.	All ages
Precipitants	No	Maybe physical or emotional precipitants	Phobic situations	Emotionally significant events
ATTACK				
Onset	Acute	Acute	Acute	Acute
Duration	Usually under 5 minutes	4–8 hours	Usually minutes	Hours to days
Behaviour	Stereotyped in the early stages	Normal	May involve "escape" behaviour	May involve aimless wandering
Personal identity	Preserved	Preserved	Preserved	May be lost
Conscious level	Impaired	Normal	Normal	Normal
Affect	Usually fearful	Perplexed	Anxious or fearful	Unconcerned or depressed
Termination	Merges into confusion	Gradual	Gradual with feeling of relief	Gradual
EEG	Abnormal	Abnormal	Normal	Normal

there is a true decrease in the conscious level, rather than a narrowing of consciousness. The features of these attacks are atypical, with some episodes being prolonged for days and sometimes involving psychotic features. The conscious level may be difficult to assess and the patient may maintain a substantial degree of contact with his surroundings, despite his disturbed behaviour. If consciousness appears to be preserved and psychotic features are absent, then the more prolonged the fugue the more likely it is to be psychogenic in origin, even if the patient is epileptic.

Epileptic seizures often occur when the patient is relaxing on his own, drowsy and away from all stresses (Marsden, 1976b), in contrast to most psychogenic disorders. However, stress can also precipitate seizures (Friis and Lund, 1974) and this may result from an anxiety provoking situation. Also, anxiety may cause hyperventilation and precipitate seizures in the predisposed, especially in those with petit mal epilepsy. Lack of sleep, tiredness and alcohol, are all potent inducers of seizures in some epileptic patients.

13.3 DEPERSONALISATION

In this condition the patient experiences an alteration in his normal level of consciousness. *Depersonalisation typically involves an alteration in the perception of one's body with a feeling of unreality and detachment.* Often the outside world seems unreal and this is called derealisation. The patient feels as if he is observing his own behaviour from outside. He feels like a "robot" and the people around him are like puppets or actors on a stage. It is an important condition because the symptoms, and the way they are described, can vary widely and may mimic many other disorders. As Ackner (1954a) has said "the phenomena accepted as those of depersonalisation (are) such that no clear cut boundaries can exist for the condition" and hence "the disagreements on aetiology have partly arisen on a semantic basis". The patient typically has great difficulty putting his experiences into words, unless asked direct questions. He may avoid attempting to describe them, as their bizarre nature makes him fear he is going insane. The essential features of depersonalisation have been described by Ackner (1954a), and are as follows:

1. A feeling that one's body and/or the outside world has changed in some way.
2. The unpleasant quality of the feeling.
3. The empathic feeling that one normally has for others is lost and there is an inability to respond emotionally to events that occur around oneself.
4. There is a feeling of unreality.
5. It is an "as if" experience (and not a delusion that one's body *really* has changed in some way).

These experiences may be chronic or recurrent. They are commonly found in a mild form in healthy, young people, particularly when they are tired.

Depersonalisation can be found in a variety of neurological and psychiatric disorders. It is the severe cases that are most likely to be seen by the physician and in some cases the patient's experiences are unusually bizarre and incapacitating.

Gabbard *et al.* (1982) differentiate between depersonalisation and *"out-of-body" experiences* (OBE). OBE involve an *"altered state of consciousness in which one's mind or awareness is experienced as separated from one's physical body"*. In contrast to depersonalisation, OBE is an enjoyable, sometimes ecstatic experience, in which the observing and functioning parts of the patient's body are felt to be outside his inactive body. This appears to be a not uncommon phenomenon and usually does not cause the person to consult a doctor. It may be perceived as a religious experience.

Depersonalisation can be one manifestation of a personality disorder, and Ackner (1954b) found that it could be a chronic state in patients with schizoid personalities, when it was sometimes the sole complaint. This was also true for a number of patients with hysterical personality types. In certain patients, the unpleasant subjective sensation may attain such a degree that they may resort to self-mutilation in an attempt to relieve themselves of it (Simpson, 1976).

Depersonalisation may be seen in the affective disorders and schizophrenia, and the diagnosis may be indicated by the presence of psychotic symptoms, or a depressed or elated affect. *If the experience of bodily change is delusional, a psychotic illness is present.* Nihilistic delusions may be seen in depressive psychosis, e.g. "my head is empty" or "my bowels have turned to stone", and there is a striking similarity between these complaints and some depersonalisation phenomena, e.g. "I'm a vacuum . . . there is a jammed up feeling in my head— it feels split in two as if my brain is peeling off . . ." (Ackner, 1954b).

If the experience is pleasant it suggests that it is caused by alcohol or drug ingestion (especially the hallucinogens or the barbiturates), or hypomania. It can be seen in any disorder producing delirium, and is also seen in association with temporo-parietal disease (including TLE). If the patient requests a particular drug such as a barbiturate, it should be suspected that the depersonalisation is a consequence of withdrawal from this drug, even if drug abuse is denied. Drug ingestion, head injury and other organic events, may act to precipitate chronic or recurrent depersonalisation, which may continue long after the original precipitant has stopped.

Depersonalisation may involve distortions of body image, with parts of the body feeling altered in size or shape, and such experiences are also found in focal brain disease. Hemi-depersonalisation is the experience of there being nothing on one side of the body, usually the left side, and clinically it shows some similarity with neglect phenomena. It is found in parietal lobe disorders (Critchley, 1953). The more bizarre the symptoms, the more organic brain disease or psychosis is likely to be present.

A high index of suspicion is needed to identify depersonalisation, in view of the difficulty these patients have in describing their symptoms and because of the bizarre nature they may assume. If there is a misinterpretation of the patients' experiences, this can may lead to inappropriate management and cause clinical deterioration. The disorder can be occasionally intractable, though the prognosis is usually good. The treatment, if required, depends on the cause and can involve just reassurance or the use of drugs, ECT and, in persistent cases, the monoamine oxidase inhibitor drugs may be effective.

The disorder often coexists with phobic anxiety (Harper and Roth, 1962) and the combination of symptoms can closely mimic temporal lobe seizure phenomena. The differentiation of these two disorders will be discussed in the next section.

13.4 PHOBIC ANXIETY AND HYPERVENTILATION

Table 14.2 shows some of the typical features of anxiety attacks. They usually occur in the first half of life, but are not uncommon in most age groups. The onset is usually sudden with a feeling of fear developing in association with the autonomic accompaniments of anxiety, i.e. choking, blushing, diarrhoea, dyspnoea, chest pain, dry mouth, dizziness, "butterfly" feelings in the stomach and palpitations. In "free-floating" anxiety these feelings may occur in the absence of any specific cause.

Hyperventilation (HV) is a commonly associated phenomenon. By reducing the level of carbon dioxide in the blood, it decreases cerebral blood flow. It may cause paraesthesiae in the hands, feet and periorally, and carpopedal muscle spasms of the hands (main d'accoucheur). In addition, there may be dizziness, depersonalisation, feelings of anxiety, blurring of vision, muscle cramps, weakness and tiredness (Riley, 1982). Symptoms produced by hyperventilation may be confined to one side of the body and suggest the presence of focal intracranial disease. Blau et al. (1983) described a series of patients with unilateral somatic symptoms resulting from HV, usually consisting of weakness, numbness or paraesthesia. They had received previous diagnoses that included multiple sclerosis, epilepsy, migraine and cerebrovascular disease. No intracranial disease was present and they concluded *"when the simple procedure of hyperventilation reproduces the patient's symptoms, no further investigation is necessary"*. It should be emphasised that the conscious level need not be altered when hyperventilation induces somatic symptoms and, in some cases, breathing exercises taught by a physiotherapist may be all the treatment that is needed.

Even when there is a specific cause (phobia) for the anxiety, the patient may not recognise the reason for his fear. When there is no obvious cause, such as a threat to his life, the patient may just describe his physical symptoms, being unable to conceptualise his experience as one of fear, in the absence of an appropriate cause, i.e. "I wasn't frightened doctor, there was nothing to be frightened of". Also some patients have difficulty verbalising their feelings in any understandable way and this is particularly likely if depersonalisation phenomena are prominent. For these reasons it is clear that episodic anxiety may prove a diagnostic problem and may be misdiagnosed as a physical disorder, e.g. palpitations regarded as indicating the presence of cardiac disease. If the anxiety is severe and prolonged, the patient may faint, but usually there is a gradual decrease in the symptoms, with relief. This may follow behaviour aimed at escaping from a phobic situation.

The attacks usually last minutes to hours and, because of the patient's high level of arousal, his subsequent recall of the episode will often be incomplete. There will be a variable sequence of events from one attack to another which will occur when the patient is exposed to some phobic situation, e.g. a crowded elevator. Such fears tend to be superimposed on a previous history of anxiety particularly in young married women, but Harper and Roth (1962) found that these patients often have a previous history of a stable, if somewhat obsessional, premorbid personality.

Depersonalisation and derealisation frequently accompany phobic anxiety, particularly in patients with agoraphobia, and the combination has been called the *Phobic anxiety–depersonalisation syndrome* (Harper and Roth, 1962). *Agoraphobia is an inexplicable and inappropriately morbid fear of open spaces*, but it is often also associated with fear of crowded places and enclosed spaces (Thorley and Stern, 1979). Depersonalisation has been discussed in the previous section and basically involves a disturbance in the patient's perception of his body image, with a subjective feeling of strangeness with regard to himself and his surroundings. This syndrome (PAD) often involves peceptual distortions, déjà vu and hallucinatory-like experiences. Because of the dramatic and episodic nature of these phenomena, clinically they can closely mimic temporal lobe seizures (TLE).

Harper and Roth (1962) found that certain features significantly differentiated between TLE and PAD attacks. A family history of neurosis, a previous history of migraine and childhood phobias, were more common in PAD. A previous history of neurological trauma (severe birth trauma, prolonged anoxia or a head injury, with loss of consciousness), neurological infection (meningitis, encephalitis or mastoiditis) and an abnormal EEG (usually epileptiform), were significantly more common in TLE.

However, it should be noted that patients with epilepsy, especially TLE, have a raised incidence of neurotic problems, especially anxiety (Trimble, 1981a). They are particularly prone to acute attacks of anxiety, in addition to their epileptic seizures. These patients may regard any brief episode involving abnormal experiences as being another form of "seizure", and report them as such. Differentiation of the two types of attacks depends on the taking of a careful history.

13.5 PSYCHOGENIC FUGUE

Psychogenic fugue states tend to be precipitated by an emotionally traumatic event, they are relatively acute in onset and involve a tendency to wander, sometimes with the patient losing his personal identity. They are characterised by amnesia of the hysterical (dissociative) type. *Hysterical amnesia typically involves "a loss of knowledge of personal identity combined with preservation of environmental information and, often, complex learned information or skills"* and it is when this amnesia is "combined with an impulse to wander" that a fugue state develops (Merskey, 1979). More mundane memories, such as how to travel from A to B, are intact, and retrograde amnesia is not present. Once memory begins to return full recovery is relatively rapid. This selective loss of memory contrasts with the more diffuse loss and the retrograde amnesia that are characteristically found in organic disorders.

During the fugue state these patients show purposeful and coordinated behaviour. The loss of memory and personal identity are incompatible with the degree of preservation of higher cortical functions indicated by the patient's behaviour on the ward and his responses on clinical and psychological testing. It is important to appreciate that there may be a preceding history of some "organic" event, particularly alcohol intake, a head injury or a predisposition to epilepsy, preceding the fugue (Berrington *et al.*, 1956; Kennedy and Neville, 1957). Head injury is also a common preceding event in psychogenic amnesia unassociated with any tendency to wander (Kennedy and Neville, 1957). However, the presence of these organic features must be balanced against other aspects of the clinical picture, as they are acting to precipitate or facilitate what is primarily a psychogenic disorder.

Exploratory interviews are necessary, not only to identify the cause of the disorder, but to provide the patient with an opportunity to abreact any repressed feelings that may have played a role in precipitating it. Depression is commonly found (Stengel, 1941; Berrington *et la.*, 1956) and will require treatment in its own right. Suggestion can be used to facilitate recovery of memory, and may be aided by procedures such as hypnosis or intravenous barbiturates.

The distinction between hysteria and malingering can be very difficult and often they are both present. Lying is common in patients who have undergone what appears, clinically, to be a psychogenic fugue (Stengel, 1941; Berrington *et al.*, 1956). Only if the patient admits to simulating mental illness or is caught in the act, can malingering be clearly separated from hysteria. However, features which would suggest the presence of malingering include a disturbed premorbid personality and a patient who is defensive, and may even be aggressive, in his behaviour, particularly when confronted with inconsistencies in the history he has given and in the level of functioning he exhibits on the ward. Such responses tend to be absent in the pure form of conversion hysteria, as the patient is not conscious of the psychogenic basis of his disorder.

13.6 TRANSIENT GLOBAL AMNESIA

Transient global amnesia (TGA) was first described in detail by Fisher and Adams (1964). It consists of an acute onset, short-lived period (a few hours) of confusion and amnesia. TGA is most commonly found in males in their sixth or seventh decade and primarily involves an inability to memorise new information. Though this has been regarded as an uncommon phenomenon, it may be more common than is currently realised, and it is a condition that easily lends itself to misdiagnosis. Corston and Godwin-Austen (1982) have described four brothers, all of whom seem to have had at least one attack of TGA, but only one of whom initially sought medical advice. Their paper also suggests that, in some cases, this disorder may have a familial basis. Some of the important features of this disorder are listed in Table 13.2.

TGA may be precipitated by certain events, such as excessive physical exertion, exposure to changes in environmental temperature, pain or a highly emotional experience (Fisher, 1982b). It has also been precipitated by flushing an intra-aortic catheter, and recurrent attacks have been seen in association with recurrent cerebral emboli (Alexander, 1982).

During the attack the patient, aware of his disability, becomes perplexed and agitated and may repeatedly ask questions of people he encounters, in order to try and understand what is happening to him. It involves a short-term memory impairment, with an inability to form new memories, and so the patient is unable to retain new information. Though this deficit in memory appears to be mainly an impairment of consolidation, retrograde amnesia (RGA) is common after the attack. This RGA may extend for years, but usually recovers with time. Attention and the ability to perform complex, goal-directed behaviour are preserved, which may suggest in retrospect that the disorder was a psychogenic fugue. Alexander (1982) has listed the main characteristics that he feels differentiate psychogenic amnesia from TGA. They are as follows:

Hysterical amnesia:
1. Is precipitated by a threatening situation;
2. Does not have a recognisable onset;
3. Involves mainly personal information;
4. Ceases abruptly.

In addition, the patient is calm and is found wandering or asking for help in conventional locations, such as a police station.

The bulk of the evidence suggests the cause of TGA is ischaemia in the distribution of the posterior cerebral arteries, resulting in impairment of hippocampal function. This evidence includes the documentation of cases of TGA associated with visual field deficits, though such deficits need not be present. In general TGA patients have an increased incidence of factors predisposing them to cerebrovascular disease, particularly involving the posterior cerebral circulation. Though the global memory impairment is of the type associated with bilateral hippocampal damage, it can occasionally be produced by vascular disease confined to the left posterior cerebral artery (Benson et al., 1974).

One EEG study carried out on a 74-year-old female during an episode of TGA showed paroxysmal bursts of sharp waves occurring independently from both mid-temporal regions. The EEG was normal 5 months later (Tharp, 1969). Following the attack 38% of cases have EEG abnormalities involving slowing in the temporal lobe regions, sometimes with spike discharges (Fisher and

Adams, 1964). It has been suggested that some cases of TGA may have en epileptic basis, but a past history of epilepsy is rare and the attacks do not involve impairment of consciousness or other features suggestive of temporal lobe epilepsy.

The prognosis is generally good, though 20% have recurrent attacks and about 5% subsequently develop more permanent cerebral deficits. Occasionally, episodes resembling TGA are the result of tumours involving the third ventricle or the limbic system, or the use of diazepam, clioquinol, or digitalis (Alexander, 1982).

13.7 ALCOHOL, DRUGS AND OTHER ORGANIC DISORDERS

Alcohol and drugs may cause altered consciousness by inducing a confusional state, particularly where there is a pre-existing history of brain damage. They may also precipitate hypersomnia with "sleep drunkenness", or attacks resembling TGA. Outbursts of aggression can occur after intake of relatively small doses of alcohol (when temporal lobe EEG abnormalities may be present) or as a release phenomenon due to disinhibition. Such responses are uncommon in people who have no pre-existing abnormality of personality or OBD.

Alcohol can cause altered consciousness as a withdrawal phenomenon, which may develop into a full-blown delirium tremens; as a result of nutritional deficiency (Wernicke's encephalopathy or the rare, Marchiafava–Bignami disease); due to hypoglycaemia; or as a result of certain neurological complications that the alcoholic is predisposed to, notably portosystemic encephalopathy, cerebral infarction or subdural haematoma. These disorders will involve delirium in many cases, but the features that characterise delirium, such as disorientation and perceptual abnormalities, may not be obvious. Altered consciousness can be caused by most drugs that have an effect on the CNS, such as the minor tranquillisers, neuroleptics and antidepressants, as well as the psychotomimetic and other drugs of abuse. In the previous section the precipitation of TGA by non-psychotropic drugs was mentioned.

Because of its effects on the brain stem neuronal mechanisms responsible for maintaining alertness, vertebrobasilar ischaemia may cause transient disorders of consciousness in the young (vertebrobasilar migraine) and the older age groups (TGA and vertebrobasilar ischaemia).

Migraine can cause episodes of altered consciousness, particularly in the first two decades of life, when headache may not be a prominent accompaniment, during the initial attacks (migraine equivalent). It may also start for the first time in those over the age of 40 years, when the attacks may mimic TIAs. In contrast to the classical scintillating scotomata aura, these attacks can involve a variety of other neurological phenomena. Fisher (1980) described a group of 120 patients who were suspected of late onset migraine. He lists the features which favour this diagnosis; they include: two or more similar episodes; visual scintillations, particularly those which exhibit a "build-up"; a "march" of paraesthesiae; a progression from one feature to the next, often with a delay in between; a duration of 15 to 25 minutes; and an associated headache (which was found in only 50% of his cases). "March" and "build-up" features are not seen in cerebrovascular disease. In addition to certain of these characteristics being present, other disorders must be ruled out, including certain blood disorders (polycythaemia, thrombocythaemia, thrombocytopenia), and cerebral angiography should be normal. This condition follows a relatively benign course, in contrast to TIA's, 30% of which will be followed by CVAs within a 5 year period (McCormick, 1983).

Other causes worth considering are hypoglycaemia, where confusion may not be marked but neurological signs will usually be present, including motor incoordination with ataxia and dysarthria. Automatic behaviour may also occur as a manifestation of the hypersomnias and parasomnias. In the former, they are usually a manifestation of subclinical sleep attacks.

CHAPTER 14

Catatonia and Stupor

14.1 INTRODUCTION

"Stupor is a condition of deep sleep or behaviorally similar unresponsiveness, from which the subject can be aroused only by vigorous and repeated stimuli. Most stuporose patients have diffuse organic cerebral dysfunction" (Plum and Posner, 1980).

"In the present state of knowledge stupor is defined in descriptive terms, the basic triad consisting of akinesis, mutism, and relative preservation of consciousness" (Joyston-Bechal, 1966).

The fundamental difference between these views is with regard to the patient's conscious level. The former definition views stupor as one stage on a continuum between clear consciousness and coma, these being called "transitional" stupors, by Berrios (1981). They are usually the result of an organic disorder. The second definition involves a relatively intact conscious level, and is usually associated with psychogenic disorders. Since one of the essential steps in evaluating the stuporose patient involves assessing conscious level, the difference in views need not hinder the diagnostic process, but *it is important to qualify the way the term stupor is being used.*

Stupor is a common component of the catatonic syndrome. "Catatonic syndrome" will be used here as a term referring to any disorder, neurological or psychiatric, where two or more catatonic signs (see Table 14.1) are prominent. The term catatonic was used in 1896 by Kraepelin to describe a subtype of Dementia Praecox (the other three subtypes being hebephrenic, paranoid and simple), a title that was changed to schizophrenia, by Bleuler in 1911, who realised that the prognosis for this disorder need not be so bleak (Sim, 1974). The term catatonic implies the presence of abnormal motor behaviour, which can be found in a wide variety of organic and non-organic disorders (Berrios, 1981; Gelenberg, 1976; Stoudemire, 1982). Catatonic schizophrenia remains a recognised diagnostic entity and is included in the DSM III. For this diagnosis the DSM III requires schizophrenia to be dominated by catatonic signs of the type listed in Table 14.1. This table describes those signs which are generally

233

accepted as catatonic phenomena. The phenomena are described as "negative" when they involve an absence of, or a reduction of, motor activity, and "positive" when motor activity is excessive in quantity and/or abnormal in quality. Evidence in support for such a separation was described by Abrams *et al.* (1979), who found catatonic signs could be separated by factor analysis into two groups, one involving positive and the other negative phenomena. The two types of phenomena are not mutually exclusive and in one series of 250 catatonic patients, 29% exhibited both retarded and excited behaviour (Morrison, 1973).

Table 14.1   Catatonic signs

POSITIVE PHENOMENA

Posturing	An inappropriate, often bizarre posture maintained for a prolonged period.
Catalepsy	Unresponsive to stimuli.
	Parts of the body can be put into positions that will be maintained for a prolonged period—however bizarre and uncomfortable they may be.
Mannerism	A particular pattern of purposeful behaviour carried out in an unusual stylised manner.
Stereotypy	Purposeless behaviour carried out repetitively (may involve speech).
Excitement	Over-activity that is not goal-directed or otherwise appropriate (may involve aggression).
Automatic obedience	Instructions are carried out automatically, irrespective of their nature.
Echophenomena	The mimicking of actions observed (echopraxia), or phrases (echolalia), words (pallilalia) or syllables (logoclonia) heard.
Verbigeration	Incomprehensible "jargon" speech.

NEGATIVE PHENOMENA

Stupor	A reduction in motor activity with preservation of normal conscious level.
Negativism	A resistance to all commands or any form of interference.
	The patient may respond by doing the opposite of what is requested.
Mutism	The absence of speech.
Ambitendency	The presence of conflicting impulses—may be manifest as tentative goal-directed movements which are not carried through to completion (such as putting out a hand to be shaken, then withdrawing it before the act is completed).

For a detailed discussion of the concepts of stupor and catatonia, the reader is referred to Berrios (1981). The remainder of this chapter will deal with the differential diagnosis of first, stupor, and then, the catatonic syndrome.

14.2 DIFFERENTIAL DIAGNOSIS OF STUPOR

Table 14.2 shows those features which will help to separate organic from psychogenic stupors. Certain signs may mislead the physician by incorrectly suggesting that the patient is deliberately producing his behaviour. They include apparently purposeful eye movements, variation over time in those parts of the body which exhibit catalepsy, abrupt changes in motor behaviour, and last minute responses. These features can be seen in organic disorders of movement (Berrios, 1981). Conversely choreiform movements may be seen in psychogenic stupor, but in such cases other catatonic signs will usually be present (Plum and Posner, 1980).

Table 14.2 Psychogenic versus organic stupor

	ORGANIC	PSYCHOGENIC
Previous Neurological Illness	+	−
Previous Psychiatric Illness	−	+
Previous Episodes of Stupor	10%	24–33%
PHYSICAL EXAMINATION		
Blepharospasm	−	+
Menace reflex	−	+
Roving eye movements	+	−
Visual fixation	−	+
Doll's Head Eye phenomenon	+	−
Henry and Woodruff's sign	−	+
Rapid eye closure after forcible opening	−	+
Coordinated movements to remove painful stimuli	−	+
Protective response	−	+
Autonomic over-arousal	−	+
SPECIAL PROCEDURES		
Abnormal EEG	+	−
Response to intravenous barbiturates	Low dose reduces conscious level and neurological signs may develop	High dose increases alertness and psychopathology may be revealed
Oculovestibular reflex	−	+
MORTALITY	35%	0–3%

+ = May be present.
− = Usually absent.

Plum and Posner (1980) found psychogenic unresponsiveness to be very uncommon, occurring in only 3.5% of 386 unresponsive patients they saw in a neurological hospital. The commonest "psychogenic" causes in their study were hysterical conversion or catatonic schizophrenia. However, severe stupor is not usually seen as a hysterical conversion phenomenon and in those occasional cases which are hysterical in origin, depression is usually present. In a study carried out on a psychiatric population, Joyston-Bechal (1966) found that 69% of a 100 stuporose patients had non-organic disorders only. Of his 100 patients 25% had depression, 34% schizophrenia and 23% organic disorders (mainly dementia). Hysterical features were present in 10%. Most of the disorders listed in Table 14.3 can cause a clinical picture dominated by stuporose behaviour.

Clarification of the cause of the condition is obviously important, especially as the potential mortality in organic stupor is 35%, compared with about 3% for psychogenic stupors (Joyston-Bechal, 1966). Also, inappropriate treatment, e.g. the use of major tranquillisers in patients with neuroleptic-induced stupor (Weinberger and Wyatt, 1978), or the use of ECT in organic stupor, can cause clinical deterioration. As the patient will be unable to give a history some other informant should be looked for. The history may reveal previous physical or mental illness, indicating that the patient is at increased risk of developing a particular disorder. Previous episodes of stupor were more frequent in psychogenic disorders (29%), in contrast to organic disorders (9%), in Joyston-Bechal's series.

The patient's behaviour preceding his presentation may indicate cognitive deterioration. The premorbid personality should be evaluated, but a history of a personality that is inclined to respond to stress with withdrawal behaviour, was found to be of no value in differentiating organic from depressive stupor, being found in 25% of each type by Joyston-Bechal (1966). However, such a premorbid personality was of value in differentiating schizophrenia (83% of them showing premorbid withdrawal behaviour) from neurotic/hysterical disorders (10%). Stupor is most common in association with catatonic signs when they are due to schizophrenia, and it was found in 75% of catatonic schizophrenics, by Abrams and Taylor (1976), compared with 51% of patients with affective disorders and 56% with organic disorders.

During the physical examination particularly, attention should be paid to the patient's eyes. A psychogenic disorder is suggested by closed eyes, which resist opening and close rapidly, when the force used to open them is released. The eyes will tend to fixate on objects in the patient's field of vision, suggesting he is alert and, to a certain extent, aware of his environment. However, the latter may be seen in the organic disorders — akinetic mutism and the "locked in" syndrome. Random roving movements of the eyes are usually only found in organic disorders.

The alert patient will usually attempt to protect himself from injury. If the physician lifts the patient's arm and allows it to fall towards his face, the patient will usually take steps to avoid it striking him. Alertness is also suggested by a blink response to visual threat, and purposeful attempts (directed specifically at the offending object) to push away any painful stimulus. Autonomic hyperarousal is usually present, with tachycardia, hypertension and pupils that are equal, dilated and which respond to light briskly and symmetrically.

Total immobility with mutism was uncommon in Joyston-Bechal's series, and was absent in neurotic/hysterical disorders. It may be possible to stimulate the patient to a degree where he will be able to respond to certain questions and procedures but, when the stimulus is removed, the patient with an organic stupor will lapse into a drowsy and unresponsive state. If the patient is only semi-stuporose, it may be possible to ask questions aimed at evaluating his level of cognition, depressive symptoms, psychotic phenomena, and other psycho-pathology. This is often possible as there is usually a diurnal fluctuation in the severity of the stupor.

Care must be taken not to mistake the "locked-in" syndrome and akinetic mutism as psychogenic disorders, despite the apparent alert and watchful nature of the patient's eye movements (vide infra). Neurological signs should be looked for in all cases of stupor.

Bedside tests which may be helpful include the oculocephalic reflex, Henry and Woodruff's sign, and an interview with the patient while giving him intravenous sodium amytal. The *oculocephalic reflex*, also called the *Doll's Head Eye phenomenon*, is a simple test that can be used in any unresponsive patient, provided there is no suspicion that a cervical injury is present. The reflex involves conjugate deviation of the eyes to the contralateral side, when the head is turned quickly to the other side. If the reflex is consistently positive then this strongly suggests the presence of organic brain disease, particularly involving the area of the frontal eye fields. It has been suggested that the phenomenon is due to this area of the brain failing to carry out its normal function of inhibiting visual fixation (Plum and Posner, 1980).

The presence of *Henry and Woodruff's sign* (Henry and Woodruff, 1978) indicates a psychogenic stupor. If this sign is positive then there is a voluntary deviation of the eyes to the ground, whichever side the patient is lying on.

The use of *intravenous sodium amytal* may be helpful. Careful evaluation of the patient should precede this procedure, as the drug may interfere with attempts to monitor the patient's conscious level, which is necessary when a progressive neurological lesion is suspected. It will also have an effect on the EEG tracing and may interfere with its interpretation. This drug tends to cause cognitive deterioration in organic disorders and, if this occurs, its administration must be immediately stopped and the patient examined for any neurological signs that may have been revealed (Plum and Posner, 1980). In the psychogenic patient psychopathology, such as the positive symptoms of psychosis, may be revealed. Psychogenic patients tend to improve with amytal, but may need a high dose of the drug. This is in contrast with the relatively low dose which will often cause sedation and confusion in patients with organic disorders (Perry and Jacobs, 1982).

The EEG is of great importance in evaluating those diagnostically difficult cases of stupor. Alpha rhythm, which becomes desynchronised on eye-opening and is maximal over the occipital region of the brain, usually indicates an alert patient. When there is an organic impairment of consciousness, diffuse slow activity will appear. Focal EEG abnormalities may indicate the presence of a focal brain lesion. Mild degrees of EEG slowing may appear to be within normal limits, particularly if a baseline recording is not available. A relatively normal

EEG in the presence of severe stupor almost excludes an organic cause, though two occasional exceptions are akinetic mutism (Wells and Duncan, 1980) and the "locked-in" syndrome (Goldensohn, 1979).

In catatonic stupor due to schizophrenia, low amplitude slow activity is particularly common, being present only during the period of stupor. The EEG is helpful in those occasional cases of petit mal status, "spike-wave" stupor, temporal lobe status, and post-ictal states. Deep lying lesions in the region of the diencephalon will tend to produce diffuse bilaterally synchronous EEG abnormalities.

Another useful diagnostic sign is the *oculovestibular reflex*. This reflex is valuable but not easy to elicit. It involves instillation of cold water into the patient's external auditory canal, though care must be taken beforehand to ensure the canal is patent and the tympanic membrane intact. The normal ocular response is a regular rhythmic nystagmus with the slow component directed towards the irrigated ear, and, if present, it indicates a psychogenic disorder is present (Plum and Posner, 1980).

In Joyston-Bechal's series (1966) 86% of stupors recovered in under a month and 36% recovered spontaneously. Those that persisted for longer tended to have a poor prognosis and were mainly patients with organic brain disease. The patient's ability to remember his experiences during the period of his stupor was of little help in differential diagnosis as both organic and psychogenic cases tended to describe experiences involving feelings of apathy, fear or a need to withdraw.

The treatment of choice in psychogenic disorders is ECT, if the patient's health is in serious jeopardy. Otherwise simple observation, major tranquillisers, antidepressants or some form of abreaction, could be used. ECT can also be effective in organic disorders and may be necessary in emergencies or in those cases resistant to other modes of treatment. It is contra-indicated in the presence of an intracranial mass and causes a deterioration in the patient's cognitive state (Clare, 1979) which, even if only transient, may be poorly tolerated by those patients who are already cognitively impaired. The presence of an intracranial infection necessitates caution as an abrupt clinical deterioration has been found in some patients with neurological syphilis, following the use of ECT (Dewhurst, 1969).

There are two neurological syndromes which can cause stupor and create diagnostic problems. The first is the *"locked-in" syndrome* where a lesion at the level of the pons renders the patient mute and quadriplegic, but fully alert and capable of communicating by conjugate movement of the eyes up and down, and by blinking of the eyelids. The second is *akinetic mutism*, where the lesion is in the reticular formation between the mid-brain and the cortex, usually involving the diencephalon or septal area. Though the patient is akinetic, mute and appears aware of his environment, it is not possible to establish communication with him. This condition is also called the Apallic state, the Persistent Vegetative state, or Coma Vigil, because these patients exhibit a persistent state of apparent alertness (Wells and Duncan, 1980).

In both akinetic mutism and the "locked-in" syndrome, neurological abnormalities are usually prominent. In brain stem infarcts the EEG may show alpha rhythm, but it will lack the occipital predominance that is seen with the normal alpha rhythm and it will show no response (desynchronisation) to external stimuli. In the "locked-in" syndrome neurological signs are occasionally minimal in the early stages and care must be taken not to miss variants of the latter condition. The EEG should be carefully examined in such cases.

14.3 DIFFERENTIAL DIAGNOSIS OF CATATONIA

Stupor is a common component of the Catatonic syndrome. The conditions that can cause this syndrome are listed in Table 14.3. Much of the previous section can be applied to those patients with catatonic features of uncertain origin. However, the separation of the psychogenic from the organic cases tends to be more difficult when stupor is associated with other catatonic signs. In

Table 14.3 Causes of the Catatonic syndrome

Alcohol* and toxins	Organic fluorides, illuminating gases
Blood vessels	Cerebrovascular disease, e.g. anterior cerebral artery anurysm, arterial malformation of the posterior cerebral vessels
Collagen and allergic disorders	Membranous glomerulonephritis
Degenerative	Parkinson's disease, focal temporal encephalomalacia, cerebromacular degeneration, cerebral atrophy
Drugs	Hallucinogens, e.g. mescaline, amphetamines,* phencyclidine,* adrenocorticotrophic hormone (ACTH), aspirin,* morphine
	Major tranquillisers — Iatrogenic catatonia — Neuroleptic malignant syndrome — Iatrogenic mutism
Endocrine, metabolic and vitamin disorders	Wernicke's encephalopathy, diabetic ketoacidosis, acute intermittent porphyria, hypercalcaemia, pellagra, homocystinuria, hepatic coma, Gjessing's periodic catatonia
Epilepsy	Petit mal status, post-ictal, "spike-wave" stupor, temporal lobe status
Functional	Schizophrenia, affective psychosis, reactive psychosis, hysterical dissociation, hypnosis
Growth	Cerebral tumours, e.g. tuberose sclerosis, subdural haematoma
Idiopathic	Stauder's Lethal Catatonia
Injury	Closed head injury Bilateral (surgical) lesions of the globus pallidus
Infection	Viral encephalitis, e.g. encephalitis lethargica
Other	Narcolepsy, hypersomnia, delirium

*High dosage or chronic use required.

psychogenic catatonia, autonomic hyper-arousal is often present and the clinical picture may involve pyrexia, choreiform jerking of the limbs, a reduced conscious level, and an absence of the blink response to visual threat (Plum and Posner, 1980).

The non-organic disorders that tend to produce catatonia are schizophrenia and the affective disorders. Catatonic schizophrenia as a diagnosis appears to be in decline and this decline dates from a period prior to the introduction of major tranquilliser treatment, suggesting that other factors are involved. These factors may be social or may reflect an attenuation in some other as yet unidentified factor, such as a virus (Mahendra, 1981). Those schizophrenic patients with prominent features of catatonia constitute no more than a few percent of all schizophrenic patients seen in the last few years, and the catatonic features are often preceded, or followed by, other psychotic features compatible with a different diagnostic subtype of schizophrenia. If one looks for signs such as catalepsy, stereotypy and automatic cooperation, individually they are a relatively frequent finding in schizophrenia and the affective disorders (Abrams and Taylor, 1976). There is some argument as to whether the excitatory and the stuporous types of catatonia should be regarded as being of a similar clinical significance, and Morrison (1973) has identified a difference in course and prognosis according to which of these features is most prominent. He found that of 250 patients diagnosed as catatonic, 110 were predominantly retarded (more often showing negativism, mutism, rigidity, catalepsy and staring); and 67 were predominantly excited (more often being impulsive, aggressive and undressing). The excited group had the better prognosis and their illness was more often acute and rapid in onset, and had a better prognosis for improvement and recovery.

A disorder that is apparently related to schizophrenia is Gjessing's *Periodic Catatonia* (Gjessing, 1974). It involves periodic episodes of catatonic excitement or stupor, associated with vegetative disturbances, including alterations in pulse rate, blood pressure and temperature. Gjessing felt that the strict periodicity of the disorder indicated that it was the result of an accumulation of some chemical substance in the body, which then acted as a stimulant and caused the psychosis. He found that thyroid medication could prevent the periodic retention of nitrogen, which characterized this disorder, and at the same time would stop the psychotic episodes, resulting in complete recovery. Other drugs that have been helpful are the steroids, major tranquillisers, and lithium.

Depression characterized by catatonic stupor is now becoming uncommon. This is probably a result of treatment being started at a relatively early stage in the illness, which prevents it progressing to this degree of severity. However, catatonic depression usually responds to the correct treatment. Individual catatonic symptoms, especially negativism, are commonly found in severe depressive illness. One study of patients with mania showed that 28% exhibited features of catatonia (Taylor and Abrams, 1977), but that these signs did not appear to have any prognostic or treatment implications.

Catatonia has also been noted in association with conversion hysteria and other dissociative disorders, but the prognosis in such cases is good provided that appropriate steps are taken. These include identifying any factors precipitating or perpetuating the disorder. The use of abreaction may also be helpful and can be facilitated by means of intravenous amytal or hypnosis. It is of interest that hypnosis itself can produce a catatonic state (Gelenberg, 1976).

Catatonic signs may be seen in association with lesions in virtually any area of the brain, including the frontal lobe, globus pallidus, temporo-limbic system, thalamus, third ventricle, and brain stem. Diffuse structural brain disease and diffuse cerebral dysfunction without structural change can also produce catatonic signs (Gelenberg, 1976). Berrios (1981) discriminates between those organic stupors which are "transitional" and represent a stage on the normal consciousness–coma spectrum, and those that result from lesions in the brain stem–diencephalon axis. Spontaneous variations in the level of consciousness are commonly seen in the former group. The latter group exhibits little variation in conscious level and these patients are particularly prone to pose diagnostic problems, as clinical features suggesting a psychogenic aetiology may be found.

14.4 CATATONIC SYNDROMES

Major tranquilliser drugs have been known to produce a variety of disorders of the extrapyramidal system including akinesia, rigidity, hand tremor ("pill-rolling"), oculogyric crises, decreased blinking, micrographia, Pisa syndrome (a tendency to tilt to one side, most noticeable during walking), Rabbit syndrome (perioral muscle tremor), dystonia, choreoathetosis and akathisia, all of which can occur from any time from 2 days onwards, following the onset of treatment. Other conditions occur after a duration of treatment of at least a few months, and this is most typical of tardive dyskinesia. In addition neuroleptics, particularly the depot preparations, can produce complications which may mimic catatonia and so create diagnostic and treatment problems. Brenner and Rheuban (1978) suggest that *neuroleptic drugs should be stopped when the patient being treated develops catatonic signs that were not previously present*, as such patients are particularly at risk of physical complications, such as pneumonia and dehydration.

Specific catatonic syndromes include Iatrogenic Catatonia, the Neuroleptic Malignant syndrome and Stauder's Lethal Catatonia. These three conditions show some clinical overlap with each other and the former two have been particularly associated with neuroleptics.

Iatrogenic Catatonia probably represents a severe dystonic reaction due to the use of neuroleptics is excessive dosage. It can also occur as an extreme sensitivity to the extrapyramidal effects of these drugs, when they are used in moderate doses. The patient becomes extremely rigid and immobile, but remains alert and responsive to his environment. Withdrawal of the responsible drug and treatment with anticholinergic medication is indicated, though the patient's response may be slow (Gelenberg and Mandel, 1977; Stoudemire, 1982; Weinberger and Wyatt, 1978).

The *Neuroleptic Malignant syndrome* is characterized by an acute onset of autonomic dysfunction, stupor, dyskinesia, rigidity, hyperthermia and pallor. A leukocytosis and an elevated serum creatine phosphoskinase level are common. It is predominantly found in young adult males and those with organic brain disease. There is no specific temporal relationship to the onset of treatment. There is a particular risk of pulmonary complications developing, especially pulmonary oedema or pulmonary emboli (Stoudemire, 1982; Weinberger and Kelley, 1977). It is a disorder which shows marked overlap clinically with *Stauder's Lethal Catatonia*. The latter had already been described before the discovery of the major tranquillisers (Stoudemire, 1982). It usually begins as a catatonic stupor, but subsequently progresses to agitation with mutism, hyperthermia and dehydration. As its name suggests, this rare condition may be lethal and it is possible that a viral encephalitis is responsible for some of these cases (Penn *et al.*, 1972). Of the survivors the majority develop schizophrenia and so it is not clear if, in some cases, the initial illness is a manifestation of schizophrenia, or if schizophrenia is a consequence of the cerebral damage sustained as a result of this disorder, whether it is due to a virus or some other cause.

In the latter two conditions it seems likely that the brunt of the pathology involves the diencephalon of the brain, especially in view of their association with hyperthermia, which results from the suppression of the central thermoregulatory mechanisms. They both have a significant mortality and treatment should be instituted urgently to avoid complications, especially pneumonia, pulmonary emboli, dehydration, thrombophlebitis, deep vein thrombosis and malnutrition. Urinary retention or incontinence, and even faecal incontinence, can occur. Treatment involves withdrawal of any aetiological agent, with the introduction of anticholinergic drugs. There is some evidence that amantadine, which acts to stimulate presynaptic dopamine release in the brain, may be particularly effective in treating these disorders (Grimes, 1983). Treatment of any physical complications should be started without delay.

CHAPTER 15

Sleep Disorders

15.1 INTRODUCTION

The Sleep Disorders Classification Committee of the Association of Sleep Disorders Centers and the Association for the Psychophysiological Study of Sleep (Sleep, 1979) has proposed that sleep disorders be classified into four categories—Disorders of Excessive Somnolence (DOES), e.g. depression, Menstrual Associated syndrome, narcolepsy, hypersomnia with "sleep drunkenness", Kleine–Levin syndrome; Disorders of Initiating and Maintaining Sleep (DIMS), e.g. neuroses, psychoses, nocturnal myoclonus, "restless legs" syndrome; Disorders of the sleep–wake schedule, e.g. "jet-lag", and Disorders associated with sleep or partial arousal, e.g. sleepwalking, sleep terrors, nocturnal epilepsy, other disorders which need not be confined to sleeping periods. Such a classification reflects an increasing interest in the research and clinical aspects of sleep disorders over the last two decades. However, some of the categories of sleep disorders that have been described are based on findings made in sleep laboratories by research workers. Though such categories are useful for the purpose of communication between specialists involved in this field, it is arguable if the patient populations investigated by such procedures are always representative of those patients with disorders of sleep who are seen by psychiatrists. There is some question of whether the use of time-consuming and expensive investigatory techniques, such as polysomnography, are worthwhile as part of the routine investigation of such patients, and if any information of practical or diagnostic usefulness is revealed by such procedures in the majority of cases (Kales *et al.*, 1983; Oswald, 1981). *Polysomnography is the continuous monitoring of the patient's EEG, eye movements (electro-oculogram), muscle potentials (electromyogram) and other psychophysiological parameters, during sleep.*

The clinical disorders of sleep vary in the effects they have on the different sleep stages, and so these stages will be briefly mentioned here. Experimental work on cats in the past revealed that if the mid-brain was sectioned just below the oculomotor nucleus (cerveau isolé), the animal entered a chronic unresponsive sleep-like state, accompanied by high amplitude delta activity on the EEG. This finding could be taken to indicate that sleep is a passive phenomenon produced by an interruption of the tonic arousal that is maintained by the activity of the ascending reticular activating system (ARAS). However, the subsequent finding that certain periods of sleep involved rapid eye movements (REM) provided evidence that sleep was an active process. REM sleep occupies 20% of the total sleep time (TST) in adults (Boddy, 1978).

REM sleep normally starts about 90 minutes after the onset of sleep and it is preceded by non-REM stage 4 sleep. The REM period is initially about 5 minutes long, but it recurs every 90 minutes and becomes increasingly longer in duration. An adult has about six REM periods in a normal night's sleep. It is characterised by a reduced muscle tone, though there is usually twitching in the distal limb muscles and penile erection. Pulse and respiration rate increase, the blood pressure varies and there is an increase in the brain's blood flow, metabolism and temperature. REM sleep periods appear to be almost entirely occupied with dreaming. Complex, vivid and detailed dreams are recalled by 75% of people who are aroused from REM sleep. Dreaming also occurs in non-REM sleep, even during the first hour after the onset of sleep, but the dreams are more mundane and unremarkable. They are recalled by only 15% of people aroused from non-REM sleep.

Non-REM sleep is classified into four stages. Light sleep is found in stage 1. Initially there is low voltage mixed frequency activity with slowing of the alpha rhythm, in the EEG. Then slow activity becomes increasingly pronounced as the sleep becomes deeper, with high amplitude delta (less than 4 c/s) activity dominating the EEG, by stage 4. The body temperature, muscle tone, heart and respiration rate all decrease during the night and carbon dioxide accumulates in the blood. Slow eye movements, each of which lasts several seconds, are confined to stage 1 and should not be confused with REM. The bulk of sleep (50%) in adults is stage 2 in type (though it is REM sleep in the first few years of life), and this is the stage containing the characteristic sleep spindles (12–16 c/s) and K complexes. This is discussed further by Boddy (1978).

It is the brain stem and diencephalon, especially the structures surrounding the third ventricle, that are of particular importance in mediating normal sleep. The prefrontal area can act to inhibit the ARAS and stimulation of this area in animals has been shown to induce sleep. The giant neurones in the pontine tegmentum appear to play an important role in maintaining REM sleep. However, not all sleep phenomena can be understood as the direct result of neuronal activity and other processes are almost certainly involved.

In order to assess and treat sleep disturbances, it is important to have some appreciation of the normal variations of the sleep pattern and the factors that influence it. TST tends to decrease from infancy until adulthood, when it remains relatively stable. However, the number of nocturnal wakenings tends to increase throughout life. The ability to sleep is influenced by numerous factors. The longer a person is awake beforehand, the shorter is his sleep latency (the time it takes to get to sleep). There are certain periods during his circadian cycle when he will be resistant to sleep. Insomnia can be produced by events such as exercise, taken irregularly, before going to bed, and factors during sleep, such as excessive noise, marked variations in the environmental temperature, excessive light and hunger. Any dramatic alteration in life style, e.g. switching from day to night shift work, can cause insomnia. After travelling from one continent to another, a period of time is required for the regular sleep pattern to establish itself ("jet-lag") and this may result in temporary insomnia.

The natural tendency is for the sleep pattern of the patient with insomnia to become normal with time, if: his complaints of insomnia do reflect a true disturbance of sleep; he is motivated to cooperate in correcting his sleep pattern; he is not obtaining any form of "gain" from his disorder; the sleep disturbance is of relatively recent onset; and providing any illness underlying the disorder is identified and treated. This assumes that adequate time is allowed and that the sleep pattern is not interfered with by incorrect treatment, e.g. the injudicious use of hypnotic drugs.

Certain conditions, such as the Sleep Apnoea syndrome, Alveolar Hypoventilation syndrome, and alcohol or drug abuse, can cause both DOES and DIMS. It is only to be expected that there is some degree of association between nocturnal insomnia and diurnal hypersomnia. In some cases the latter develops as a compensatory phenomena for nocturnal insomnia. It is clear that an assessment of any sleeping problem requires the careful evaluation of a patient's typical sleep patterns over a 24 hour period. This can be obtained by means of simple techniques, such as the patient using a diary to record his pattern of sleeping throughout each day.

For a more extensive discussion of sleep and related disorders, the reader is referred to Mendelson *et al.* (1977) or Williams and Karacan (1978).

The rest of this chapter will be concerned with the causes and differential diagnosis of, firstly, narcolepsy and hypersomnia, and then, insomnia. It will close with a brief discussion of disorders of the sleep–wake schedule and certain sleep-related phenomena.

15.2 NARCOLEPSY AND HYPERSOMNIA

In contrast to insomnia, where a satisfactory diagnosis may not be arrived at, a clear history of hypersomnia will usually be found to result from some specific disorder(s).

Hypersomnia and narcolepsy both involve pathological, recurrent episodes of diurnal sleeping, but they are classified separately because they differ in certain important respects. *In hypersomnia sleep is more gradual in onset, more prolonged in duration, always involves non-REM sleep only, and the patient has difficulty becoming fully awake and does not feel alert and refreshed* (Sleep, 1979). In the case of narcolepsy, the reverse of these is true except that when the other features of the Narcoleptic syndrome are absent, the sleep episodes can involve non-REM sleep only.

Table 15.1 lists the causes of narcolepsy and hypersomnia. Narcolepsy, the Kleine–Levin syndrome, and Hypersomnia with "sleep drunkenness", all have features which may lead to their being initially diagnosed as being due to a psychiatric disorder. In some cases the psychiatric symptoms may be such as to overshadow the hypersomniac component of the illness. Table 15.2 compares and contrasts the main features of these three disorders (and psychogenic hypersomnia). From this table it can be seen that certain features make these three conditions unlikely to be present. These features are—a sleep disorder that starts after the age of 40 years and a prolonged latency before the onset of normal nocturnal sleep. In addition it is usually relatively easy to wake the patient during the episodes of pathological sleep. If, despite the greatest effort the patient cannot be roused, then this raises a real doubt if this is a sleep attack or some other form of impaired consciousness.

Table 15.1   Causes of narcolepsy or hypersomnia

Blood vessel disease	Cerebrovascular disease (especially in the region of the diencephalon), vertebrobasilar migraine
Collagen disorders	Vasculitis
Degenerative	Multiple sclerosis, hydrocephalus
Endocrine and metabolic	Apathetic hyperthyroidism, hypothyroidism, hypo-adrenalism, Cushing's disease, diabetes mellitus, hypoglycaemia (e.g. hyperinsulinism), hypercapnia, hyperosmolar state, hyponatraemia, menstrual associated hypersomnia
Failure	Renal, hepatic
Functional	Depression
Growth	Frontal lobe meningioma, tumour in the diencephalic region
Hypoxia	Sleep apnoea syndrome, cardiac failure, Alveolar Hypoventilation syndrome
Idiopathic	Narcolepsy, Kleine–Levin syndrome, hypersomnia with "sleep drunkenness"
Infection	Tuberculous meningitis, encephalitis, e.g. encephalitis lethargica, "Sleeping Sickness"—African trypanosomiasis
Injury	Closed head injury

Depression or anxiety may become superimposed on top of a sleep disorder, particularly if there is a prolonged delay before the correct diagnosis is made and the appropriate treatment initiated. Emotional factors may alter the duration, frequency, nature of onset, and after effects, of sleep attacks, even if they were originally due to an organic cause, e.g. anxiety developing in association with a primary sleep disorder may cause a prolonged sleep latency.

Narcolepsy is a disorder characterized by a recurrent compulsion to sleep, that usually occurs several times a day. The duration of the sleep is usually a matter of minutes, though the pathological sleep attack may appear more prolonged by merging into a state of "normal" sleep. After, the patient characteristically feels refreshed and alert. Onset is usually in the second decade of life, it is a life-long condition and it has a familial incidence, apparently involving a dominant mode of inheritance with partial penetrance (Fenton, 1975). The term appears to cover a spectrum of disorders. At the severe end of the spectrum is the patient who experiences the full narcoleptic syndrome, otherwise known as Gelineau's syndrome, which involves cataplexy, sleep paralysis and hypnagogic hallucinations, as well as the compulsive sleep attacks (Gelineau, 1880). At the other end of the spectrum is the patient who merely experiences a recurrent tendency to excessive drowsiness (Idiopathic hyper-somnolence), which may not lead to sleep and is not associated with the other features of the syndrome. The full syndrome occurs in about 10% of cases, but narcolepsy and cataplexy occur together in 70%. There may be a matter of years between the onset of narcolepsy and other components of the syndrome, but narcolepsy is usually the first to develop (Parkes, 1982).

In *cataplexy* there is a sudden reduction in muscle tone, usually only lasting a few seconds, and often precipitated by emotion, especially laughter, or sudden movement. The muscle weakness may be localized, only involving the head falling forwards, for example, or generalized, causing the patient to fall to the ground. The patient remains fully alert at all times. This sign may occur as a symptom of organic brain disease.

Sleep paralysis involves a reduction in muscle tone that usually occurs when the patient is waking up, and results in an inability to move. It can last 15 minutes, but is usually less than a minute in duration, and it may be possible to bring the patient out of the attack by touching him. Consciousness is preserved and hypnagogic hallucinations may be associated with the paralysis, this combination tending to make the experience even more frightening for the patient. This condition can occur as a benign familial disorder, unrelated to narcolepsy (Sleep, 1979).

Hypnagogic hallucinations differ from those seen in the normal population by being more vivid and having a dream-like quality. They consist of complex visual, auditory or somatosensory illusions or hallucinations, and are often unpleasant in quality. In some cases these perceptual disturbances may occur independently of the other parts of the syndrome and so create diagnostic problems.

Psychosis is more frequent in narcoleptic patients and does not appear to be entirely explicable on the basis of stimulant drug usage. The evidence is that the abuse of stimulants is uncommon in this disorder (Lishman, 1978). There is a raised incidence of other types of psychiatric illness, which appears to be the result of its psychosocial effects (Kales *et al.*, 1983).

When narcolepsy is associated with at least one of the other features of the syndrome, the sleep attacks will consist mainly of dream (REM) sleep. In such cases nocturnal sleep is characterized by an early onset of REM sleep, a normal sleep latency, and restless sleep with frequent wakenings. The hallucinatory phenomena can be understood as an abnormal tendency for REM sleep to intrude into the wakeful state. When narcolepsy alone is present the attacks may consist of non-REM sleep, they are often hypersomniac in quality, the nocturnal sleep pattern is usually normal, and there is no early REM onset during sleep. The mechanism underlying this variant of narcolepsy may be different from that involved in the Narcoleptic syndrome and involve an abnormality of the non-REM sleep mechanisms (Parkes, 1982). An underlying organic cause for narcolepsy is rarely found.

The narcolepsy responds to treatment with stimulants, e.g. methyl-phenidate, but the other features of the syndrome may require treatment with other drugs, e.g. imipramine (Murray and Pryse-Phillips, 1983). Minor tranquillisers can be used to relieve the insomnia.

The *Kleine-Levin syndrome* usually occurs in male adolescents and involves recurrent episodes during which compulsive sleeping and abnormal behaviour alternate, each episode lasting up to several weeks. At the onset of the illness, the episodes occur with a frequency of about three to four times a year. Unlike narcolepsy, which remains a lifelong disorder, these episodes tend to become less frequent and severe with time, gradually ceasing after a few years. During each episode the patient shows a pattern of social withdrawal, dysphoria and compulsive sleeping, that lasts the majority of the day. After a period of sleep, pathological overeating and, sometimes, hypersexuality, occur. Other features that are seen include dream-like experience, hallucinations in different modalities, delusions, thought disorder and restlessness. Some of these features can continue for weeks after the hypersomnia has ceased. Marked alterations of mood can occur, with the symptoms of severe depression or mania being seen. Disturbances of eating, sleeping and body temperature (pyrexia) may occur, and suggest that condition is caused by a disturbance of hypothalamic function, but no clear cause has been found. There is no evidence of any increase in neuropsychiatric morbidity in between the attacks. The EEG may be abnormal during the attack, and show a pattern of high amplitude delta activity (Gilbert, 1964). Sometimes treatment with stimulant drugs is used, though the fluctuating and ultimately benign course of the disorder, makes it difficult to assess their efficacy. A similar disorder may occasionally be seen in women at the time of menstruation (Sleep, 1979).

In *hypersomnia with "sleep drunkenness"* (HSD) there is a defect in the patient's ability to make the transition from the sleeping state to the fully awake state. The onset of the disorder is in the first half of life, it is a life-long condition and there is a family history in 30% of cases. There is some evidence that this condition may be quite common (Roth *et al.*, 1972), unlike the narcoleptic and Kleine-Levin syndromes. Rapid onset of deep and prolonged nocturnal sleep is usually present, and the patient remains drowsy and in a "drunken-like" state for a period of up to four hours after waking. Daytime sleep episodes often occur and though they are not compulsive in type, they are also associated with "drunkenness". HSD has a high psychiatric morbidity and has been found in association with most psychiatric disorders, including psychosis.

The *Sleep Apnoea syndrome* is the result of inadequate ventilation of the lungs and/or obstruction of the upper respiratory tract. Apnoea can be defined as occurring when air exchange at the nose and mouth stops for over 10 seconds (Kales *et al.*, 1983). This may cause insomnia, though there is evidence that it is common and clinically asymptomatic in many people, particularly in the elderly. In one study it was found in 25% of the normal population over 65 years of age (Sackner *et al.*, 1975). Sleep apnoea may also cause hypersomnia. It is often found in association with gross obesity, heavy smoking and excess alcohol consumption. There may be an obstruction to airflow, e.g. due to congenital or acquired obstruction of the upper airways, or a goitre. A central form of recurrent apnoea may be seen and it is discussed in the next section, because it tends to cause insomnia rather than hypersomnia. However, a combination of central and peripheral components is commonly found. A disorder of respiration during sleep should be considered in patients who fall asleep easily, snore loudly and sleep restlessly, with frequent nocturnal wakenings and apnoeic periods.

Clinically significant sleep apnoea has been particularly associated with early morning headache, secondary enuresis, personality change and a deterioration in work performance. The patient may be unaware of his apnoeic spells and it may be his spouse who describes his periods of prolonged apnoea (these may last almost a minute), which culminate in sudden loud snorting sounds. Treatment is aimed at correcting the underlying cause(s), and drugs, such as medroxyprogesterone, protryptylline or acetazolamide, have been tried with variable results. In severe cases a permanent tracheostomy may be needed because serious complications, such as cardiac dysrhythmias, may develop (Kales *et al.*, 1983; Murray and Pryse-Phillips, 1983).

Alvoeolar hypoventilation may result from many central and peripheral neurological disorders, thoracoskeletal abnormalities, or obesity. During sleep hypercapnia and hypoxaemia develop. Apnoeic periods are not present. This condition can cause hypersomnolence and/or insomnia (Sleep, 1979).

Organic brain disease usually does not cause episodic hypersomnia, prolonged sleep or drowsiness being more usual, and on waking the patient does not feel refreshed. In some cases, where drowsiness becomes severe, the patient may be incontinent of urine. This is uncommon in the sleep disorders described in Table 15.1, where the patient will usually arouse himself and attend to his toilet activities.

Two particular causes of hypersomnolence are communicating hydrocephalus, where it may be an early sign; and as a delayed consequence of head injury, developing 6 to 18 months after the traumatic event. The latter disorder shows a variable course over time (Sleep, 1979).

Vertebrobasilar migraine is a benign condition found in adolescent girls. There is usually a previous history of typical migraine. It is characterised by a gradual onset of sleep-like episodes, preceded by the clinical features of vertebrobasilar insufficiency, e.g. vivid teichopsia, diplopia, vertigo. On waking there is a severe occipital headache. The prognosis is good and the attacks usually abate over the ensuing years (Alexander, 1982).

Cerebral tumours, cerebral infarcts or cerebral infection may all produce a syndrome closely similar to narcolepsy, if they involve the posterior hypothalamus or the mid-brain tegmentum. In such cases evidence for

Table 15.2 Comparative features of certain disorders of excessive sleep

	NARCOLEPTIC SYNDROME	KLEINE–LEVIN SYNDROME	HYPERSOMNIA AND "SLEEP DRUNKENNESS"	PSYCHOGENIC
Age of Onset (in years)	10 to 40	10 to 20	Under 30	Any age
Males only affected	–	+	–	–
Family history of hypersomnia	30% of cases	–	30%	–
FEATURES OF PATHOLOGICAL SLEEP EPISODES				
Compulsive onset	+	+	–	–
Duration	10 to 15 mins.	18 to 24 hrs.	1 to 4 hrs.	Variable
Refreshed and alert on waking	+	–	–	–
EEG during	Early onset REM sleep, Phasic REM bursts	Persistent high amplitude delta activity or normal	Normal sleep reading	Normal sleep reading
BETWEEN ATTACKS				
Drowsiness	+	–	+	–
NOCTURNAL SLEEP				
Prolonged latency	–	–	–	+
Insomnia	+	–	–	+

+ = Usually present.
– = Usually absent.

diencephalic dysfunction should be looked for, including obesity (which is commonly found in idiopathic narcolepsy), diabetes insipidus with polydipsia and polyuria, memory impairment, amenorrhoea or impotence, hyperphagia, or abnormalities of the body temperature. These features may be seen in the acute and convalescent phases of encephalitis lethargica, and appear to be related to the tendency for the inflammatory process to involve the midbrain and diencephalon. Also, tuberculous meningitis can produce a similar picture, presumably due to hypothalmic damage.

Drowsiness, responding to a sweetened drink, first thing in the morning, is characteristic of hypoglycaemia due to an insulinoma (Turner *et al.*, 1981). The differential diagnosis of hypersomnia also includes hypothyroidism (Murray and Pryse-Phillips, 1983), epilepsy, myasthenia gravis and multiple sclerosis (Kales *et al.*, 1983).

A reversal of the sleep–wake cycle is characteristic of a variety of neurological conditions and in view of the association between insomnia and hypersomnia, the differential diagnosis of both conditions should be considered when either of these disorders is found to be a clinical problem.

Psychogenic hypersomnia

It is unusual for hypersomnia to be a presenting or prominent complaint, in primary psychiatric disorders. In such cases it is more likely for the sleep pattern to be disrupted, with a prolonged sleep latency and intermittent nocturnal wakenings. Some degree of compensatory daytime drowsiness, possibly exacerbated by the use of drugs, may occur. Complaints of fatigue and physical exhaustion are common and when the "hypersomniac" patient is examined during "sleep" he will often be found to be awake but merely withdrawing from social contact. Intermittent stupor with or without other catatonic features being present, may mimic hypersomnia. In some cases sleep offers an "escape" from environmental stresses and these patients show a relatively "light" pattern of sleep (Murray and Pryse-Phillips, 1983).

Hypersomnia is not uncommon in psychotic depression (Hartman, 1972), but it can also be seen in neurotic depression. In the former the REM sleep latency is shortened, the sleeping lacks a compulsive quality, and the patient does not feel refreshed after. Psychomotor retardation will usually be present during the waking periods and there should be a history of waking in the early hours of the morning. The mood will be depressed, with guilt feelings, loss of libido, anorexia and weight loss (Sleep, 1979).

15.3 ORGANIC VERSUS PSYCHOGENIC HYPERSOMNIA

Drowsiness is a normal phenomenon at certain times of the day, for example, after lunch or during relaxation at home in the evening. It is at these times that pathological hypersomnia may be most evident. To clarify the clinical significance of such drowsiness it is necessary to know to what extent it occurs in inappropriate circumstances, for example, has the patient fallen asleep while driving his car for a short distance, in the middle of a meal, or during a conversation. Enquiry should also be made about any periods for which the patient is amnesic and during which he may have behaved in a somewhat automatic manner, as a result of an episode of subclinical sleep.

Almost any psychiatric disorder can be found in association with the primary sleep disorders and, because of their early age of onset, the psychiatric features may be regarded as being an understandable consequence of the social and other stresses that are particularly prevalent at this period of life. This is particularly true when the patient is an adolescent. When the sleep disorder has been present for a prolonged period of time a secondary disruption of personality functioning may result and be misinterpreted as the primary problem. Emotional factors may affect the clinical features of the disorder, e.g. stress may provoke an exacerbation in the symptoms of narcolepsy. Also, cataplectic attacks can be provoked by emotionally charged situations.

When drowsiness occurs during the day time the patient may be suspected of drug or alcohol abuse. In HSD the ataxic, drowsy and dysarthric state of the patient may be ascribed to such causes and this disorder can be made more severe, or even precipitated, by the use of alcohol or drugs. Even in the absence of primary HSD, excessive use of sedative drugs or alcohol, or withdrawal from stimulant drugs, may cause hypersomnia.

A reduction in alertness may occur due to subclinical "sleep" attacks and result in automatic behaviour which may mimic a hysterical fugue state or some other cause of altered consciousness. However, unlike the fugue, the episodes will be relatively brief and lack the "selective" amnesia and the loss of personal identity that are characteristic of hysterical dissociative states.

Psychotic symptoms may suggest that a non-organic psychosis is present or the patient has been using psychotomimetic drugs. The compulsive sleep attacks will usually dominate the clinical picture in narcolepsy and the Kleine–Levin (K-L) syndrome. In the former, disorders of thought content (delusions) or of the process of thinking are not a feature. In the latter, though these features may be present, they will exhibit a marked periodicity. The intermittent nature of the K-L syndrome may suggest a diagnosis of periodic catatonia, but catatonic signs should not be present, though the episodes of sleeping should not be confused with stupor. If affective features are prominent an affective psychosis may be suggested, particularly of the rapid cycling type. However the young age of the patient, and the features of hypersomnia and bulimia, are against such a diagnosis.

Bulimia has been defined as the "rapid consumption of large amounts of food in a short period of time" (Casper *et al.*, 1980). It is typically seen in association with anorexia nervosa and is a poor prognostic sign, frequently reflecting a more profound disturbance of personality than that found in the non-bulimic anorexic patient (Garfinkel *et al.*, 1980). These patients fear that they will be unable to stop eating when they start. However, the sleep disturbance in anorexia nervosa typically involves a reduced TST, but psychotic symptoms and a marked periodicity, are not features of this disorder. Bulimia is also found in association with the Klüver–Bucy syndrome, diencephalic lesions, phencyclidine intoxication (Jacob *et al.*, 1981), chronic schizophrenia (Arieti, 1974), and as a manifestation of socially inappropriate eating behaviour in patients with organic brain disease. Neurotic patients may eat excessively, using food as a "comforter", but this overeating does not usually attain the level of bulimia.

If an incorrect diagnosis is made and inappropriate drug treatment instituted then the patient's response may be misleading. Use of antidepressant drugs with a stimulant effect can produce symptomatic improvement in the hypersomnias. Inappropriate use of sedative or hypnotic drugs may be dangerous, especially when the sleep apnoea syndrome is present, when they can cause respiratory depression. Such drugs may also cause deterioration in patients with HSD, as well as precipitating this disorder.

15.4 INSOMNIA

When a patient complains of insomnia it is important to find out if this refers to an excessively long sleep latency period, a short total sleep time (TST), a tendency to wake frequently, or any combination of these sleep abnormalities. In general, complaints of insomnia tend to increase in frequency with age, and patients who complain of insomnia tend to be emotionally disturbed, females from poor socio-economic and educational backgrounds. They also tend to be inaccurate in their assessment of their duration of sleep latency and TST, tending to overestimate the former and underestimate the latter. Stress factors are commonly present and should be looked for (Kales *et al.*, 1983).

Organic causes of insomnia

Table 15.3 lists the common causes of insomnia. Conditions that have been associated with this disorder are the Sleep Apnoea syndrome, myoclonus, and the "restless legs" syndrome. However, even when they have been associated with insomnia, they have not always been proven to be responsible for the sleep disturbance (Oswald, 1981).

The *Sleep Apnoea syndrome* (SAS) has been demonstrated to be particularly frequent among elderly patients, though they do not always complain of any difficulty sleeping (Kramer, 1982). In this condition there are repeated periods of apnoea during nocturnal sleep, which result in insomnia, and sometimes hypersomnia during the daytime. The two possible causes of this disorder have been mentioned: the obstructive type, where there is an interference in the passage of air through the upper respiratory tract, and the central type, where there is a periodic depression of the activity of the medullary respiratory centre. It is the latter condition which usually causes insomnia, whereas the former tends to cause hypersomnia during the daytime, though the two causes often coexist.

The features that should cause the physician to suspect SAS in the elderly patient with insomnia, are obesity, pulmonary or muscle disease, and restless sleeping, with a tendency to snore loudly. When the disorder is causing problems, treatment should be aimed at any contributory factor, a reduction of weight, a trial of drugs, or even a tracheostomy (Murray and Pryse-Phillips, 1983).

Table 15.3   Causes of insomnia

Alcohol	
Blood vessel disease	Angina, cardiac dysrhythmias, left ventricular failure, aortic incompetence, cerebral infarction, "Cluster" headaches, occipital neuralgia
Drugs	Sedatives, caffeine, propanolol, steroids, bronchodilators, stimulants
Epilepsy	Nocturnal seizures
Functional	Neurosis, psychosis, personality disorder
Gastrointestinal	Duodenal ulcer, oesophagitis and gastric reflux
Growth	Intracerebral mass
Hypoxia	Sleep apnoea, asthma, alveolar hypoventilation
Idiopathic	
Injury	Post-traumatic neurosis
Neurological	Mycolonus, "Restless Legs" (Ekbom's) syndrome

SAS is a particularly important condition, not only because of its psychiatric implications, but also because the injudicious use of sedative drugs in these patients may produce a potentially dangerous depression of the respiratory centre. It may be relevant to the pathophysiological basis of this disorder that there is evidence of a raised incidence of "Sudden Infant Death syndrome" or a history of an unexplained death in a young adult, among the relatives of these patients. Sleep apnoea has been implicated as the cause, in some cases, of the former (Sleep, 1979).

Psychiatric disturbance is frequent in these patients and they can show a wide spectrum of neuropsychiatric problems, including impairment of cognition, mood disturbance, aggression, and automatic behaviour which may last up to several hours and for which the patient is totally amnesic. Hypnagogic hallcuinations may be present.

The *"Restless Legs"* syndrome involves a feeling of discomfort and restlessness in the legs at night, with an urge to move them. It has been seen in a variety of disorders, especially following withdrawal of sedatives after long-term usage. It has also been seen in motor neurone disease, uraemia, hypocalcemia, vitamin E deficiency, pregnancy, and in association with a low serum iron. Some cases may be familial and it is found as an idiopathic phenomenon in 5% of the population.

Nocturnal myoclonus consists of brief muscular jerks of the legs, usually at the onset of sleep. It may involve one or both legs and the jerks can occur repeatedly for periods of up to an hour or two. It is usually a normal phenomenon. It can become clinically significant if it is persistant or occurs frequently, during the night. There is usually no apparent cause, though other conditions, e.g. uraemia, should be considered. If treatment is required the benzodiazepines are often effective. The condition is possibly due to neuronal discharges in the pyramidal system, resulting from a reduction in neuronal inhibition (Murray and Pryse-Phillips, 1983).

A profound disruption of sleep can occur as a result of *alcohol abuse or alcohol withdrawal*, and may persist despite many months of sobriety. *Sedative or hypnotic drugs* are frequently used to induce sleep and prolonged use of such drugs can cause insomnia, the patients developing withdrawal effects as the action of the drug wears off before the morning. Though such drugs may be effective in correcting insomnia in the early stages of use, after about a couple of weeks the patient tends to go back to his original sleep pattern, with the insomnia becoming worse as a rebound phenomenon. Barbiturates tend to maintain their effects on sleep for only a few days, benzodiazepines for 2 to 3 weeks, and sedative drugs in general are not effective for more than 1 month (Mullen, 1980). So what may have been used initially as a treatment for insomnia, may eventually act to perpetuate the insomnia. A whole variety of non-sedative preparations, including such drugs as propanolol, caffeine and aspirin, may have a disrupting effect on sleep, and if the physician is in doubt he should consult the appropriate literature and, if possible, encourage the patient to take a trial period off the medication.

Sleep can be a potent activator of *epileptic seizures*. They are probably caused by a reduction in pyramidal neuronal inhibition. Sleep-related epilepsy is most commonly found in children. The seizures may be tonic, tonic–clonic, myoclonic or temporal lobe in origin (TLE). Most common are the tonic seizures seen in the Lennox–Gastaut syndrome. In about 20% of epileptics seizures remain confined to sleep. 35% of epileptics experience seizures during sleeping *and* waking hours. TLE should be considered in the differential diagnosis of sleepwalking, and when a ''recurrent and stereotyped dream content'' is experienced (Sleep, 1979).

Cerebral tumours and many acute and chronic cerebral infections may cause insomnia, particularly if the brain stem or hypothalamus are involved. Degenerative, vascular and traumatic disorders of the CNS, may also be responsible. For a more detailed list the reader is referred to Sleep (1979).

Psychogenic insomnia

Insomnia is a complaint most frequently associated with the middle or later part of life and is more common in females. It can be divided into the primary and secondary types. The primary type is usually associated with a long history which may go back to childhood, and extensive investigations, including polysomnography, usually shows no causative abnormality. Treatment is difficult and sedative or hypnotic drugs are of limited value. A shorter history and a better prognosis characterise the secondary type.

Insomnia is a common accompaniment to most psychiatric disorders, though the patient does not always complain of it. Sleep disturbance in the initial half of the night tends to be related to mood disorders, particularly anger and tension (Crisp, 1980). Neurotically anxious patients frequently have a prolonged sleep latency and lie awake at night preoccupied with their problems. If autonomic symptoms develop, e.g. dyspnoea or palpitations, this can lead to a vicious cycle of further anxiety, as a result of the patient's concern about his physical health, and further autonomic over-activity, sometimes culminating in a panic attack. Characteristically these patients dread facing the world on waking in the early morning and experience an exacerbation in their anxiety at that time. A disturbance of sleep with frequent waking during the night can often also be seen.

Patients with endogenous depression do not show consistent differences in the quality of their insomnia, when compared with neurotic patients. The insomnia in the former group tends to be more marked in the later part of the night, a prolonged sleep latency may not be present and they may have early onset REM sleep. Patients with this type of depression tend to wake in the early hours of the morning experiencing profound feelings of misery and having difficulty getting back to sleep. Such a symptom may be an early sign of severe depression, and in the initial stages of a "masked depression", may be the only sign, particularly in the elderly. Severe weight loss is often associated with depressive illness, but weight loss of any type, whether or not it is associated with an affective disturbance, tends to cause insomnia, particularly affecting sleep in the later part of the night (Crisp, 1980). This has been noted in patients with anorexia nervosa, who rarely complain of their insomnia.

The behaviour exhibited by a patient who gets up in the night will often give some indication of the cause of his insomnia. Patients with anorexia nervosa characteristically exhibit motor over-activity. Similarly, patients with mania, though they often have a normal sleep latency, tend to require only a few hours of sleep before they get up and about, leaving their bed and engaging in a variety of jobs. They do not complain of their sleep disturbance. In contrast, the patient with organic brain disease tends to wake at night and exhibit disorganised behaviour that is not appropriately goal-directed. He often exhibits disorientation for time and place, at such times.

A prolonged sleep latency, with frequent wakenings, is also common in acute schizophrenia, acute exacerbations of chronic schizophrenia, and obsessional neurosis. Obsessional patients often have difficulty in relaxing sufficiently to initiate sleep at night and this may be made worse by the presence of obsessional ruminations. Such patients often find it easier to sleep away from their beds, as they feel compelled to engage in rituals when in their own bedrooms. Stable chronic schizophrenics tend to have no disturbance of their sleep pattern.

15.5 DISORDERS OF THE SLEEP–WAKE SCHEDULE

Transient disturbances of sleep, of this type, are experienced by most people who have had a disturbance of their circadian rhythm. Such a disturbance may occur as a result of "jet-leg", after travelling across a time-zone, or as a result of working irregular hours. It takes a short period of time to recover.

More persistent reversal of the sleep–wake cycle is characteristic of certain neurological conditions, e.g. encephalitis, senile dementia, uraemia, diabetes mellitus, trypanosomiasis, hepatic encephalopathy, and it may be a presenting feature in primary polycythaemia (when the patient may also complain of a fullness in the head, dizziness and pruritis). Some disturbance of sleep pattern is to be expected after any neurological insult, such as a head injury, that affects the nervous system above the level of the foramen magnum.

15.6 DYSFUNCTIONS ASSOCIATED WITH SLEEP, SLEEP STAGES, OR PARTIAL AROUSALS

Sleep walking (somnambulism), sleep terrors (pavor nocturnus), head banging (jactatio capitis nocturna), sleep talking (somniloquy), and enuresis, are sometimes referred to as parasomnias. They are usually found in children, occur in the early part of the night, during non-REM sleep (the reduction in muscle tone that characterises REM sleep, precludes motor activity), and the patient is usually amnesic for the event. Because of the sleep stage involved these disorders may respond to the benzodiazepines (e.g. flurazepam), which suppress stage 3 and 4 sleep.

If the patient is woken by pain, this is a significant finding. *It is unusual for psychogenic pain to wake the patient from sleep.* Nocturnal head pain is most characteristic of cluster headaches, occipital neuralgia, and intracranial tumours. Cluster headaches consist of paroxysms of severe pain in one eye and the adjacent part of the face, associated with rhinorrhoea and lachrymation. They may last up to 2 hours and occur in periodic bursts, for a few weeks at a time. This pain characteristically wakes the patient in the early hours of the morning. Occipital neuralgia tends to be found in the elderly and results from cervical spondylosis causing pressure on the sensory nerve roots. Intracranial tumours cause pain mainly due to traction on cerebral blood vessels and the pain is initially periodic and made worse by anything that increases intracranial pressure, such as coughing and stooping. This pain may wake the patient at night or may be present on waking, and is typically associated with vomiting and papilloedema. Pain elsewhere in the body may occur during sleep, e.g. in the chest (angina), or in the abdomen (oesophageal reflux or duodenal ulcer). Other physical disorders may occur during sleep and wake the patient, including asthma and cardiac failure.

CHAPTER 16

Disorders of Perception

16.1 INTRODUCTION

A physically and mentally healthy person can produce an image, in any modality, in his mind. This ability is under his control and the image is capable of being altered at will. The images are experienced as being in subjective space (in his mind), as opposed to objective space (in the outside world). The ability to create images varies with different people and it is children who particularly have the ability to create very vivid (eidetic) images of previous visual perceptions, sometime after the visual percept is no longer present. These images differ from after-images, which involve a true perception remaining in the mind for a brief period immediately after the stimulus is no longer present. The "photographic" memory is a different phenomenon and involves a person being able to create an image in his mind of a previous perception that was experienced some time (possibly years) previously. In this rare condition, the image is remarkable for the accurate detail it involves.

An illusion occurs when a real perception is distorted in some way. We are all capable of such misperceptions given the appropriate state of mind and circumstances, e.g. when sitting alone at night watching a frightening film on television, a creaking floor may be misinterpreted as the footsteps of an intruder. Illusions can also be morbid phenomena and frequently co-exist with hallucinations.

It is difficult to define a *hallucination* in a satisfactory way. The DSM III (1980) describes it as *"a sensory perception without external stimulation of the relevant sensory organ"*. Such a description could include dreams. If we exclude such phenomena by specifying that clear consciousness must be present, then hallucinations, by definition, do not occur in delirium! Mullen (1979) suggested that hallucinations "proper" are false perceptions and that the criteria for their presence requires that they occur in objective space, concurrently with true perceptions (thus excluding dreams), are not under voluntary control, and have the features of true perceptions, i.e. qualities such as vividness, wholeness and immediacy. However in many cases perceptual abnormalities will have some, but not all of these characteristics, and these can be described as pseudohallucinations.

The *pseudohallucination* has some of the properties of a mental image, lacks the qualities of a normal perception and occurs in subjective space. They are usually experienced in clear consciousness. Though they are not under voluntary control, they tend to be experienced as one's own thoughts and are not accessible to others. Hare (1973) felt that the most important distinguishing point between true hallucinations and pseudohallucinations is the fact that only in the former is the patient convinced of the reality of his perceptions and expects other people present to be having the same experience. An example of the latter can be seen in the normal course of a bereavement reaction, when the bereaved person sees the deceased person or hears him talking. Such a view clearly imparts a greater morbid significance to true hallucinations. To a certain extent hallucinations can be regarded as the opposite and more pathological end of a spectrum of perceptual disorders, with illusions being at the other end and pseudohallucinations being somewhere in between.

When a patient has a hallucination, it is a subjective experience. The lack of an objective stimulus that is responsible, can be confirmed, in many cases, by the report of a secondary informant who was present at the time, or by the very nature of the percept (which may have been impossibly bizarre). Whether the cause of the phenomena is organic or psychogenic, is another problem. When such an experience is entirely subjective it raises the question of whether it is a delusion or an hallucination. Berrios (1982) rejects the importance of such a separation and says that the absence of a sensory stimulus, the quality of the morbid percept, and the relationship of this percept to (the) contextual field of normal perception, are of little significance in the recognition or diagnosis of hallucinations.

For the purposes of this chapter there will be no attempt to discriminate between true hallucinations and pseudohallucinations. The author will be concerned with those phenomena that can be reasonably described as hallucinations, on the basis of the patient incorrectly regarding them as the result of some sensory stimulus. As Baldwin and Hofman (1969) put it, probably the most practical differentiation of pathological from non-pathological hallucinations, is whether they are "totally absorbing experiences, inseparable from reality, or . . . quite clearly distinguished from immediate reality at the time of occurrence and never so confused in subsequent recollection."

Perceptual abnormalities are particularly prone to occur when consciousness is impaired, either pathologically, as in delirium, or as part of normal experience, as in hypnagogic hallucinations. *Hypnagogic hallucinations are disorders of perception occurring at the onset of sleep or on waking.* In the latter case they are called hypnapompic (Parkes, 1982). They may occur in any sensory modality, are experienced as alien and intrusive, and have a "dream-like" quality. These experiences may be relatively simple, e.g. a sudden feeling of falling (often accompanied by myoclonic jerking), hearing one's name being called, or seeing coloured designs. They can be more complex though, involving frightening faces or landscapes. They tend to be evanescent in quality, changing from one moment to the next and involving an element of movement. They are probably common experiences, but are often not recalled (Oswald, 1969). They can occur in neuro-psychiatric disorders and are particularly vivid and frightening in narcolepsy, in contrast to the unremarkable content of these patients' dreams (Roth and Bruhova, 1969). Hypnagogic hallucinations are also seen in chronic alcoholism, delirium (Lipowski, 1980) and other organic brain disorders.

Organic hallucinosis is one of the DSM III organic mental disorders, and *the criteria for this diagnosis include hallucinations occurring in clear consciousness, intact cognition (a diagnosis of dementia should not be appropriate) and no prominent mood disorder or delusions. In addition, an organic cause should be present*, and it will usually be alcohol or drugs (LSD, mescaline, bromide, cocaine, amphetamines, etc.).

Many varied factors have been implicated in contributing to the development of hallucinations, and in some cases several of them are interacting together. These factors include disturbances of affect (especially anxiety), age, organic brain disease, suggestion, sleep deprivation, sensory overload, sensory deprivation or sensory monotony (a lack of variation in sensory stimulation), immobility, and impairment of the primary sense organs, e.g. blindness or deafness (Lipowski, 1980).

In the following sections, the causes and differential diagnosis of abnormalities of perception will be discussed, and particular attention will be paid to those found in *temporal lobe epilepsy* (TLE). Unless otherwise stated, reference to the occurrence of a phenomenon in TLE will mean that it is the direct behavioural or experiential result of an actual seizure discharge, i.e. it is ictal. The emphasis on TLE is because of the importance of this disorder in neuropsychiatry and because the symptoms and signs resulting from a focal epileptic discharge increase our understanding about brain–behaviour relation-ships. In some cases of focal brain lesions the nature of the perceptual abnormality may suggest the site of the focus. Focal seizures originating from the primary sensory cortex tend to produce simple hallucinations, e.g. unformed flashes of light or tinnitus. Those arising from the cortical association areas tend to cause more complex phenomena, e.g. detailed visions of people or music. One case reported by Penfield and Jasper (1954) experienced seizures involving visual hallucinations of coloured triangles, which then gradually changed to a vision of a man approaching the patient with a gun. The increase in complexity of this hallucination was felt to reflect the spread of the seizure discharge away from the primary visual cortex in the occipital lobe, to the temporal lobe. However, subcortical disease and even brain stem disorders can produce hallucinations which may be highly complex and not explainable as the result of an altered conscious level.

Table 16.1 shows the relative frequency of different types of ictal experiences in a population of 666 patients with TLE (Currie *et al.*, 1971). Many of these phenomena may also be seen as a result of a focal seizure discharge without impairment of consciousness, in which case they can be described as simple (as opposed to complex) partial seizures. Alternatively, perceptual abnormalities may occur as a result of focal brain disease but unassociated with an ictal discharge, e.g. palinopsia. *Palinopsia is "the persistence of a visual sensation after viewing an object or a setting within the environment"* (Feldman and Bender, 1970), e.g. in one case, 7 days after looking at the number "29" on a tin can, the image recurred to such a degree and with such vividness, that the patient was unable to read a newspaper. Palinopsia usually involves part of an object that has just been seen beforehand and occurs in a defective field of vision, usually with other abnormalities of visual perception, e.g. hallucinations. It is particularly associated with right parieto-occipital tumours. The hallucinations may be multiple, can last from seconds to hours, are recurrent, and usually do not occur in a field where vision is totally lost. They may be ictal or precede epileptic seizures; they may resemble "after-images" (persistence of an image after the responsible stimulus is no longer present); in other cases none of these explanations are satisfactory and the experience is regarded as some other type of organic hallucination, or a psychogenic phenomenon of the type seen in the psychoses. A similar somatosensory experience may be seen with parietal lobe lesions and is called palisomaesthesia (Feldman and Bender, 1970).

The patient's level of consciousness may have been impaired during his experience and this may be indicated by the report of an observer, or by the manner in which the patient describes his experiences. There will usually be an impaired memory of some or all of the event. Delirium or TLE should be suspected in such cases. A high level of emotional arousal can interfere with conscious awareness (Antoni, 1946) and this may occur in phobic anxiety attacks, where perceptual distortions, including déjà vu, body image disturbances

Table 16.1 Components of seizures in a sample of 666 patients with TLE

COMPONENT OF ATTACK	% OF PATIENTS
Visceral	40
Thought disorder	27
Déjà Vu	14
Other time disorder	3
Speech disorders	22
Vertigo	19
Special sensory components	
Visual	18
Auditory	16
Olfactory	12
Gustatory	3
Motor phenomena	14
Adversive	0.5
Masticatory	10
Sensory phenomena	2
Emotional disorders	19

From S. Currie *et al.* (1971). *Brain*, vol. **94**, pp.173–90. Reproduced by permission of Oxford University Press.

(depersonalisation) and even hallucinations may sometimes occur (Harper and Roth, 1962). Hyperventilation can cause a dreamy state, "formication" and even visual hallucinations on occasions (Pincus, 1978; Riley, 1982). The subject of altered consciousness is discussed further in Chapter 13.

The patients reaction to his experiences will depend on their content, the circumstances under which they arise, his previous experiences, his affective state and his premorbid personality. Fear is a normal response when any unusual experience occurs for the first time and the patient is unaware of the cause. Pleasure is commonly experienced with "Lilliputian" hallucinations or when the perceptual distortion has been deliberately induced by drugs, especially stimulants or psychotomimetics. Depression or elation will be present when an affective illness is responsible, and the content of the experience will usually be consonant with the patient's mood. The depressed patient may see visions of hell or hear voices accusing him of crimes. The manic patient may see visions of angels and hear voices acclaiming him as an important and special person. Indifference to such experiences may be found in chronic schizophrenia, hysteria and advanced dementia. In some cases the depressed or schizophrenic patient may attempt to harm himself in response to hallucinatory "commands" to do so. The alcoholic, schizophrenic or delirious patient may attack those who he feels are responsible for auditory hallucinations that are insulting or persecutory. In TLE, an affective disturbance, usually dysphoric, commonly occurs during the seizure, and such dysphoric states sometimes remain for several days after the seizure has ceased. However, the seizure may have the effect of relieving an unpleasant mood that has developed for several days prior to the seizure, until the "build-up" of dysphoria occurs again before the next seizure.

16.2 VISUAL HALLUCINATIONS AND ILLUSIONS

Table 16.2 shows the important conditions associated with visual hallucinations. *Visual hallucinations are frequently caused by organic brain disease*, evidence of which will usually be found, though it may be necessary to look carefully for it (Bell and Hall, 1977).

In temporal lobe epilepsy visual perceptual abnormalities are common. Illusions may occur involving distortions of size, shape or distance. Alterations in the form of objects is called dysmegalopsia, e.g. this may involve objects appearing larger (macropsia) or smaller (micropsia) than they really are. These illusions have little value as localising signs. When micropsia involves hallucinations of people, they are called Lilliputian and are typically associated with a pleasurable affect. They can be found in delirium, often due to alcohol, and in peduncular hallucinosis. When hallucinations are associated with such an affect, deliberate drug abuse, for the purpose of inducing perceptual and affective distortions, should be considered.

If visual hallucinations are brief, stereotyped, and acute in onset and cessation, epilepsy should be suspected. Less often focal brain lesions may produce these phenomena without an associated epileptic discharge, but such cases are often associated with a visual field defect and the hallucinations are "seen" in the "blind" area of vision. This has been mentioned with regard to palinopsia.

In *delirium* any sensory modality may be involved, though visual hallucinations are the commonest type and are found in 40 to 75% of cases (Lipowski, 1980). Illusions are a feature of the early stages of delirium and they are usually associated with the experience of fear. In delirium tremens (DT), which develops in the chronic alcoholic patient, usually on the third or fourth day of withdrawal from alcohol, the patient is usually frightened and over-active and the delirium conforms to the "hyperactive" type. When examining the patient it should be remembered that the DTs may be precipitated by a head injury or an infection, and alcohol withdrawal is not always essential for its development.

In the early stages of the DTs the patient may experience an increase in dreaming, with nightmares and hypnagogic phenomena. The hallucinations vary in their content and may include complex scenes or Lilliputian hallucinations. Visions of rapidly moving small animals are particularly characteristic. Alcohol supresses REM sleep and withdrawal leads to a rebound increase of REM activity, and it is probably the intrusion of this activity into non-sleep periods that causes these perceptual abnormalities. The clinical picture seen in the DTs is not pathognomomic, and other causes of delirium should be considered in such cases. Visual hallucinations are less marked in the hypo-active type of delirium, especially in the elderly patient (Lipowski, 1980).

If epilepsy and delirium are excluded there is no clear relationship between either operative removal of a part of the brain or a localised lesion in the brain, and subsequent hallucinations (Baldwin, 1970). This contrasts with the work of Wilder Penfield who produced hallucinations by *electrical stimulation of the exposed cortex of the temporal lobe,* during surgery. The conscious patient would describe his psychic experiences during the period of stimulation and Penfield mapped out the functions of different areas of the brain based on this data. He found visual hallucinations produced by stimulation in the region of the primary visual cortex were simple, and if the posterior temporal association areas were stimulated, they were complex (Penfield and Perot, 1963). Penfield felt that the electrical stimulation produced hallucinations by activating records of past experience. However, Horowitz and Adams (1970) found that the hallucinations they produced by depth stimulation of the temporal lobe, could not always be explained as prior perceptual experiences and were sometimes related to the patient's mental content pre-operatively. They felt that some of these hallucinations were products of the patient's imagination and that previous perceptions were revived "in order to construct representations of ideas and affects".

Non-organic disorders less often cause visual hallucinations. Visual hallucinations in delirious patients were found to differ from those found in the non-organic psychoses by more often involving moving objects, by preferentially occurring at night, by being briefer in duration, and because their content had less personal significance (Frieske and Wilson, 1966). In the affective

Table 16.2 Causes of perceptual abnormalities in the visual modality

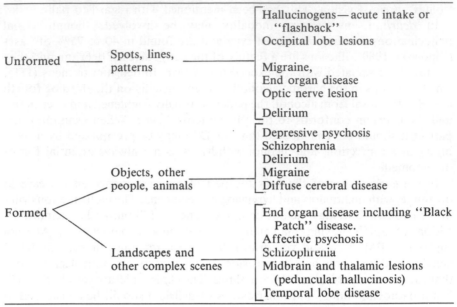

Unformed	Spots, lines, patterns	Hallucinogens—acute intake or "flashback" Occipital lobe lesions Migraine, End organ disease Optic nerve lesion Delirium
Formed	Objects, other people, animals	Depressive psychosis Schizophrenia Delirium Migraine Diffuse cerebral disease
	Landscapes and other complex scenes	End organ disease including "Black Patch" disease. Affective psychosis Schizophrenia Midbrain and thalamic lesions (peduncular hallucinosis) Temporal lobe disease

psychoses the content of the hallucinations is more consistent with the patient's affective state.

Cerebral ischaemia may produce visual perceptual abnormalities confined to one part of the visual field. *Migraine* should be suspected when such phenomena are followed by a severe throbbing headache, which is unilateral for at least part of the attack, lasts many hours, incapacitates the patient, and is associated with nausea, vomiting and photophobia. The headache is due to vasodilation and the initial visual "aura" to cerebral vasoconstriction. The most typical aura, when the vasospasm involves branches of the internal carotid artery, is the fortification spectra. This is an irregular coloured crescent of light with multicoloured edges, which develops close to the centre of the visual field and gradually expands, decreasing in intensity, into one half of the visual field, leaving an area of darkness in its wake. The progression lasts 15 to 30 minutes and diagnostic difficulties may arise if the headache does not develop or is only very slight. Other visual phenomena include small bright dots (teichopsia) or large scotomata with scintillating edges (Gawel, 1983).

In vertebrobasilar migraine the aura lasts 10 to 45 minutes and involves vivid teichopsia and the loss or impairment of vision in part or the whole of the visual fields. Its association with menstruation, adolescent girls, brain stem signs (e.g. dysarthria etc.), impaired consciousness and the subsequent development of a severe occipital headache, should suggest the diagnosis (Bickerstaff, 1961).

The migrainous aura usually occurs in clear consciousness and so could be described as a hallucinosis. Drug ingestion is a common cause of visual hallucinosis and it is usually due to the hallucinogens (LSD and mescaline). Other perceptual distortions occur with these drugs and they particularly involve the body image. *Synaesthesiae are characteristic of hallucinogen use.* In this phenomenon a real percept in one modality (e.g. hearing a knocking sound), evokes a hallucination in another modality (e.g. seeing a flash of light). Such hallucinogen-induced hallucinations usually do not last over 48 hours and are associated with the signs of sympathetic over-activity (mydriasis, hypertension, tachycardia, sweating and tremor). Other drugs that can produce visual hallucinosis include the stimulants (amphetamines) and alcohol, and it may occur as an idiosyncratic effect of psychotropic and other drugs.

Hallucinosis is not usually the result of a focal brain lesion. However, it may be seen as a manifestation of lesions of the mid-brain tegmentum or in the region of the diencephalon, when it is called *"peduncular hallucinosis"*. This condition typically involves vivid and complex hallucinations, e.g. detailed visions of people, animals or landscapes, which are often "Lilliputian" in type. The hallucinations may last for years, are particularly found in the elderly and associated with vertigo and visual impairment. The cause of the latter symptom is not clear (Benson and Geschwind, 1975).

Hallucinogenic drugs can cause perceptual alterations in any of the sensory modalities. They also cause the phenomenon of *"flashbacks"* which *are the return "of imagery or recurrence of psychedelic drug effects"*, though these may occur with other drugs as well (Alarcon *et al.*, 1982). They are found in about a quarter of drug abusers. The natural course is for these phenomena to become less frequent with time, though they may occur on a daily basis initially. A number of drug abusers experience an increasing frequency of these attacks, over a period of time, and they may continue to be affected despite not using drugs for over a year. These flashback phenomena are usually visual and have been found to be facilitated by alcohol and stress (Matefy *et al.*, 1978), by the frequency and amount of drug used, and by cannabis (which can itself produce flashback experiences). The cause of "flashbacks" is unknown but may be related to organic brain disease (Alarcon *et al.*, 1982). It is a condition that can cause diagnostic confusion as it can involve a variety of experiences including depersonalisation and confusional episodes. It may be misdiagnosed as TLE, though the episodes have a more gradual onset and cessation than those of TLE. Treatment is by reassurance, avoiding precipitating factors, and major tranquillisers may be helpful. Many of these patients have underlying personality disturbance or psychosis (Breakey *et al.*, 1974).

A curious phenomenon is the discolouration of visual perceptions, which may appear yellow or green, for example. This has been found as a side effect of digitalis and other glycosides. Santonin, an anti-helminthic drug found in oil of wormwood, can produce purple vision.

End-organ disorders can result in hallucinations. Visual hallucinations that can be simple or complex can result from damage to the structure of the eyes, e.g. as a result of disease or surgery. It is not clear how important a role cerebral impairment may play in predisposing the patient to hallucinate in many of these cases. However, in "black-patch" disease (post-operative delirium following cataract surgery), organic brain disease often appears to be present (Hamilton, 1974). Lesions of the visual pathways between the eye and the thalamus do not usually cause hallucinations.

Visual hallucinations can occur in *schizophrenia and other non-organic psychoses*. In the former they are usually associated with auditory hallucinations, delusions and thought disorder. Illusions are common at the onset of schizophrenia, and the socially withdrawn chronic schizophrenic is particularly predisposed to develop pareidolic illusions, e.g. seeing faces in the clouds or in the flames of a fire.

Hallucinations can occur as *hysterical conversion phenomena* and their aetiology may be indicated by a dramatic quality to their description, the details of which may be changed from one occasion to the next, possibly being susceptible to alteration by suggestion. They may resemble emotionally disturbing events from the patient's past and be related to the doctor in the manner of a story, often without any evidence of the appropriate accompanying emotional distress, though they may be disturbing to the patient when they are experienced (Fitzgerald and Wells, 1977; Modai *et al.*, 1980).

16.3 AUDITORY HALLUCINATIONS AND ILLUSIONS

Auditory hallucinations in clear consciousness are most commonly associated with schizophrenia. Probably the most important exception to this generalisation is the organic hallucinosis that is associated with *chronic alcohol abuse*. The hallucinations usually start within 12 hours of ceasing alcohol intake. They are often simple unformed sounds initially, which then develop into voices which tend to be insulting and threatening. The voices may be recognised as friends or relatives. In 90% of cases they stop within a week, but they continue as a chronic phenomenon in about 5%. Recurrent alcoholic hallucinosis seems to predispose to chronicity. If they are present after 6 months of sobriety they are probably going to remain chronic and these patients may be difficult to differentiate from chronic schizophrenics, particularly as the voices may be phenomenologically identical to Schneider's first rank symptoms of schizophrenia (see below). These patients with chronic hallucinosis, differ from chronic schizophrenic patients in lacking a schizoid premorbid personality and a genetic predisposition to the disorder, but they do develop paranoid delusions and emotional withdrawal (Victor and Hope, 1958). However, they should be differentiated from those patients with pre-existing schizophrenia who drink alcohol in order to try and get rid of their auditory hallucinations. Withdrawal of alcohol in schizophrenic patients may cause an exacerbation of their psychosis.

Organic disorders should be suspected if the auditory hallucinations are only simple (clicking, buzzing, ringing, etc.) of if they are associated with impaired consciousness. Common causes of such auditory experiences are listed in Table 16.3. Simple auditory hallucinations are associated with a lesion of Heschl's gyrus, salicylates, and disease of the middle ear and auditory nerve. More complex phenomena suggest involvement of the association areas of the temporal lobe. Either simple (tinnitus) or complex (phrases or passages of music) hallucinations, may occur as epileptic phenomena. In TLE auditory perceptual abnormalities are common and may involve the illusion of sounds changing in intensity or pitch.

In delirium, auditory perceptual abnormalities are common. Hallucinations may be simple or complex, and are often combined with visual hallucinations.

Drugs may produce auditory hallucinosis, particularly amphetamines which can produce persistent hallucinoses with a paranoid content. This drug can also produce flattening of affect.

Table 16.3   Causes of perceptual abnormalities in the auditory modality

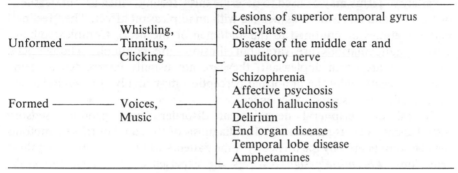

Unformed	Whistling, Tinnitus, Clicking	Lesions of superior temporal gyrus Salicylates Disease of the middle ear and auditory nerve
Formed	Voices, Music	Schizophrenia Affective psychosis Alcohol hallucinosis Delirium End organ disease Temporal lobe disease Amphetamines

Schizophrenia is the commonest cause of auditory perceptual abnormalities in clear consciousness, and though all varieties of hallucinations or illusions can occur, certain types are particularly characteristic. Schneider (1957) described four characteristic, though not pathognomonic, types of hallucinations particularly associated with this diagnosis and which form part of his first rank symptoms. These are—voices discussing the patient and referring to him in the third person, voices commenting on the patient's actions, and voices repeating the patient's thoughts immediately after he has experienced them (giving the impression of his thoughts being spoken aloud inside his head). The latter is also called "écho de la pensée" or "gedankenlautwerden". Other Schneiderian first rank symptoms are autochthonous (primary) delusions, passivity experiences, and thought-withdrawal, insertion and broadcasting.

Functional hallucinations are sometimes seen in chronic schizophrenia and consist of a true perception causing and being experienced at the same time as, a hallucination (such as hearing a clock ticking and hallucinating a voice at the same time, the voice stopping when the clock is removed). This type of hallucination does not seem to have any particular importance except in so far as it offers a way of stopping a particular hallucination.

Auditory illusions may be seen in the neuroses, and hallucinations can occasionally occur as hysterical conversion phenomena (Fitzgerald and Wells, 1977; Modai *et al.*, 1980). As mentioned in the previous section, the affective psychoses should be suspected if the content of the hallucinations is consonant with the patient's predominant affect.

16.4 DISORDERS OF SOMATIC AND VISCERAL PERCEPTION

The term somatic is used here to refer to the body, excluding the internal organs (viscera) and the nervous system (Drever, 1964). *Visceral experiences are probably the commonest perceptual abnormality found in TLE* and the commonest aura consists of a "feeling" in the abdomen, rising up into the head. A variety of terms may be used to describe this "feeling" such as "butterflies" or "pain", and it is usually associated with an unpleasant affect. The "feeling" may sometimes be confined to the abdomen or the head. Complex somato-sensory hallucinations are rare, but illusions are common. Though ictal experiences are often unpleasant, they are not usually interpreted as being painful. Occasionally the abnormal perception may involve the genitalia and have quality of a sexual experience.

Central or peripheral neurological disorders may produce sensory disturbances, such as paraethesia. The diagnosis of the cause of these symptoms may be complicated by the difficulty some patients will have in describing these sensations. *Lhermitte's sign* involves the experience of electric shock-like sensations radiating down the body and limbs. It is produced by a lesion in the medullary region of the brain stem, it is usually triggered by neck flexion, and it is commonly found in subacute combined degeneration of the cord and multiple sclerosis (Jones, 1964). It is mentioned here because it demonstrates the problems encountered in evaluating such experiences. In a study of how this phenomenon was described by patients who had experienced it, terms such as "pain", "ripple or shiver", "hair standing on end", and "fizzing", were used (Kanchandani and Howe, 1982). In this series, it was found to be a common symptom in the first attack of multiple sclerosis and could occasionally be the first. Under such circumstances it is possible to see how a psychogenic cause for it could be considered, particularly in view of the psychiatric problems and diagnostic difficulties associated with disorders, such as multiple sclerosis and vitamin B_{12} deficiency. Mullen (1979) emphasised that "care must be . . . exercised to distinguish odd ways of expressing true sensory disturbances from the delusional elaborations of false perceptions" and that "a bizarre interpretation . . . of a somatic sensation in a schizophrenic may mask the symptom of a physical disorder."

Formication is a disagreeable creeping sensation in the skin. It is a tactile hallucination that is usually associated with cocaine intoxication (15% of cases) and typically occurs in clear consciousness (Berrios, 1982). Cocaine-induced formication tends to be preceded by visual hallucinations and pruritis (Siegel, 1978). They are more common after the prolonged (over 6 months) intravenous use of cocaine. Other causes for tactile hallucinations include the belladonna alkaloids, chloral, amphetamines, diabetes mellitus, hypophyseal tumour, brain damage, dementia, and hyperventilation (Berrios, 1982; Riley, 1982).

In depressive psychosis *nihilistic delusions* of bodily change (Cotard's syndrome) may be confused with somatic hallucinations. They can be expressed in terms such as "there is nothing inside my head" or "my bowels have turned to stone". This disorder is usually found in the middle-aged or elderly, two groups who are particularly prone to develop delusions of parasitic infestation, otherwise known as delusional parasitosis or delusional zoopathy. In one sample of 46 cases of delusions of infestation, abnormal EEGs were found in 61%, evidence of organic brain disease in 50%, and 12% had malignant disease (Skott, 1978, quoted in Berrios, 1982). Such figures emphasise the importance of being careful before assessing the diagnostic significance of a delusional elaboration of tactile hallucinations, e.g. "crawling of ants". Fish (Hamilton, 1974) described a case of a person who, for 7 years, thought he was infested by a small animal, until he died and post mortem examination revealed a thalamic tumour. A sensory deficit will usually be present when an organic lesion is responsible for somatic hallucinations, but not necessarily in epilepsy or parietal lobe lesions.

Pain is not perceived at the cerebral cortical level and is not usually experienced as an ictal phenomenon. The parenchyma and pia-arachnoid tissues are insensitive to pain, and it is the cranial sinuses, the dura mater and the vessels of the brain, that are the pain sensitive structures above the level of the thalamus. Pain is seen in association with thalamic lesions, when it has a "burning" quality and is poorly localised. It is also seen with lesions of the central nervous system caudal to the thalamus.

The quality of the description of the pain is of little use in determining whether it is organic or non-organic in origin, in the absence of other information. Attempts to identify differences in the pain experiences of patients with or without organic lesions, have not been successful (Trimble, 1981a).

Complaints of pain are frequently seen in neurotic and non-organic psychotic conditions, and can be a manifestation of masked depression. The experience of pain is subjective and in chronic cases, where the cause is not clear, the psychological contribution can be difficult to evaluate, particularly as superimposed depression or anxiety are only to be expected as reactive phenomena.

16.5 OTHER DISORDERS OF PERCEPTION

Disorders of both olfactory and gustatory perception can be ictal phenomena and are particularly associated with a lesion in the region of the uncus. *Hallucinations of smell are common in TLE* and are usually experienced as unpleasant and unrecognisable. Such ictal experiences may occur as simple partial seizures, and the patient may search in vain for the source of the odour. Illusions in this modality are also common in TLE, but hallucinations of taste (gustation) are uncommon, and illusions rare. The taste is usually described in mundane terms, such as "salty" or "bitter".

These phenomena may be seen in non-organic psychoses, particularly paranoid psychoses, and sometimes in depression. Schizophrenia should be suspected if there is a bizarre quality to the description or if it is associated with other psychotic symptoms. Often these experiences represent delusions rather than hallucinations.

Distortion of memory, with events becoming abnormally familiar or unfamiliar, is common in TLE. This may involve a feeling of familiarity with scenes witnessed (déjà vu) or sounds heard (déjà entendu), or conversely a feeling of strangeness (jamais vu or jamais entendu, respectively). Other ictal experiences may be coloured by this distortion of memory. Déjà vu-like experiences can occur as normal phenomena, but they will then lack the intensity and other qualities of an ictal experience. Similarly phenomena involving distortions of body image (derealisation and depersonalisation) and altered time perception (time passing too fast or too slow), are common as ictal experiences, as well as being part of normal experience and occurring frequently in many non-organic disorders.

Other disturbances of body image may be seen in association with *parietal lobe lesions*. They can involve parts of the body being experienced as altered in some way, e.g. a limb feeling too heavy or large. The illusion of bodily movement is common in TLE and to a lesser degree may involve a sense of loss of balance. A feeling of rotation of oneself or one's surroundings (vertigo) can also be found. This experience is symptomatic of a variety of *disorders involving the vestibulo-cerebellar system* and must be differentiated from the mélange of less specific symptoms, usually described by psychiatric patients under the title "dizziness". The sensation of falling or flying particularly suggests an organic disorder and is frequently experienced in delirium.

16.6 POLYMODAL HALLUCINATIONS

Combined auditory and visual hallucinations are usually associated with TLE, organic brain syndromes, and schizophrenia.

In *autoscopy* the patient sees an hallucination of himself, but the experience is not just visual and involves distorted perception in somatic and other modalities, interacting to produce his awareness that it is truly himself he is seeing. It may not have all the qualities of a true hallucination, e.g. it may lack the depth or colour of a real visual perception. This phenomenon is sometimes called a phantom mirror-image and the hallucinated double called a doppelgänger. Autoscopy is most common in delirium and as a result of a lesion in the parieto-occipital region. It also occurs in TLE and schizophrenia. It should be distinguished from depersonalisation/derealisation and "out of body" experiences. Patients with a tendency to dissociation, especially those with histrionic tendencies, may elaborate their description of their depersonalisation episodes into an autoscopic-like experience.

Religious conversion experiences can include auditory hallucinations and visions of God and the devil, and are particularly associated with TLE. They are not ictal phenomena, but short-lived psychoses that may be inter-ictal or post-ictal. If recurrent, they may progress to the picture of a chronic schizophreniform psychosis of the type associated with epilepsy (Slater *et al.*, 1963). Such experiences may occur in schizophrenia, or alternatively can be within the realms of normality, being culturally sanctioned phenomena in the setting of certain religious rituals.

CHAPTER 17

Case Studies in Neuropsychiatry

Sixteen cases will now be presented in order to illustrate and, in some cases, elaborate on certain parts in the preceding text. The length of the presentation, and subsequent discussion, will vary according to its relevance to the text. Literature references will be kept to a minimum and will mainly involve those which have not been previously used. For other references the reader is advised to consult the relevant chapters.

Where a urine or blood screen for drugs is referred to, unless otherwise stated, this refers to the following drugs:

Amphetamine, glutethimide, phenobarbitone and intermediate barbiturates, chlordiazepoxide, diazepam, chlorpromazine, morphine, codeine.

CASE 17.1
EPILEPSY AND PERSONALITY CHANGE

Mr. V. G., a 36-year-old man, was admitted to hospital for assessment of epilepsy and psychosis.

He was well until the age of 21, when he began having episodes of impaired consciousness. During these episodes he would have a brief (lasting a few seconds) feeling of intense familiarity with his surroundings (déjà vu) and was noted by observers to make repetitive chewing movements. This was followed by either a grand mal convulsion or a tendency to wander aimlessly off, during which he occasionally muttered a few words or asked people mundane questions, such as "what time is it?". This disorganised behaviour could last up to 15 minutes and was followed by confusion. His attacks became more frequent and 2 years later he was investigated with bilateral carotid angiography, the results being normal. His EEGs consistently showed bilateral, independent, paroxysmal spike discharges in the temporal lobe regions.

His attacks became less frequent with adjustment of his anticonvulsant treatment. He was having one attack a month until the age of 28, when they became more frequent again. Some of his seizures were now being followed immediately by short-lived psychoses. During one psychotic episode, while recovering from his seizure, he saw a flash of light, became elated and felt a great strength spreading over him. This was followed by a feeling of great sadness and he heard a voice, which he thought belonged to God. The voice told him to go out into the streets and proclaim the existence of God which, to his wife's distress, he did. These psychotic episodes lasted several hours and occurred at monthly intervals, initially. They were always post-ictal. Though they were not identical, each one had prominent religious features, was associated with a marked disturbance of affect and involved little impairment of his conscious level.

In between these episodes he did not have any psychotic experiences, but his personality gradually changed. He lost his sense of humour, ruminated retrospectively about most of his actions and analysed them in the light of religious values. He would write extensively about God and religion, often in a ritualistic manner. His sexual drive decreased and he developed feelings of guilt about sex, believing it should only be used for reproduction. He began to make statements such as "epilepsy is the hand of God in one's heart".

Over the years he had been treated with barbiturates, phenytoin, and carbamazepine, and on admission was taking the latter two drugs.

Personal history

His grandfather had suffered from post-traumatic epilepsy after a head injury in the First World War. He had one sibling who was well. There was no other family history of neuropsychiatric significance. His birth and early development were normal. His interpersonal relationships with his peers were normal, as a child, and he had no difficulty making friends. He was academically average at school. He was heterosexual and had been enjoying a normal active marital sex life, prior to the age of 28 years. He had no children. He had always been steadily employed.

Past medical history

He had meningitis as a child, but with no apparent sequelae. There was no other history of significant medical or psychiatric illness. Premorbidly he had been a cheerful, socially outward-going person. He had not had any particular interest in religion. There was no history of antisocial behaviour, or drug or alcohol abuse.

Mental state and physical examination

He behaved normally on the ward, though exhibiting the traits previously mentioned. He appeared intelligent and was orientated in all three spheres. On giving his history, gaps were found in his memory for past events, and he complained of a poor memory of 2 years duration. No psychotic symptoms were found. There was no evidence of affective illness, and his appetite, weight and sleeping pattern were within normal limits.

On physical examination he was found to be right-handed for most motor activities. No abnormality was found, except for a slight facial asymmetry.

Investigations

Routine blood tests including fasting glucose and calcium levels were normal, as were his serum anticonvulsant levels. An EEG showed bilateral and independent spike discharges in his temporal regions. Psychological testing showed intact memory functions and his WAIS full scale IQ was 92 (verbal IQ = 94, performance IQ = 90). A CAT head scan showed a small calcified nodule lateral and anterior to the right frontal horn, with mild cortical atrophy.

Discussion

The occurrence of visual and auditory hallucinations following immediately after an epileptic seizure, would conform to what the DSM III describes as an organic brain syndrome. The hallucinations in clear consciousness would favour a diagnosis of organic hallucinosis. In view of the disorder of mood that occurred, an alternative diagnosis that might be considered would be an organic affective syndrome, but hallucinations are not prominent in this syndrome.

This patient gives a history of complex partial seizures of 15 years duration. His aura involved a déjà vu experience and oral movements. The seizure discharge would, on occasions, generalise to produce a grand mal convulsion and on other occasions a period of automatic behaviour would follow the aura. The cause of the seizures in this case was probably a calcified hamartoma in the right frontal lobe. Other contributory factors that may have facilitated the development of seizures in this patient are an inherited tendency to epilepsy and covert brain damage due to his childhood "meningitis".

It is possible that this patient's seizures originated from the right side of his brain when they first started at the age of 21 years. Though his EEG showed bilateral independent seizure discharges, this can be caused by a unilateral focus. This is thought to be a result of the formation of a "mirror" focus. Theoretically the primary ictal site causes repeated nervous impulses to pass via the interhemispheric commissural fibres, to a mirror image site in the opposite cerebral hemisphere. The mechanism of kindling is thought to be involved in this process whereby an independent epileptic focus develops at a secondary site. Kindling is a process which has been demonstrated in animal studies involving periodic electrical stimulation of the brain. The effect of this stimulation is initially of an intensity insufficient to produce behavioural effects, but it becomes more effective over time, producing seizure discharges and eventually causing an ictal focus to develop (in this case the "mirror" focus), that can produce spontaneous epileptic discharges (Goddard et al., 1969).

Theoretically this "secondary" discharge is initially dependent on the primary ictal site and the EEG shows the "mirror focus" discharge occurring immediately after, and as a consequence of, the "primary" discharge. However, with time this "mirror focus" becomes independent and its discharge unrelated to the activity of the primary focus.

Mr. V. G. developed short-lived post-ictal psychoses with a religious content, in the setting of an increase in his seizure frequency. These episodes were associated with a change in his personality so that he became morbidly preoccupied with religion. Such religious conversion experiences have been described in association with temporal lobe epilepsy (Dewhurst and Beard, 1970).

In a study of transient psychoses in patients with epilepsy, Dongier (1959) described three types. In one type, the psychosis followed a grand mal convulsion and was characterised by post-ictal confusion lasting less than 3 hours, but psychotic features or marked changes in affect were not a feature. The EEG in such cases shows a diffuse slowing.

The second type of psychosis is petit mal status and is usually found in children, being associated with the characteristic 3 c/s spike and wave EEG discharge. Clinically they resemble post-ictal confusional states, with the patient appearing to be stuporose, and they usually last under 3 hours.

Mr. V. G.'s psychoses conform more to the third type, in which affective change and psychotic symptoms are present, and the conscious level is relatively normal. In these psychoses the epilepsy is usually focal in type (usually a temporal lobe focus) and is associated with either EEG evidence of an increase in the activity of the ictal focus, or a normal EEG. The latter is sometimes referred to a "forced normalisation" (described by Landolt, 1958) and has been regarded as reflecting an antagonistic relationship between the psychosis and the seizure frequency. This normalisation can be seen in the affective, as well as the schizophrenia-like psychoses. The inverse relationship between epilepsy and psychosis has implications for patient treatment; for example, it may be efficacious to use electroconvulsive treatment in the management of such cases.

The group of psychoses associated with an increase in focal epileptic activity appears to result from an increase in seizure activity in the temporo-limbic structures, which may fall short of causing a clinical temporal lobe seizure. In such cases better seizure control using anticonvulsants would be logically indicated, as in this case, where an increase in seizure frequency preceded the onset of the psychosis.

The importance of the transient psychoses of TLE is not only in recognising them and instituting the appropriate treatment, but in differentiating them from the chronic schizophrenia-like psychoses and the affective psychoses. The affective component and their periodic nature may result in the latter diagnosis being made and inappropriate drug treatment used. Antidepressant drugs or lithium may lower the seizure threshhold, and complicate the management of the epilepsy (Reynolds, 1983). A prolonged psychosis (these transient psychoses can last several weeks), associated with clear consciousness, may result in the use of neuroleptic drugs, which not only lower seizure threshhold, but can cause neurological damage (Marsden et al., 1975), and may be continued for an unnecessarily long period of time, if the self-limiting nature of the psychosis is not recognised.

Following the onset of his psychoses this patient then developed hyposexuality, which is found in the majority of patients with TLE (Blumer and Walker, 1975), and other personality changes that have been described as part of the inter-ictal personality syndrome of TLE, notably hyper-religiosity, hypergraphia (a compulsion to write) and humourless sobriety (Bear and Fedio, 1977). It has been suggested that such personality change may result from neuronal hyperconnection, and kindling has been invoked to explain the mechanism by which such hyperconnection occurs (Bear, 1979b).

These personality traits are not unique to TLE and many of them are also found in psychiatric patients without epilepsy (Mungas, 1982). However, in this case the diagnosis of TLE is not in doubt and though his change in personality is profound, he has not developed the chronic schizophrenia-like picture that is associated with TLE—he does not exhibit any delusions, hallucinations or thought disorder, except for the period of his transient psychoses. Moreover, it appears that such chronic psychoses are more often associated with left-sided or bilateral temporal lobe foci (Flor-Henry, 1969; Trimble, 1981a), though this association has been disputed (Stevens and Herman, 1981).

CASE 17.2
CHRONIC POLYSYMPTOMATIC ILLNESS IN A YOUNG WOMAN

Miss B. E., a 26-year-old girl, was admitted for investigation of a 12 year history of multiple fluctuating somatic complaints.

The history was obtained from the patient and her mother. At the age of 14 years she suddenly developed complaints of difficulty in raising her head, tremor of her head and neck, and neck stiffness. This was followed by attacks of feeling cold, light-headed and unreal, which could last for over an hour. Over the next few weeks she developed blurred vision, slurred speech, weakness of her legs and muscular spasm of her hands and fingers. She became unable to continue attending school at this time and remained confined to her home for prolonged periods, as a result of her physical disability. At the age of 17 years many of her complaints decreased, though she continued to have difficulties with her vision and neck stiffness.

She began to work as a receptionist, but had to leave after a year because the heating at her place of work caused her to develop "asthma". She subsequently began working as a dental nurse, but stopped this after a few months because she "became upset at seeing people being given anaesthetics". She then began to study at night school for a short time.

At the age of 22 she developed generalised muscle weakness and episodes of hyperextension of the neck and blurred vision. This was followed by intermittent pains in her joints. During the last 3 years she had spent most of her time in bed. Her current problems included attacks of blurred vision, following which she would develop dizziness and fall to the ground, but without loss of consciousness. She was having difficulty swallowing all types of food and developed a "bloated" feeling in her stomach, when she did succeed in eating. She had lost 1.5 kilogrammes in weight in the 3 months prior to this admission.

Personal history

Her great aunt and grandmother (on her mother's side) had suffered from Parkinson's disease. Her father had had meningitis for 6 months before her illness began, but had made a full recovery. There was no other family history of neurological or psychiatric illness. She had one sibling and he was fit and well.

She was born "face down" and was difficult to feed initially, but her subsequent developmental milestones were normal. She attended school from the age of 5 years until 14 years. Her illness began just before she was due to attend grammar school. Academically she was above average and had had no difficulty making friends with her peers.

Menarche was at the age of 13 years and her periods were regular. She had had several boyfriends before becoming engaged at the age of 19 years to a boy she had known for only a couple of months. She broke off this engagement because she was unwell and did not wish to "saddle any man with my illness". She had had no disturbing sexual experiences, had not experimented sexually, and felt that sexual relations should only occur between man and wife. She had no girlfriends currently and said that she had to prevent boys from visiting her because they tired her.

She was described by her parents as an independent person, studious, and interested in mathematics and music. She hardly ever expressed anger no matter what the situation. There was no history of obsessional traits, mood swings, drug or alcohol abuse, or antisocial behaviour.

Past medical history

She had suffered from asthmatic attacks from early childhood until her teens. There was no other history of childhood illnesses. She had been investigated at several hospitals since this illness began and she had been seen by psychiatrists on several occasions, after extensive medical investigations had proved normal. She had taken her own discharge several times, usually after being informed of her normal test results and her referral to a psychiatrist. She had had no surgery in the past but was under treatment with eleven different drugs.

Mental state and physical examination

She gave her history in a clear and detailed manner, usually talking rapidly but with no disturbance of the process of thinking. She was somewhat flirtatious in her behaviour, and appeared much younger than her age, in her behaviour and appearance. Her affect appeared inappropriate as she seemed relatively unconcerned at her current situation, but at other times her mood was labile. She said "if they don't know what is wrong they say it is psychological, (that) means you are imagining things". No evidence was found of anxiety, either free-floating or phobic.

Her sleep pattern was normal and she denied any change in her appetite. No psychotic features were elicited and she was fully orientated in all three spheres, with no evidence of an attentional deficit and no impairment of 5 minute memory.

On physical examination she was found to be right-handed for most motor activities. She exhibited a bizarre gait, walking in a tandem fashion, frequently almost falling, but managing to regain her balance without sustaining any injury. On Romberg's test she fell backwards, abducting her arms. On extending her arms she externally rotated them and exhibited a rapid flapping tremor. Neurological examination was otherwise normal and she was observed to walk normally and show normal coordination of her arms and legs when she was not aware that she was being observed. The rest of her physical examination was normal.

Investigations

The results of a full blood count and other routine tests, serology for syphilis and antinuclear antibody, thyroid function tests and fasting blood sugar levels, were within normal limits. A standard EEG, CAT head scan, serum copper and serum caeruloplasmin were also within normal limits. When overbreathing during her EEG, she developed tremors of her head and limbs, light-headedness and a "drunken" feeling. Neuro-opthalmological assessment revealed no abnormality. Visual evoked responses were normal. Psychological testing revealed a WAIS full scale IQ of 107 (verbal IQ = 108 and performance IQ = 107). Visual and verbal memory were normal and there was no evidence of cognitive impairment.

Discussion

When considering the diagnosis of a young patient with multiple, poorly defined neurological symptoms, it is necessary to consider the following possible causes:

A. Psychogenic disorders.
B. Multiple sclerosis.
C. Other disorders (SLE, Wilson's disease, etc.)

A. Psychogenic disorders

Miss B. E. exhibited an unusual personality with a tendency to overdramatise her descriptions of events and other people, using terms such as "lovely", "wonderful", and "brilliant". She showed a relative lack of concern over her illness (la belle indifférence), emotional lability, and a tendency to produce physical signs that could not be understood on an organic basis (there was a discrepancy between her performance when being examined and at other times). She had little interest in heterosexual relationships, appeared to be emotionally shallow and excessively dependent on her parents, considering her age. In addition her history suggested a tendency to over-react to certain events, e.g. leaving dental nursing because the use of anaesthetics upset her, and a predisposition to repress unpleasant emotions (she virtually never became angry). These features conform to those found in the *histrionic personality type*. Such a personality type appears to be at an increased risk of developing hysterical conversion disorders, though the majority of patients with conversion disorders do not have a premorbidly histrionic personality type (Merskey, 1979).

However, care should be taken before attributing this illness to psychogenic factors, as it started at an age when her personality was in the process of developing. To a certain degree her current behaviour can be viewed as an understandable reaction of a person who finds that she is suffering from an illness that is not responding to medical treatment and cannot be explained to her satisfaction, by the doctors. Under such circumstances a tendency to exaggerate her symptoms, in an attempt to draw attention to her plight, is understandable. Her initial illness in her teens may have been organic in origin, but as it may have conferred certain advantages on her at that time, such secondary gain may have predisposed her to perpetuate her symptoms. In this case the illness enabled her to remain at home with her parents and continue to function without the responsibilities or strains of adult life. However, such gain can also be found in association with chronic physical illness, and so it has a limited diagnostic significance, and limited weight should be attached to it in the absence of other more reliable features of hysterical conversion.

Any chronic physical illness may interact with, influencing and being influenced by, the patient's personality. This may affect the clinical picture to an extent where the psychological features are more prominent than the physical features.

Trimble and Grant (1982) have drawn attention to those patients who have a long history of neurological disability, but who exhibit few objective neurological signs, despite their incapacity. This appears to be a relatively malignant form of hysterical conversion disorder, and they emphasise the importance of carefully evaluating the patient's previous behaviour and personality traits.

The picture of a chronic fluctuating illness with multiple recurrent somatic complaints, for which no adequate physical cause has been found, is suggestive of *Briquet's hysteria*, otherwise known as Somatisation disorder (DSM III, 1980). This typically starts in adolescence, is associated with the use of multiple medications and "shopping around" among various doctors in different medical specialities. These features are found in this case, but there is no family history of hysteria, antisocial personality or alcoholism, that might be expected in association with Briquet's hysteria (Merskey, 1979). Neither is there a history of multiple operations.

Patient's with Briquet's hysteria are also prone to develop affective disorders. One of the diagnostic problems in those with hysterical personality disorders is that the presence of depression may not be obvious, because of the patient's inability to express emotion in any but the most superficial way. The symptoms of depression may thus be complained of without the appropriate affect, or may be manifest by the development of conversion phenomena. In this patient the loss of weight and inability to eat were felt to be manifestations of a superimposed depression.

Chronic anxiety can produce somatic symptoms of a neurological type. Such an illness may have an intermittent course and mimic a fluctuating neurological disorder, such as multiple sclerosis. A similar picture has been described in association with recurrent "masked depression" where somatic complaints are the most prominent feature of the affective disorder (Trimble and Grant, 1982). Somatic complaints such as these may result from overbreathing. When Miss B. E. was encouraged to hyperventilate during her EEG recording, this resulted in her developing many of her presenting complaints. Overbreathing has been used as a diagnostic test in neurological patients for whom no other physical cause was found for their symptoms, despite full investigation (Pincus, 1978). If the test reproduces all the patient's symptoms then the *Hyperventilation syndrome* (HVS) is suggested as the cause of the illness. Overbreathing can reduce cerebral circulation by 40% (Plum and Posner, 1980) and can produce a myriad of symptoms involving most body systems and including dizziness, depersonalisation, perceptual alterations, visual disturbance, anxiety, paraesthesia, headache, muscle cramps and weakness. In addition, globus (the sensation of a "lump" in the throat and difficulty swallowing) and a "bloated feeling" (usually attributed to the swallowing of excess air) can be produced, both of which were prominent among Miss B. E.'s presenting complaints. The spasm and clawing of her hands probably indicated the development of "main d'accoucheur" as a result of tetany secondary to hyperventilation-induced alkalosis, as her serum calcium level was found to be normal.

HVS has been found to be particularly common in women in the 15–30 year age group (Pincus, 1978) and was found to be the only apparent cause for their complaints in 29% of women of this age referred for neurological assessment in Pincus' study. There is evidence that some of these patients are particularly sensitive to the metabolic effects of hyperventilation and that they develop a hypocapnia that remains low significantly longer than in patients who do not tend to hyperventilate so easily (Lum, 1981). Hyperventilation may occur as a manifestation of the hysterical personality, and as a feature of Briquet's hysteria (Trimble, 1981a). Whatever the cause, explanation of the mechanism by which the symptoms develop and reassurance and advice on simple measures to take during such episodes, such as breathing in and out of a paper bag (which results in the patient rebreathing his own carbon dioxide and counteracts the hyperventilation-induced hypocapnia), can be very effective. Sometimes breathing exercises or minor tranquillisers may be helpful. In cases where there is a specific anxiety provoking event, other treatment such as desensitisation should be considered.

In *malingering* the patient is deliberately feigning illness in order to gain some advantage. In practice these features are difficult to confirm unless the patient is caught in the act of deception or admits to it. There is often overlap between hysteria and malingering, with features of both co-existing. However, a chronic illness of this type, which has considerably incapacitated the patient and led to numerous investigations, some of which are very unpleasant (e.g. lumbar puncture), without a clear gain of the type (often financial) seen in malingering, makes this diagnosis unlikely. The only comparable condition involving malingering is *Munchausen's syndrome*, also known as Chronic Factitious Disorder with physical symptoms (DSM III, 1980). In this condition the patient, usually male, feigns illness to gain admission to hospital. Once in hospital they are usually found to be extremely disturbed personalities, attempting to manipulate the staff, often using repeated lying, sometimes to a degree which defies belief (pseudologia fantastica). Sadomasochistic behaviour is characteristic of these patients. These features were not present in this case.

B. Multiple sclerosis

Organic disease frequently co-exists with conversion disorders in neurological patients (Merskey and Buhrich, 1975). *Those neurological disorders that are especially associated with hysterical conversion phenomena are epilepsy, cerebrovascular disease, multiple sclerosis, head injury and dementia* (Merskey, 1979).

A chronic, fluctuating, polysymptomatic disorder with "neurological" symptoms predominating, in a young adult, should always suggest multiple sclerosis (MS) as a possible diagnosis. In its early stages, transient symptoms and signs with complete recovery are common. Also, brief and inexplicable emotional fluctuations may occur and a sense of physical well-being (eutonia), that is often seen in this condition, may be misinterpreted as a manifestation of la belle indifférence (Pratt, 1951; Trimble and Grant, 1982). However, in this patient the history lasts 12 years, and some significant neurological signs, or an abnormality revealed by the CAT brain scan or EEG, would be expected. In view of her history of visual symptoms an abnormal response in her visual pattern evoked potentials (PEP), would also be expected, but her PEP's were normal.

It is uncommon (about 6% in one study) for patients who have had optic neuritis in the past, to have normal PEPs (Lueders *et al.*, 1980). However, in general, those MS patients who follow a relapsing and remitting course have inconsistent PEP results, which do not correlate with the clinical state at the time (Halliday, 1980).

C. Other disorders

In any chronic fluctuating neuropsychiatric disorder *systemic lupus erythematosis* must be considered, but the absence of objective evidence of multiple system involvement, the normal ESR and the negative antinuclear factor test, effectively eliminates this diagnosis.

A high percentage of patients with *Wilson's disease* present with a psychiatric picture, often hysterical in type. Also, a tremor of the arms is commonly seen, which is described as "wing beating" in type. However, in this case the absence of definite neurological or hepatic abnormality, and normal slit-lamp microscopy (with no evidence of a Kayser–Fleischer ring), rule it out. The normal examination and investigations after repeated neurological assessments and an illness of this duration, make other organic diagnoses relatively unlikely.

It should be emphasised that in those neurological patients where no organic disease is found at the time of discharge, follow-up may reveal neurological disorder even after a prolonged time (Slater and Glithero, 1965) and therefore, where possible, follow-up and further assessment of such cases should take place at regular intervals.

Summary

The diagnosis of Briquet's hysteria is the diagnosis which manages to bring together the history, findings on examination and investigation, and the patient's premorbid personality, most effectively. The initial illness at the age of 14 years in this patient may have been organic or non-organic, but it is impossible to say at this late date, with the limited information available. If it was organic it may have functioned as a "release" mechanism, setting in motion an hysterical illness to which the patient was predisposed by her personality, possibly with the illness being perpetuated by factors such as secondary gain. The diagnoses of Briquet's hysteria and hyperventilation are not mutually exclusive. Also HVS may follow a physical illness.

The prognosis in Briquet's hysteria is poor with a tendency to chronicity and in this case the patient was unlikely to accept a purely psychological explanation of her illness. She was treated by graded exercises to improve her physical state, advice on control of her breathing and an explanation of how overbreathing contributed to her symptoms. Hypnotic suggestion and antidepressant treatment were also used. She was discharged after improvement in her appetite, weight and mobility, with a reduction in her other symptoms.

CASE 17.3
RECURRENT SLEEPING ATTACKS IN A YOUNG MAN

Mr. F. R., a 23-year-old university student, was admitted to hospital for investigation of a 5 year history of recurrent episodes of depersonalisation and hypersomnia.

At the age of 18 he was knocked unconscious briefly while boxing and, though he recovered without any apparent sequelae, 1 month later he developed a feeling of dullness in his head "as if I had not woken up properly". He noticed that he felt strange, his surroundings seemed unreal and his sense of time was altered. He was unable to work and wanted only to lie down and be left alone. He felt a compulsion to sleep and other people noticed that he appeared to be in a dreamy state. During these episodes, which lasted 1 to 2 weeks, he would remain in bed most of the time, getting out only in order to eat voraciously and to attend to his basic toilet needs. He experienced strange ideas during these episodes, though they were never truly delusional, such as thinking that he was responsible for all the events in the outside world, to such a degree that he felt uncomfortable looking at newspaper reports of morbid events. At one time he thought that he could stop the clock with his thoughts, and time seemed to go too fast or too slow. He found that he would have particularly vivid daydreams about things that had happened in the past. His concentration was markedly impaired and towards the end of these episodes he would become sad and feel that life was hopeless. These attacks would end gradually and be followed by 1 to 2 days of an excessively cheerful mood, when he was capable of large amounts of work and required little sleep.

These abnormal experiences would occur four times a year, but they had become monthly during the last year, though less intense in severity. He was relatively well in between his attacks and had total recall of all the events that occurred during them, when he was not sleeping. They were unpleasant experiences and, when well, he would dread the thought that he might become ill again.

His parents noticed that since the onset of his illness he had become less cheerful and more socially withdrawn. His academic performance had deteriorated and he was behaving irresponsibly at times. However, these changes were relatively mild and his sleeping pattern between attacks was quite normal.

Personal details

There was a family history of several relatives suffering from neurotic illness, on his father's side. His father had had a "nervous collapse" as a young man and was also prone to hypnagogic myoclonic jerking, but there was no other family history of epilepsy, hallucinations, cataplexy, sleep paralysis or hypersomnia. His father was otherwise physically and mentally well, and so were the patient's three siblings.

His birth and early development were normal and he had had no neurotic traits in his childhood. He was academically above average at school and had developed good peer relationships. He was in the army for 3 years until the age of 21, when he entered university. He was heterosexual and there was no history of sexual problems. He was not the nervous type, nor was he prone to mood swings. He was normally full of energy, engaging in outdoor pursuits, such as skiing and gliding, and had a cheerful and generous nature. He had not abused drugs or alcohol, and had no history of antisocial behaviour.

Previous medical history

At the age of 4 years he was ill with dysentery for several months while spending a year in Persia with his parents, and was delirious for part of this illness.

There were no apparent sequelae though. He had had asthmatic attacks inter-mittently from the age of 8 years until the age of 16 years, when they had stopped. There was no history of febrile convulsions, epilepsy, head injury or migraine.

Mental state examination

He was admitted during one of his attacks and the nursing staff noticed that he was tense and irritable. He would remain curled up in bed, drowsy and resent-ful of any interference. He slept most of each day, but could be woken. His sleep was not restless or associated with snoring or apnoeic episodes. He would wake only to eat food voraciously. He was not refreshed by his episodes of sleeping. When he was interviewed, he said that he felt "I am not here and all this is part of what I am imagining". He felt the examiner was "part of myself to whom I am talking". He felt insecure and that things "might not be right", but was not deluded or hallucinated. He exhibited no abnormal sexual behaviour.

His concentration was poor, but his memory for past and recent events was good. He was orientated in all three spheres and his immediate and 5 minute memory were normal. There was no evidence of aphasia, apraxia or agnosia.

A detailed neurological examination was normal, he was right-handed and was found to be physically healthy. He was not obese. His blood pressure was 105/60 mm.Hg, and his pulse rate was 68/minute and regular. There was no evidence of upper respiratory tract obstruction or cardiovascular disease.

Investigations (during the attack)

Routine blood tests, chest and skull radiographs, were normal. Examination of his cerebrospinal fluid showed 2 cells/cu. mm and a normal glucose and protein level. Lumbar air encephalography showed mild ventricular asymmetry. An EEG was abnormal and showed moderate voltage slow waves, which became less marked after the attack, though the EEG remained abnormal and was thought to reflect a lesion in the region of the third ventricle. Psychological testing was difficult in view of his attentional difficulties, but provided evidence indicating that he had a high average intellectual endowment.

Progress

After about 10 days he became markedly excited with restlessness, insomnia, and expressed bizarre ideas about his health. He discharged himself and fully recovered from his attack at home over the next 1 to 2 weeks.

Discussion

The diagnoses that must be considered in a young patient subject to recurrent attacks of compulsive sleeping, dysphoric mood and bizarre ideas, include the following:

A. Kleine–Levin Syndrome.
B. Psychogenic disorder.
C. Other causes of hypersomnia/narcolepsy.

A. Kleine–Levin Syndrome

The combination of periodic hypersomnia, irritability and bizarre ideas, with intermittent overeating, in a young male patient, suggests a diagnosis of the Kleine–Levin Syndrome. Though there are a number of other conditions that should be considered, it is the combination of features in this case which make this almost certainly the diagnosis. However, this syndrome normally has a good prognosis and the attacks become less frequent with time, but in this patient's case they were becoming more frequent, though less severe. Also, the personality is usually unchanged in between attacks, but in this case there was some evidence of a change in personality. This change may well reflect the impact of recurrent, disturbing episodes of altered behaviour on a patient whose personality is still in its formative period. Certainly the illness itself, as well as the effect it had on others, had had a significant impact on this patient's life. Any more sinister significance underlying this change, would require further follow up before its true nature became clear.

B. Psychiatric disorders

Most psychogenic causes of "hypersomnia" are usually not true sleep episodes, but are manifestations of either *hysterical dissociation* or some disorder causing *stupor* (usually associated with a psychotic illness). In the former there maybe a clear precipitating cause, and observation and careful enquiry could indicate that the patient is simply withdrawing from a stressful situation. A past history and current evidence of conversion features may be present. This will tend to occur in females (the Kleine–Levin syndrome is virtually confined to young males) and will not show the other features of the syndrome.

The hypersomniac patient can be roused, in contrast to the patient in a catatonic stupor, who should show other features of catatonia, e.g. negativism, disorders of movement and posture. A periodic catatonic picture may be seen, but these cases tend to show a precipitating factor and a pattern of attack involving an ordered sequence of events (Crammer, 1959). A *periodic psychosis* is suggested by the presence of bizarre ideas expressed during his attack, and the evidence of change in his personality and behaviour in between attacks. But there was no hard evidence of positive psychotic phenomena or any genetic predisposition, to support the presence of a psychotic illness.

There is evidence of an affective disorder in this case, as indicated by the features of depression and elation, and patients with severe depression may develop hypersomnia. In view of this a *rapid cycling manic/depressive illness* should be considered. However, hyperphagia and bizarre ideas (not consistent with a disorder of mood) are not a feature of depression, and there was no depressive ideation exhibited by this patient. Mood swings have been described in diencephalic disorders (Lishman, 1978) and this is probably the cause in this patient, as the Kleine–Levin syndrome is felt to be the result of diencephalic dysfunction (Critchley, 1962).

C. Other disorders

Narcolepsy commonly starts at a similar age and may involve psychotic features, notably hypnagogic and hypnapompic hallucinations. However, narcoleptic attacks, though compulsive, usually only last about 15 minutes and characteristically the patient is refreshed after his sleeping. Overeating is not a feature of narcolepsy, though the patients are sometimes obese. Also there was no family history of a sleeping disorder. There was no cataplexy or sleep paralysis, and his sleeping pattern in between these episodes of hypersomnia was undisturbed.

Alveolar hypoventilation is associated with obesity and the signs of chronic hypoxia may be present, with heart failure (right-sided), cyanosis and polycythaemia. Insomnia and nocturnal myoclonus may also be present. None of these features were present in this case. This condition, like any hypersomnia, may be associated with brief periods of abnormal behaviour due to subclinical sleep episodes, but the behaviour involved is not goal-directed, and is followed by a degree of amnesia for the event. In contrast, F. R. would actively seek out food and would have full recall for his actions in between his sleep episodes.

In *hypersomnia with "sleep drunkenness"* a compulsion to sleep is not typically present, but it primarily involves a need for prolonged periods of sleep, with difficulty waking to a level of full alertness. However, episodes of sleeping followed by confusion may occur during the day and all types of psychiatric disorder may be associated, but hyperphagia and a marked periodicity are not usually found.

"Sleep-like" episodes in young adults should always raise the suspicion of *vertebrobasilar migraine*. However, this condition is typically found in females, the sleep episodes are short-lived, vertebrobasilar symptoms arc prcscnt, and occipital headache is a prominent feature. None of these features are present in this case.

Other causes of hypersomnolence should be considered. *Structural brain disease in the region of the diencephalon* is suggested by the combination of sleep disorder and overeating. In such conditions drowsiness may be present, but there is usually not the episodic compulsion to sleep. Also, there was no evidence of neurological abnormality on examination, lumbar puncture or lumbar air encephalography. The EEG suggested a diencephalic abnormality, but such findings may be present in the Kleine–Levin Syndrome (Critchley, 1962) and probably reflect a disorder of function in this area, rather than a structural lesion.

Damage to this area of the brain may have been sustained during the patient's childhood illness. Marked disorders of sleep were common sequelae to encephalitis lethargica, and neuropsychiatric sequelae could take years to develop after the acute illness (Yahr, 1974). However, the periodic nature of this illness, the 19 year interval and the absence of extrapyramidal features, make this diagnosis unlikely.

The prominent depersonalisation/derealisation features, a "dreamy-like" appearance, bizarre ideas occurring episodically, and change in personality, are all compatible with a diagnosis of *temporal lobe epilepsy*, but the attacks in this patient do not have the acute onset or cessation, short duration, or stereotyped quality, seen in TLE. The EEG was not epileptiform and did not show any abnormality localised to the temporal lobe. Also, there was nothing in the patient's past history to suggest a predisposition to epilepsy.

CASE 17.4
MENTAL RETARDATION, EPILEPSY AND PSYCHOSIS

Miss W. C., a 19-year-old intellectually retarded girl, was admitted for investigation of abnormal behaviour.

She was a normal full term birth, following an uneventful pregnancy, and her subsequent development was normal until the age of 18 months. She walked at 10 months, was controlling her bladder at 11 months, and began to say words a few months later.

At 18 months she had a generalised convulsion. During the ensuing years she had repeated convulsions of different types for which she was treated with anticonvulsants. She had three types of seizure, all involving impaired consciousness and, in some cases, progressing to a grand mal convulsion. At the age of 5 she was noted to be consistently overactive in her motor behaviour, with a limited attention span. At this time she was found to have a rash on her face and it was thought that she might be developing a drug reaction, but the lesions took on a nodular form and proved to be unrelated to her drug intake. At the age of 6 years she was investigated, and chest and skull radiographs were found to be normal. A sleep EEG, following rectal pentothal, showed aynchronous spiking from the left and right parietal regions. Psychological testing (Stanford Binet Form L–M) demonstrated an IQ of 71.

Her behaviour deteriorated and she became aggressive and irritable, and it became necessary to transfer her to a residential school for disturbed children, at the age of 7 years. She remained there until 13 years old. Her mother was not satisfied with her treatment at that time and brought her back home.

Her behaviour changed at the age of 16 years. She began talking to imaginary figures and would at times become agitated and frightened. On one occasion she complained that there were elephants in her room. She became terrified of the pictures of pop stars she had put on her bedroom wall. She began locking her window and bedroom door, and on one occasion threw her shoe through the window saying there were people looking through her window at her, though this was not true. Psychological testing at the age of 16 years demonstrated a verbal IQ of 48 and a performance IQ of 46. Her reading age was 9 years.

Three months before her current admission she began to eat less and started to lose weight. She was sleeping poorly and would talk to herself during the night.

Personal history

An uncle on her mother's side of the family, and one of her father's great uncles, had had epilepsy, but neither were intellectually retarded. There was no other family history of neurological or psychiatric illness. She had one older sibling who was attending a technical college. Both her brother and her parents had been examined by doctors, but no stigmata consistent with an inheritable cause for Miss C's condition could be found.

Menarche was in her early teens and her periods were regular. She was not sexually active. There was no history of alcohol or drug abuse. She was currently living with her parents and brother. It was a caring family and there were no financial problems.

She had a tonsillectomy at the age of 4 years but apart from her afore-mentioned problems, had no previous history of note. Her current medication was the anticonvulsants, sulthiame and ethotoin.

Mental state and physical examination

Miss W. C. smiled inappropriately and laughed to herself during the interview. She gave one-word answers to questions she was asked, except for admitting that she did hear a voice talking to her when there was no one around to explain it, but would give no more details. She was orientated in all three spheres and her attention was within normal limits. She appeared euthymic and there was no evidence of psychomotor over- or underactivity. Her behaviour on the ward was consistent with her behaviour in the interview and suggested that she was experiencing auditory hallucinations.

On physical examination she was found to have an erythematous papular rash in the shape of a butterfly, bilaterally over the maxillary region of her face. On each leg she had an irregular area of depigmentation about 5 to 7 cm in diameter. Physical and neurological examination was otherwise normal. She was right handed. Her pulse was 80 beats/minute and regular. Blood pressure was 160/90 mm. Hg.

Investigations

Routine blood tests and anticonvulsant blood levels were normal. An EEG showed right posterior temporal spikes on a background of widespread slow activity. A CAT head scan, with infusion of contrast media, showed discrete masses in three different areas of the brain tissue, all close to the lateral ventricles. One tumour appeared as an enhancing isodense mass in the region of the foramen of Monro.

Discussion

The history of a normal birth and development, until 18 months of age, with subsequent intellectual and behavioural deterioration associated with epileptic seizures, suggests that some progressive organic brain disease is present. The EEG indicated the multifocal nature of the disorder and this was confirmed by the subsequent CAT head scan. The combination of the facial rash, patches of hypopigmented skin, epilepsy and mental subnormality, strongly indicated a diagnosis of tuberose sclerosis (epiloia). Tuberose sclerosis is one of the *phakomatoses* (disorders of the ectodermal tissue). The other important disorders of this group are: neurofibromatosis, Sturge–Weber syndrome (a craniofacial vascular naevus, with an underlying ipsilateral cerebral atrophy, "tramline" calcification of the cerebral cortex and mental retardation), and von Hippel-Lindau disease (cerebellar and retinal haemangioblastomas, and polycythaemia). They are all inherited as autosomal dominant disorders (Solomon, 1980).

The presence of an erythematous butterfly rash on the face in epiloia is usually associated with intracranial tumours (Dyken and Miller, 1980), and the characteristic findings in such cases are tumours situated just below the surface of the cerebral ventricles. Malignant transformation may occur and the enhancing, isodense cerebral mass, seen in this patient's scan, was thought to be a glioma, developing from a tuberous nodule. This is of importance as the causes of death in epiloia include status epilepticus, cerebral tumour and renal disease (Lishman, 1978).

The absence of a family history is not unusual in this condition, though it is inherited via an autosomal dominant gene, and indicates that the risk of occurrence in a further child is very low. Formes frustes of this disorder may occur without the external stigmata, e.g. the gene may only be manifest clinically as epilepsy or even diagnosed incidentally at autopsy. So the family history of epilepsy may indicate a relatively covert form of tuberose sclerosis, manifesting as seizures only, or may have simply reflected a genetic predisposition to seizures, in this patient interacting with the gene for tuberose sclerosis.

It is notable that she had a relative preservation of her reading ability and such select preservation of intellectual ability in the setting of generalised mental retardation is not unusual. If it is social skills that are relatively preserved, the patient's intellectual level may be over-estimated, and conversely a lack of social skills may lead to under-estimation of a patient's intellect. For example, a person of normal intellect and a schizoid personality may be regarded as mentally subnormal, because of his lack of social skills and disinterest in certain aspects of academic work at school, if careful evaluation of his intellectual abilities is not carried out. Many people with mental deficiency show a particular skill in some area of functioning, and if such an individual shows a prodigious skill, he is referred to as an "idiot savant", and this skill commonly involves remembering dates or numbers, or performing other rote tasks (Hill, 1978).

Miss W. C.'s IQ was in the 40's when she was 16 years old and this puts her in the range of moderate mental retardation (IQ 35–49, DSM III).

The DSM III discriminates between several levels of retardation depending on IQ score, but intellectual ability is only one aspect of mental functioning. Also important are educational potential and social ability. However, an IQ score two standard deviations below the mean (70 IQ points on the WAIS) is arbitrarily taken as the separation between normal and retarded intellect; 2.5% of the population score below this level and, of this group 80% are mildly retarded (IQ 50–70). It is in the more severely retarded group (below 50 IQ points) that gross cerebral pathology and a specific pathological cause are likely to be present. In one study these were found to be divided as follows, in a severely retarded population (Corbett *et al.*, 1975):

26% Down's Syndrome
19% Inherited or congenital malformations (such as tuberose sclerosis)
18% Perinatal injury
14% Infection (such as rubella)
 4% Inherited biochemical errors
15% Unknown
 4% Other causes

20% of this group had epilepsy. They tend to show correlation between their intellectual, social, and educational limitations, unlike many of the mildly retarded, and their limitations are usually identified before they have completed their schooling.

Psychotic illness is a frequent, but not invariable, accompaniment of tuberose sclerosis and is not necessarily related to the level of intellect. The change in behaviour in Miss W. C., with suspiciousness, auditory hallucinations, and generally bizarre behaviour, for the last 3 years, indicated that she had developed a psychotic illness. In many cases, the psychosis resembles a process schizophrenia (Critchley and Earl, 1932).

The diagnosis of *schizophrenia* can be difficult in the presence of mental retardation. In general such combinations typically involve a poverty of thought content, childish and silly behaviour, and primitive and monotonous hallucinations (Pfropfschizophrenie). The retarded patient is limited in his ability to give an account of his experiences and may have difficulty separating fantasy from reality, a finding which should not be mistaken as indicating psychosis. Mannerisms and sterotypes are frequent accompaniments of retardation and should not be confused with the motor abnormalities seen in catatonic schizophrenia. In catatonic schizophrenia other features of psychosis should be present, frequently involving a fluctuating and deteriorating course.

Similarly, the affective psychoses may be masked by the intellectual deficit, mania manifesting itself primarily as over-activity, and depression as withdrawal or the development of obsessional behaviour. In the diagnosis of the latter, the dexamethasone suppression test may be helpful. It is also important to be aware that depression in the presence of mental retardation is particularly likely to mimic dementia. The diminished self-criticism and poor emotional resources of many with limited intellect, will predispose them to develop hysterical conversion phenomena under stress.

It is in the mildly retarded group where problems of diagnosis are particularly likely to arise. Many of them make a good adjustment socially and become independent and self-supporting, though in their earlier years they are more at risk of problems with the police, in gaining employment, and coping with interpersonal relationships. However, because their intellectual limitations often remain undetected (even at school), they may cause some degree of diagnostic confusion when psychiatric illness develops.

This patient improved substantially on the addition of major tranquillisers to her anticonvulsants, she became more cheerful, active, less suspicious and autistic, and began eating and sleeping properly. It was not thought that the malignant change in her cerebral tumour was affecting her current clinical state.

CASE 17.5
POST-ENCEPHALITIC BRAIN DAMAGE

Mrs. B. K., a 60-year-old lady, was admitted to hospital for evaluation of a severe memory deficit and bizarre behaviour.

She was unable to give a history, but her husband described an illness 2 years beforehand. At that time she had been in good health, when she developed a headache, fever and increasing confusion, over a period of 48 hours, and had been subsequently admitted to a local hospital, where a diagnosis of herpes simplex encephalitis was made.

Further details were obtained from this hospital and it was found that during her previous illness a CAT head scan had demonstrated an area of low attenuation in her left temporal lobe, and an EEG had shown a diffuse abnormality with focal slow wave activity over the left temporal region. In addition, on screening her blood for viral antibodies a rise, and then a fall, in the titre of herpes simplex antibodies, had been found. She was treated with steroids and made a partial recovery, but was so severely disabled that her husband had to give up his job to look after her at home.

Mental state and physical examination

On this current admission she was noted by the nursing staff to eat any food put in front of her, to the point of excess, and on occasions would eat inappropriate objects, e.g. the flowers in her room. She would make inappropriate sexual advances to other patients and attempted to kiss other female patients. She would constantly reiterate certain phrases, such as "I hope I am worth it" and "I hope the weather improves". Recent memory impairment was evident and she would forget a meal a few minutes after eating it.

During her first interview with the physician, she exhibited an inappropriate emotional lability. She was continually looking in her handbag and on occasions took out a photograph of herself and her husband, and looked at it, but was unable to recognise him.

She was disorientated for time and place. She was totally unable to remember a name and address after 5 minutes, saying "I don't remember", though she was able to repeat it back immediately after hearing it. She spoke fluently, but usually conveyed little useful information in her speech, though she seemed unconcerned at this difficulty she had in communicating. No psychiatric phenomena were elicited.

Other responses were as follows:

> Question (Q): "What is 3 + 5".
> Answer (A) 1: "35".
> Q: "What is 15 + 7".
> A2: "57".
> Q: "What is that" (pointing at a wrist watch).
> A3: "Watch to tell the life thank you".
> Q: "What is that" (ballpoint pen).
> A4: "That's a watch for writing".

(She was able to demonstrate the correct use of the objects she was shown).

> Q: "How have you been getting on at home".
> A5: "Bed—I suppose". (She had misunderstood the question as— "What are you getting on at home".)
> Q: "Write—a pair of robins nested in the tree".
> A6: She wrote: A pare of robins nesded in the tree.
> Q: She was asked to read what she had written, 5 minutes later:
> A7: "A pair of L . . . O . . . K . . . I . . . N . . . S . . . lokins N . . . E . . . S . . . D . . . E . . . P . . . in the T . . . R . . . E . . . E . . ."
> Q: "Repeat the sentence—Snow White looked after the seven dwarfs".
> A8: "Snout wite".
> Question repeated.
> A9: "The snow wife".

She was asked to draw a clock face and then put in the numbers (see Figure 17.1).

A clock face with the correct numbers inserted, was then drawn by the examiner and she was asked to put in the clock hands pointing at 9.30 (see Figure 17.2).

On physical examination she was found to be obese. She was right-handed and neurological examination was within normal limits (there was no visual field defect or sensory inattention).

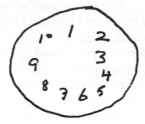

Figure 17.1 Drawing of a clock face (Case 17.5)

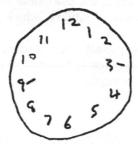

**Figure 17.2 Drawing of a clock face (Case 17.5).
Note the small marks next to the 9 and the 3**

Investigations

A CAT head scan showed severe generalised cerebral atrophy, with a low attentuation area in each temporal lobe, both changes being more pronounced on the left side. An EEG was normal. Her WAIS verbal IQ = 70 and performance IQ = 76.

Discussion

This lady shows evidence of damage to the posterior part of the left cerebral hemisphere of the brain. She exhibited fluent dysphasia and impairment of verbal comprehension (see answer A5). Paraphasias were present, with her misusing the word "life" instead of "time" in A3, and nominal aphasia — "watch" instead of "pen" in A4. The word "watch" was used correctly in A3, but is repeated inappropriately in A4. This phenomenon of using a response that was previously correct, to inappropriately answer another question, is called perseveration. It is not only seen in dysphasic speech, but may be seen in other aspects of motor behaviour, for example, in testing for apraxia. She also exhibited dyscalculia (A1 and 2), dysgraphia (spelling errors in A6), and impairment of verbal repetition (A8). Dyslexia is shown in A7, where the patient was unable to read the words she had written (verbal dyslexia), but could read most of the individual letters and then say the words. A constructional apraxia of the left parietal type was suggested by her drawings (see Figures 17.1 and 17.2), which showed organisation, but an absence of detail.

Damage to the occipital lobes was indicated by her difficulty in recognising her husband's picture (prosopagnosia). She exhibited a short-term memory deficit, with no recall of material after 5 minutes, but insight and no denial or confabulation (hippocampal amnesia).

Bilateral cerebral damage was indicated by this memory deficit and by the features of the Klüver–Bucy syndrome which she exhibited (hyperphagia and hypersexuality, with inappropriate choice of food and sex objects). The other features of the syndrome, visual agnosia, the tendency to examine objects using the mouth, and a loss of appropriate emotional responses, were not present. However, there was an emotional lability, which is a feature of an organic personality change.

These findings were compatible with a diagnosis of post-encephalitic (herpes simplex) brain damage that is bilateral, but maximal in the posterior region of the left hemisphere (dyscalculia, sensory aphasia, verbal dyslexia, dysgraphia).

CASE 17.6
PERSONALITY CHANGE IN A MIDDLE-AGED MAN

Mr. D. A., a 43-year-old man, who owned his own business delivering bread, was referred to the psychiatric department with history of personality change.

Two years prior to his admission his behaviour changed and he began to exhibit sexually disinhibited behaviour, making sexual approaches to his 17-year-old niece, even in the presence of his wife, laughing inappropriately when his wife complained about this. His behaviour began to deteriorate even further, so that he was playing with the local children in a manner which had sexual overtones, and on one occasion actually made sexual advances to a 7-year-old girl. When he was approached about this he ran away giggling and apparently unconcerned.

His social behaviour had also changed and on one occasion while in the middle of entertaining visitors he walked out of the room and left the house without explanation. On other occasions he would speak to relative strangers about personal details of his marriage.

Other changes in his behaviour included restlessness, a penchant for eating candy, a loss of interest in sex with his wife, and the development of impotence. There was a deterioration in attention to his personal hygiene, so that he was only bathing once a week, with encouragement, as opposed to his previous daily routine. He spent increasing periods of time in bed, sometimes lasting up to 15 hours a day, though he was usually not sleeping.

Personal history

There was no family history of psychiatric or neurological disease. His birth and early development was relatively normal, though he had a poor relationship with his father, who tended to drink alcohol to excess. He was the sixth of eleven siblings. Academically he was average at school, attaining grade 11 and leaving at the age of 17. He subsequently held a series of jobs of semi-skilled type, before starting his own business delivering bread, which he had done for the past 4 years (until this admission to hospital). He showed a normal level of sexual activity, was heterosexual and had been happily married for 20 years, with three healthy children. His premorbid personality was that of an extravert man, able to form mature interpersonal relationships, up until his current illness. There was nothing of note in his previous medical history. There was no previous history of trouble with the police, drug or alcohol abuse. He had had no previous psychiatric treatment.

Mental state and physical examination

He was restless, inattentive and inappropriately left the examining room on a number of occasions, though he returned when requested to do so. He appeared to be somewhat suspicious and his speech consisted of stereotyped phrases such as "my wife is coming to fetch me this evening". He would run off the ward on occasions, but would make no serious attempt to leave the hospital, subsequently being found nearby, giggling in a childish manner. At no time did he attempt to explain the inappropriate behaviour he had exhibited before his admission. When examination was possible he exhibited orientation in all three spheres and his cognitive functions were normal. No psychotic phenomena were evident.

On physical examination his appearance was normal. His blood pressure was 100/70 mm.Hg, pulse 72/minute and regular. There was no abnormality of his thyroid gland or cardiovascular systems. Neurological examination was normal, with no evidence of primitive reflexes. He was right-handed.

Investigations

Normal investigations included skull radiography, EEGs (including one sleep deprived recording with nasopharyngeal leads and chlorpromazine activation), EKG, cerebrospinal fluid examination (including culture, cells, protein, glucose, and protein electrophoresis). Full blood count, ESR, fasting glucose and serum cortisols, were all within normal limits. Serum B_{12} and copper, serum caerulopasmin, serology for syphilis, serum calcium and thyroid function tests were all normal. Urine and blood drug screens were normal. A CAT head scan showed mild uniform ventricular dilatation. Chest x-ray was normal. Neuropsychological test battery showed a borderline expressive aphasia, with a WAIS verbal IQ of 66, a performance IQ of 84, and a full scale IQ of 72. No aphasia, apraxia or agnosia, were found.

Discussion

The presence of a gradual personality change in the setting of a well-adjusted premorbid personality, involving sexual disinhibition, attentional deficits and deterioration in social behaviour, strongly suggest organic brain disease, especially impairment of the frontal lobe. The presence of an expressive aphasia implicates the left frontal lobe. These findings strongly suggested a diagnosis of presenile dementia, notably primary degenerative dementia, in view of the absence of any focal abnormality in the CAT scan or EEG. As there was little evidence of memory impairment, apraxia or agnosia, *Pick's Presenile dementia* was more likely to be present, than dementia of the Alzheimer's type. The presence of a normal EEG also favoured the former diagnosis. Minimal changes on the brain scan are compatible with this diagnosis, as the "focal" atrophy of Pick's disease is frequently not evident on brain scanning. In the later stages of this disorder it may become indistinguishable from Alzheimer's.

Personality change with the silly fatuous affect and childlike behaviour, is also seen in *hebephrenic schizophrenia*. In this disorder there is a shallowness and coarsening of emotional responsiveness, with positive psychotic symptoms (notably thought disorder). These patients may also show sexual preoccupation. *Simple schizophrenia* is characterised by gradual deterioration of personality, involving social behaviour, but the affective change in these cases is more of a cold, callous and affectionless type. Hebephrenic features and positive psychotic symptoms may also be present in such a disorder (Sim, 1974). However, both these types of schizophrenia are disorders of the younger adult and this patient did not show any evidence of positive psychotic symptomatology.

Recurrent affective illness sometimes leads into a state of *chronic mania*, with a shallow and facile euphoria, but in this case there was none of the expected genetic predisposition and no preceding history of psychiatric illness.

Covert *alcohol abuse* can lead to damage to the frontal lobes of the brain and there is a genetic loading for alcoholism in this patient, but there is no history to suggest this and there was no evidence of memory deficit or any of the physical signs of alcohol abuse, such as peripheral neuropathy, hepatomegaly and splenomegaly.

Follow-up

After 6 months in institutional care, the patient was reassessed and found to have deteriorated, being even more restless, preoccupied with waiting for his meals and uttering stereotyped phrases such as "is it suppertime yet", though exhibiting a marked reduction in verbal fluency otherwise. He had a greatly reduced attention span, which precluded adequate testing of his memory functions, though he appeared able to find his way around the ward adequately and was continent of urine. No psychotic phenomena were evident.

Physical examination showed him to have lost 15 pounds in weight since his last admission. His gait was normal, but his tendon jerks were hyperreflexic and there was a grasp reflex on the right side, with a pronounced snouting reflex. Extrapyramidal rigidity, presumably drug induced, as he was receiving treatment with neuroleptics, was present. A CAT head scan showed further enlargement of the lateral ventricles, with an increase in the width of sylvian fissures, anteriorly. An EEG showed minimal slowing of the alpha rhythm, compared with his previous EEG, but was otherwise normal. Repeated blood tests were all normal. Neuropsychological testing was not possible due to his over-activity.

The diagnosis of presenile dementia of the Pick's type seems to be confirmed by this evidence of organic deterioration, primarily involving the frontal lobes, as indicated by his decreased verbal fluency, personality change (despite relative cognitive preservation), brain scan results, and the presence of primitive reflexes, especially a grasp reflex. This organic deterioration is against the diagnosis of schizophrenia or chronic mania.

CASE 17.7
MYASTHENIA GRAVIS, STEROIDS AND PSYCHOSIS

Mr. S. G., a 42-year-old civil engineer, was admitted for assessment of disturbed behaviour and persecutory ideas, of recent onset.

He had been diagnosed as suffering from myasthenia gravis at the age of 15, and had remained reasonably well controlled on drug treatment, since a thymectomy at the age of 26 years. Two weeks prior to this admission he was put on an increasing regime of prednisolone to control a worsening in his myasthenic weakness, with an apparently good response. He was otherwise, mentally and physically, functioning quite normally at this time.

Ten days before admission he began to complain of feeling tired and 1 week later was noted to be behaving bizarrely, expressing ideas of persecution, believing that a plot was going on to harm him, unable to sleep, and incorrectly identifying strangers he saw in the street, as being familiar people.

Personal history

There was no family history of neuropsychiatric illness and his birth and early development were normal, with no evidence of neurotic traits. He was academically successful at school, subsequently entering university. There were no difficulties in his interpersonal relationships. He was heterosexual in orientation, unmarried and had no history of sexual problems.

His premorbid personality was that of a somewhat introverted, hard working man, intelligent and with several close friends. There was no history of drug or alcohol abuse or antisocial behaviour.

Past medical history

There was no history of any other illnesses of note, except for the removal of a rodent ulcer from his face, under local anaesthetic, 1 month beforehand. He had no previous history of head injury, epilepsy, febrile convulsions, neurological or severe ear infections. He was currently under treatment with prednisolone 45 mgm on alternate days and mestinon 240 mgm/day in divided doses.

Mental state and physical examination

He was extremely perplexed, suspicious, frightened and restless. His clinical state was noted to fluctuate throughout the day. He initially denied that he had had any difficulties and said that he had merely come into the hospital for a period of rest, but later he expressed ideas that a number of disturbing events had been going on and he was unable to explain them, though he felt that they concerned him in some way. Several times he had seen people he knew in a number of situations where they should not have been, e.g. he had seen a friend who he knew was supposed to be in another country at that time, who had looked at him in a strange way that he felt had some form of significance. He expressed delusions, e.g. he felt as though his muscles were being monitored and that people had been making notes about him. These beliefs fluctuated with time, having an evanscent quality.

He was emotionally labile and would abruptly, and inappropriately, burst into tears, for a few minutes, during the interview. This crying would clear up equally dramatically. He had a prolonged sleep latency and would frequently wake during the night, but remained in bed and orientated on these occasions. There was no other evidence of psychotic phenomena and he was fully orientated in all three spheres, though his attention tended to wander.

On physical examination he was found to be right-handed. He had a mild left ptosis, a blood pressure of 140/90 mm.Hg and a pulse 80/minute and regular. There was no other abnormality on physical examination, except for the scar of his thymectomy operation.

Investigations

Routine investigations were normal, including a chest radiograph, thyroid function tests, blood serology for syphilis, full blood count, ESR, plasma osmolality, urea and electrolytes, liver function tests, serum glucose, serum calcium and B_{12}. No amphetamines or other drugs were detected on screening his urine. His chest radiograph and CAT head scan were normal. His EEG was within normal limits and revealed a symmetrical and responsive alpha rhythm, with a small amount of fast activity.

Discussion

Mr. S. G. described a series of disturbing events that he had experienced and that he felt had a persecutory quality, but that he was unable to explain. He had experienced the misrecognition of people in his environment as familiar figures. He was emotionally labile and suffered from insomnia and restlessness. These events had disrupted his ability to function normally and had developed abruptly, 2 weeks beforehand. These features, with his fluctuating delusions, were typical of the clinical pattern seen in non-systematised delusional syndromes (Detre and Jarecki, 1971).

Diagnoses that require consideration in such cases include the following:

A.   Drug induced psychosis.
B.   Other causes of delirium.
C.   Acute non-organic psychoses.
D.   Transient psychosis of epilepsy.

A. Drug induced psychosis

The acute onset of a psychotic illness in a man of stable premorbid personality, without a previous psychiatric history, who is taking a high dose of prednisolone, strongly suggests a diagnosis of steroid-induced psychosis. Patients are particularly at risk of this psychosis if they are taking *high* doses of steroids. Pre-existing personality problems, or a history of previous psychiatric disorder, were not present in this case, and are not particularly associated with the development of steroid psychosis (Hall *et al.*, 1979). A normal EEG is a frequent finding in steroid psychosis.

The onset of delirium induced by steroids is usually sudden, with initial symptoms including euphoria, anxiety, depression, insomnia, tension, and depersonalisation, which then progress into a heterogenous and fluctuating psychosis. The incidence of psychosis appears to be less frequent with the new preparations of prednisolone, in contrast to drugs such as cortisone and adrenocorticotrophic hormone (ATCH). The evidence suggests that steroids do not release a latent predisposition to psychosis and improvement in symptoms occurs in a few weeks, following their discontinuation, even when other medications, such as major tranquillisers, are not used (Lipowski, 1980). What is characteristic is the polymorphous quality of the illness, with shifts in the type, intensity, subjective meaning, and behavioural response, to auditory and visual hallucinations, and rapid shifts in the type of psychosis, e.g. from affective to schizophrenic. It has been said that there is no such thing as a steroid psychosis, but rather "steroid psychoses". There is some evidence that tricyclic antidepressants are contra-indicated (Hall *et al.*, 1979), as several psychotic patients who were started on this medication showed a rapid clinical deterioration in their condition.

75% of patients who have psychiatric problems on steroids are receiving more than 40 mg of prednisolone each day, and only 1% of patients taking less than this dose have psychiatric problems, compared to 18% in those taking over 80 mg a day. The majority of psychoses develop within 6 days after the onset of these doses. However, in this case there was a gradual increase of dosage over time, up to his current dosage of 40 mgm. on alternate days, though it is not clear exactly how long the patient had been taking his current dosage.

In this case the diagnosis of steroid-induced psychosis was supported by his clinical response to a reduction in his steroid dosage and the use of chlorpromazine, which led to his mental state improving over a matter of days. Such psychoses are sensitive to neuroleptic treatment, as well as to a reduction in steroid dosage. A past history of steroid-induced psychosis has not been shown to be a contra-indication to further treatment with steroids.

Where psychosis may be a major problem is when steroids are used in the treatment of systemic lupus erythematosus (SLE), where it may not be clear which is causing the psychosis, the drug or the SLE. In such cases the use of technetium head scanning (which is abnormal in 90% of cerebral SLE cases) and the EEG may be helpful. The value of CAT head scanning is less clear (Carette *et al.*, 1981). If there is doubt and the steroids need to be continued, a major tranquilliser should be used also, e.g. haloperidol.

Other drugs need to be considered when this type of psychosis develops acutely, notably the amphetamines or "similarly acting sympathomimetic" drugs (DSM III), such as methylphenidate. Cocaine can produce a similar picture, but recovery occurs within a day. However, clinical features implicating these drugs, such as tachycardia, hypertension, perspiration, nausea, vomiting, elation, tactile and olfactory hallucinations, often in the presence of clear consciousness, were not present in this case. Such a delirium rarely lasts over 6 hours, unless the drug is used chronically, when a persistent paranoid delusional state may occur, sometimes with formication (Lipowski, 1980). Also, there was no other evidence for drug abuse in this patient's case. Though this cannot be ruled out as a cause, it seems unlikely. Phencyclidine can produce a more prolonged psychosis lasting a week or more, but in addition to the other autonomic features described, tends to produce dysarthria, nystagmus and ataxia (Jacob *et al.*, 1981).

B. Other causes of delirium

Diurnal fluctuation in the clinical state involving impaired attention, perceptual disturbances, misidentifying the unfamiliar for the familiar, insomnia and restlessness, were present, and so this condition could be regarded as a mild delirium. The normal EEG is against this, though there was no previous baseline EEG for comparison.

Delirium is uncommon in this age group and when it occurs the causes that should be considered include, not only drugs, but alcohol, endocrinopathies and auto-immune diseases. The history, normal examination and investigations, make these causes unlikely.

Myasthenia gravis itself is unlikely to be the cause. Though neurotic anxiety and depression may occur in association with this disorder, psychoses are uncommon (in the absence of steroid treatment), to an extent where it has been suggested there is an inverse relationship between psychosis and this disorder (Gittleson and Richardson, 1973). However, emotional influences may play an important part in bringing the illness to light and causing exacerbations in the muscle weakness, even to the extent of a "cataplectic-like" (sudden dramatic onset of weakness) response to extreme emotion. Anxiety attacks are associated with an increased mortality (about 50%) in this disorder. Anxious patients are more likely to die as a result of their myasthenic illness, than those without emotional problems (Lishman, 1978).

It seems likely that when psychosis does occur in association with myasthenia gravis, but does not appear to be a consequence of drug treatment, then some degree of premorbid predisposition in the patient should be looked for.

C. Acute non-organic psychoses

The patient's experience that something was going on which referred to him, is similar to the delusional mood experienced by schizophrenic patients, prior to the development of a primary (autochthonous) delusion (Mullen, 1979). When the primary delusion develops, in such cases, it provides the patient with what he feels is an explanation for his experiences. However, this did not occur in this patient, and his illness resolved within a few days of admission to hospital.

As the total duration of the illness lasted a few weeks only (rather than the 6 months required by DSM III criteria for a diagnosis of schizophrenia), it was more in keeping with a schizophreniform psychosis, if it manifested the clinical features otherwise associated with schizophrenia. However, true delusions, auditory hallucinations, and thought disorder, were not present, and there was no evidence of any genetic or personality predisposition to such an illness. These prominent psychotic phenomena would also be expected in a Brief Reactive psychosis (which by DSM III criteria lasts less than two weeks), but there was no evidence of any preceding psychosocial stress which could have precipitated such an illness. As there was no marked depression or elation of mood, the patient's symptoms were unlikely to be the result of a mood disturbance, making an affective psychosis unlikely to be the cause, especially in view of the rapid response to treatment.

D. Transient psychosis of epilepsy

Epilepsy is not likely to be present in view of the lack of evidence for this disorder in his past history, but this condition is mentioned to emphasise that a transient psychosis may occur inter-ictally in association with temporal lobe epilepsy, with a normal EEG ("normalisation" pattern), relative preservation of consciousness, prominent hallucinations, delusions and affective changes (Dongier, 1959).

CASE 17.8
MEMORY IMPAIRMENT, ANXIETY AND HEART DISEASE

Mr. W. F., a 57-year-old chartered accountant, was admitted to hospital for investigation of memory impairment.

He described being hospitalised for "heart attacks" at the ages of 44, 52, 53 and 55 years. Following each of his last three episodes, he had noticed an increasingly marked deterioration in his memory, with poor concentration and difficulty coping with familiar routines at work. His wife had noticed that he had become intellectually slower each time, and that he needed to be told when to bathe and given other instructions concerning his personal care. Also, he worried excessively about minor problems, and when she sent him out to the shops to get something, he brought back either the wrong thing or nothing at all, having forgotten what he was supposed to be getting. His sleep was disturbed with a prolonged latency and frequent wakenings, and his appetite and libido had decreased. He was currently taking diazepam 5 mgm at night. Otherwise there had been no marked change in personality.

Personal history

There was no family history of any neurological or psychiatric disorder, but his mother had had seven miscarriages in her earlier years and a heart attack when 75 years old. Both his parents had been dead for several years.

His early development and peer relationships, were normal. He was academically above average and left school at the age of 18 years to become a chartered accountant. He had been in steady employment since then. He had had no sexual problems, had been happily married since his 20's and had three healthy children.

He had always been an anxious individual, inclined to worry over many things, and had obsessional traits in his premorbid personality. There was no history of drug or alcohol abuse, or antisocial behaviour.

Previous medical history

In his 20's he had had pulmonary tuberculosis and a few years later haematuria, which was investigated by a renal biopsy, but the cause remained undiagnosed. There was no history of transient neurological episodes suggestive of cerebrovascular disease.

During his admission to hospital, 4 years beforehand, he had become distressed to find out his serological tests for syphilis (including fluorescent treponemal antibody test and treponema pallidum immobilisation test) were positive on two occasions, though he denied ever having had extramarital sexual relations. His wife and brother were found to have negative serology for syphilis at that time. He did not show any of the physical stigmata of syphilis, and corneal microscopy had found no evidence of interstitial keratitis. He had been treated with a course of penicillin.

The following year his daughter had had marital problems which had led to him developing an anxiety state, for which he was treated with minor tranquillisers.

Mental state and physical examination

His behaviour on the ward was appropriate and normal. He was found to be an anxious man, worried about his inability to cope with things he had previously been able to manage. He gave his history in a reasonably coherent manner. His concentration was impaired, but 5 minute memory and orientation in all three spheres were normal. No psychotic features were found and no specific phobias identified.

On physical examination he was found to be right-handed and to exhibit minimal unsteadiness on tandem gait, a reduced visual acuity (6/9 in his right eye and 6/12 in his left eye), and slight drift of his left arm when both arms were held out and his eyes were closed. The rest of his examination was normal and he was not pyrexial.

Investigations

Routine blood tests, serum B_{12}, and thyroid function tests, were all normal. Fluorescent treponemal antibody test was positive, and cerebro-spinal fluid contained a normal quantity of sugar and protein, but no cells. Pandy test was negative and the Lange test showed no change. A skull radiograph was normal. A chest radiograph showed multiple fibrocalcareous areas in both upper zones, with atelectasis of the upper lobes. There had been no significant change from previous films taken on his previous admission 2 years before. Sputum showed no acid fast bacilli on film or culture. An EEG showed a responsive 12.5 c/s alpha rhythm, with diffuse fast activity. A CAT head scan showed minimal widening of the frontal lobe sulci. Psychological testing revealed normal memory functions and a WAIS verbal IQ = 133, performance IQ = 117. An EEG showed T wave flattening in leads III and AVF.

Discussion

The diagnosis in this case rests primarily between the following disorders:

    A.   Presenile dementia.
    B.   Affective illness.

A. Presenile dementia

The subjective deterioration in memory and difficulty in managing familiar routines, increasing in severity over the past 5 years, is superficially compatible with a dementing process. In addition, features of anxiety are present and this is frequently found in the early stages of senile dementia of the Alzheimer's type (DAT). However, the absence of any objective signs of cognitive impairment, after a 5 year history, without any neurological signs or any features of cerebral cortical disease (aphasia, apraxia, or agnosia), and normal psychological test results, makes any progressive dementing process unlikely. The fast activity of his EEG is probably due to the diazepam effect, and the preservation of his alpha activity is unusual in presenile DAT of such a long duration (Saunders and Westmoreland, 1979). DAT would be the most likely presenile dementia to be present in such a case. Though this performance IQ is 16 points below his verbal IQ, a discrepancy in this direction is not particularly abnormal in people of above average intelligence.

In view of his history of cardiovascular disease a multi-infarct dementia might be considered initially but the absence of a history of hypertension or neurological symptoms, a normal neurological examination and the relatively normal CAT brain scan, virtually rules this out.

The positive serology for syphilis indicated that he had been infected by the spirochaete, but if he had not had extramarital relations, or been infected by his wife, then congenital transmission was likely and his mother's history of repeated miscarriages would support this diagnosis. The brain scan suggested frontal lobe atrophy and syphilis has been noted, in the past, to attack the frontal lobes particularly. But in this patient's age group, mild atrophy on the brain scan cannot be taken as significant without other confirmatory evidence of organic brain disease. Moreover there are no signs to suggest neurological syphilis on examination (Argyll–Robertson pupils, dysarthria or ataxia) or in the CSF (lymphocytosis, increased pressure, raised level of globulin, or paretic Lange curve).

B. Affective illness

He showed some of the features of pseudodementia. He and his wife appeared to exaggerate his deficits, his complaints about his impairment are out of keeping with more objective assessment of his cognition and his level of functioning. In addition, his mood change was not the type usually associated with organic cerebral disease, that is to say, he did not show apathy or emotional lability, and his social impairment had developed at a relatively early stage in his illness.

A *post-myocardial infarction neurosis* is much more likely to explain these findings, in the light of his premorbid personality, the temporal relationship between his mental and cardiac states, and other contributory psychosocial stresses, including the diagnosis of syphilis that had been made 4 years beforehand. An affective neurosis would explain his impaired concentration, resulting in the subjective experience of memory impairment. Persistent psychological disturbance is common after myocardial infarction and occurs in about 30% of cases. It usually involves neurotic symptoms, particularly anxiety and depression. The effects can also be pronounced on other members of the family. Such problems can continue for over a year after the infarction (Mayou, 1979).

A vicious circle of anxiety leading to an impaired ability to cope, which in turn results in more anxiety and depression, and so on, was felt to be the cause of his current problems. Reassurance and the use of sedative antidepressant treatment was initiated on this basis.

CASE 17.9
EPILEPSY, TETANY AND PSYCHOSIS

Mr. H. T., a 39-year-old unemployed electrician, was admitted to hospital for an investigation of psychosis and epilepsy.

At the age of 20 years he developed a psychotic illness involving the delusion that he was being followed by the secret service and that the Russians were trying to harm him. His delusions decreased after a course of ECT and treatment with neuroleptics, and a diagnosis of paranoid schizophrenia was made. Over the ensuing years he had seven admissions to psychiatric units and on each admission was found to be overactive, aggressive, deluded and experiencing auditory hallucinations. He responded to treatment on each occasion. He never regained his premorbid level of functioning, but became withdrawn and socially isolated, lacking insight into his illness. He was also found to be extremely sensitive to treatment with neuroleptics and would rapidly develop severe extrapyramidal side effects.

At the age of 29 years he had a grand mal convulsion. He continued to have frequent seizures and was having two each month, just prior to his current admission. For 10 years he had also been experiencing what he described as "whimsies". These involved episodes of muscle twitching in both arms and a "cramp-like" discomfort in his legs. His hands would go into carpopedal spasm and he had difficulty in speaking. They lasted up to 30 minutes and, sometimes, directly followed some form of stressful situation.

On admission he was receiving anticonvulsant treatment with phenytoin and phenobarbitone.

Personal history

There was no family history of epilepsy or any other neurological or psychiatric illness, except for his mother who had been diagnosed as suffering from "toxic hydrocephalus" many years before. She was quite well now and receiving no treatment. Examination of her previous notes indicated she had been suffering from benign intracranial hypertension. He had two sisters who were mentally and physically healthy.

He was jaundiced at birth, but his subsequent development and early interpersonal relationships, were normal. He was academically average at school and left at the age of 15 years. He subsequently worked as an electrician's mate until the age of 36 years, when he was unable to continue working effectively, because of his mental illness. His sexual orientation was heterosexual.

His premorbid personality was that of a "worrier", but he was sociable and had plenty of friends. There was no previous medical or psychiatric history otherwise. He had not abused drugs or alcohol, and had not been in trouble with the police.

Mental and physical examination

On the ward he appeared orientated and aware of his environment. His behaviour was unremarkable during the interview, but he gave little history and was guarded in his answers, denying many of his previous hospital admissions. His attention, immediate and 5 minute memory, were normal. His speech reflected a lack of logical connection in his thought processes, but there was no evidence of hallucinations or delusions. His affect was markedly flat.

On physical examination he was found to be right-handed and exhibited a marked orofacial dyskinesia, tic-like movements of his left arm, and hypoactive tendon reflexes. There were bilateral early cataracts and grooving of his nails. Trousseau's and Chvostek's signs were negative.

Investigations

Routine blood tests, including a full blood count, protein electrophoresis and serum proteins, were within normal limits. His fasting serum calcium was 1.3 mmol/L (NR = 2.15 to 2.65) or less, on three occasions. His 24-hour urinary excretion of calcium was 0.71 mmol (NR = 2.5–7.5). Serum inorganic phosphorus was 1.93 mmol/L (NR = 0.8 to 1.5) or greater, on three occasions. Serum magnesium was within normal limits. Thyroid, gastric-parietal, and non-organ specific antibodies were absent from the blood. Chest radiographs were normal. Radiographs of the hands and spine suggested metabolic bone disease, but no features typical of hypoparathyroidism were seen. His metacarpal and phalangeal bone lengths were normal. Urinary creatinine clearance and an intravenous pyelogram were normal. An EEG tracing was normal, except for minimal central theta activity. Psychometric testing was unreliable, because of this thought disorder. A CAT head scan showed a remarkable picture of multiple areas of dense calcification that were bilaterally symmetrical, involving the caudate nuclei, thalamus, dentate nuclei, and, to a lesser extent, other areas of subcortical gray matter.

Discussion

This patient developed a chronic psychotic illness, followed by grand mal seizures 9 years later. There are several possible relationships between these two disorders. They are the following:

A. The psychosis is secondary to the epilepsy.
B. The epilepsy is secondary to the psychotic process or related variables such as drug treatment.
C. Their presence together is coincidental.
D. They are both the result of another underlying disorder.

A. Secondary psychosis

Chronic schizophrenia-like psychosis has been associated with epilepsy of the temporal lobe type, and it has been suggested that this is a cause and effect relationship. These patients typically develop their psychosis, on average, 14 years after the epilepsy has started. Unlike chronic schizophrenic patients they tend to have a history of a normal premorbid personality, no family history of schizophrenia, an absence of personality deterioration, and a preserved affect (often with a deepening of emotions and other features of the inter-ictal personality syndrome of TLE). Also, the prognosis is better, with deterioration occurring in only one-third (Slater *et al.*, 1963). However, in Mr. T's case his seizures *followed* his psychosis by 9 years, he had shown marked deterioration in his personality in association with his psychosis, and his affect was flat.

B. Secondary epilepsy

In some cases process schizophrenia is associated with evidence of organic brain disease (OBD) on CAT head scanning, neuropsychological testing, and neurological examination. This OBD could, theoretically, interact with the neuroleptics (which can lower the seizure threshhold), and predispose the patient to develop epileptic seizures. However, there is no evidence of any significantly increased risk of epilepsy developing in patients with established process schizophrenia, in the absence of other predisposing factors, such as a head injury or a family history of epilepsy.

C. Coincidental epilepsy and psychosis

The finding of hypocalcaemia which, in view of the history and the gross cerebral calcification, is clearly long-standing and understandable as the cause of the patient's symptoms, makes a coincidental association between epilepsy and this patient's psychosis unlikely.

D. Secondary epilepsy and psychosis

A chronically low serum calcium, probably due to idiopathic hypoparathyroidism, was responsible for causing the bone changes, tetany, lens cataracts, and nail changes. The "whimsies" this patient experienced were episodes of tetany with muscle cramps, muscle twitching, tetanic spasms of his hands ("main d'accoucheur") and spasm of the muscles responsible for speech. Though seizures can occasionally occur during tetany, they did not appear to do so in this patient, but occurred at other times and were probably a result of neuroleptics and brain damage due to extensive calcium deposition in his brain. This brain damage was probably a factor in predisposing him to his chronic psychosis, though, in general, there is no marked increase in the prevalence of psychotic illness among patients with hypoparathyroidism (Lishman, 1978).

Tetany in psychiatric patients is usually due to hyperventilation, but in such cases the total serum calcium remains normal, the alkalosis, secondary to overbreathing, causing a reduction in ionised calcium and the blood carbon dioxide level. The former causes neuronal excitability with the features of tetany resulting. As stress preceded some of these episodes, and he was of an anxious personality type, hyperventilation may have played a secondary contributory role. The anticonvulsant drugs may have made his calcium deficiency worse as they hydroxylate vitamin D and so interfere with its functions, including the facilitation of calcium absorption and bone formation.

His sensitivity to major tranquillisers, the tic-like movements of his left arm, and his oro-facial dyskinesia, were probably mainly due to the basal ganglia damage, secondary to calcium deposition (Schaaf and Payne, 1966). In some cases his episodes of tetany may have been mistakenly reported as drug-induced dystonic reactions. Schizophrenia-like psychosis is unusual in hypoparathyroidism, and episodes of delirium and neurotic emotional disorders are more common and are the neuropsychiatric disorders which respond best to the appropriate replacement treatment.

CASE 17.10
EPISODES OF ALTERED CONSCIOUSNESS

Mr. K.W. was a 26-year-old male bartender. He was admitted for investigation of recurrent episodes of altered consciousness which he had been experiencing for over 10 years, but which had become more frequent during the last few months.

His "attacks" had started at the age of 15. Initially they only lasted a minute or two, and occurred once or twice a year. Gradually they became more prolonged and now they could last up to an hour, and during the last few months had been occurring on a daily basis. Each attack consisted of a number of symptoms including a feeling of impending doom, with extreme fear, and a "numb" feeling in his head. He felt that he was in a dream world, separated from others by a barrier and unable to respond emotionally to events around him. Also, the world around him seemed to have changed, and he experienced palpitations, sweating and déjà vu experiences. There was no clear precipitating cause for these attacks and these symptoms did not follow a regular sequential pattern. The attack would start and end gradually, with a feeling of fatigue, but he was able to remember all the events that had taken place. There was no history of hunger, sweating or headache, his heart rate did not change rhythm or become excessively fast, during or in between these attacks. This was his first psychiatric assessment and he had had no treatment for these episodes.

Personal history

There was no family history of note except that his father was currently under psychiatric treatment for anxiety. His birth and development were unremarkable, though he was an anxious child, prone to nightmares and nail biting, and wet his bed until the age of 10 years. He had no difficulty in establishing or maintaining interpersonal relationships with his peers and elders. His academic level was average at school. Since leaving school at the age of 19, he had held numerous unskilled jobs, usually leaving them because of his lack of interest.

His level of sexual activity was normal and he was heterosexual. He was prone to premature ejaculation, during the past few years. His premorbid personality was that of a highly anxious insecure person, who was fearful of heights and crowds.

There was no history of febrile convulsions or any other form of epilepsy. He had had no medical illnesses of note. He had used LSD and marihuana in his teens, but had only used the latter about once a month over the last few years. He did not abuse alcohol and had had no problems with the police.

Mental state and physical examination

His behaviour on the ward was normal, but he was somewhat anxious and frightened that he was "going out of his mind". There was no evidence of depression. Cognitive examination was normal and no psychotic symptoms were elicited. Physical examination was normal except for his height, which was 1.98 metres, his span was 1.93 metres, his lower segment was shorter than his upper segment, and he had a high arched palate. Examination of his eyes, cardio-vascular system (BP = 130/70 mm.Hg, pulse 72/min regular, heart sounds normal), and nervous system, were normal. No ligament laxity or abnormality of the thyroid gland were found.

Investigations

Normal results were found on evaluating thyroid function, serum calcium, fasting glucose and a 5 hour glucose tolerance test, vanillyl mandelic acid (VMA) and metanephrines in a 24-hour urine sample, skull radiograph, EKG and echocardiography, standard and sleep deprived EEG with nasopharyngeal leads, and unenhanced CAT head scan. Chromosome keryotyping was normal (46 XY). Urine screening for drugs was negative.

Discussion

Paroxysmal attacks of automatic arousal can be found in a number of physical conditions, most notably temporal lobe epilepsy, hypoglycemia, phaeochromocytoma, and thyrotoxicosis.

In this case *temporal lobe epilepsy* (TLE) is unlikely, despite the presence of déjà vu and depersonalisation/derealisation experiences, because the attacks last up to 1 hour, are not stereotyped, do not have a well defined progression of the phenomena experienced, and do not cease abruptly, with subsequent confusion. The gradual onset and cessation, the prolonged duration and the features of anxiety, with normal EEG investigations, make the diagnosis more likely to be that of *phobic anxiety–depersonalisation syndrome* (PAD). Harper and Roth (1962) compared the profile of patients with PAD and patients with TLE and found that the former group were characterised by a family history of neurosis, a history of neurotic behaviour in childhood and normal EEG's; all of which were present in this patient. However in Harper and Roth's cases the patients were selected for one or the other of the diagnoses and in practice separation of the two diagnoses becomes difficult if a patient with pre-existing TLE develops episodes of anxiety, but this patient shows no evidence of having a seizure disorder.

Acute hypoglycemia can produce depersonalisation and anxiety. But it also produces hunger, sweating and focal neurological signs, which were absent in this case. Also there was no temporal relationship to food intake or fasting, which, taken with the normal fasting glucose and prolonged GTT, virtually rule out "fasting" or "reactive" hypoglycaemia.

Catecholamine-secreting adrenal tumours, or *phaeochromocytomas*, can produce episodic attacks of fear and automatic arousal, but hypertension is always present during these attacks, usually with a marked headache. A variety of emotional or physical precipitants can produce these attacks, and 80% of these patients are hypertensive in between. This diagnosis is unlikely in view of the absence of headaches as a feature of the attacks, and the absence of hypertension on physical examination. It is almost ruled out by a normal catecholamine content in the 24-hour urine sample.

This patient did not demonstrate heart intolerance, diarrhoea, tachycardia, increased appetite and loss of weight, which are associated with *thyrotoxicosis* (as well as being occasionally seen in phaeochromocytomas), a condition that can also produce episodic anxiety attacks. Moreover his physical examination, including examination of the thyroid gland and thyroid function tests, were all normal, ruling out this diagnosis.

Other organic disorders that can produce depersonalisation include angina pectoris and cardiac dysrhythmias (there was no history of chest pain and a normal EKG) mitral valve prolapse (no midsystolic click followed by a late systolic murmur, a normal echocardiogram), hypoparathyroidism (no tetany and a normal serum calcium), and hyperadrenalism (no obesity, hypertension, or hyperglycaemia). Recurrent pulmonary emboli can cause acute episodes of anxiety and may be associated with few signs. Chest pain or syncope on exertion, with EKG or chest radiography features of pulmonary hypertension, in a young woman, should alert the physician to this possible diagnosis; and a ventilation–perfusion lung scan carried out (Dietch, 1981; Hickam, 1971).

His height and his high arched palate raised the question of his having a connective tissue disorder. However, he had no dislocation of the lens, no abnormality of chest development (pectus excavation or carinatum) and his body proportions were inconsistent with Marfan's syndrome, which is a relevant consideration in view of its association with cardiac valvular abnormalities, including mitral valve prolapse (Braunwald, 1980).

CASE 17.11
POST-TRAUMATIC BRAIN DAMAGE

Mr. L.F., a 59-year-old man who was training to be a teacher, was admitted to hospital for investigation and treatment of depression.

At the age of 55 years he was involved in a car accident in which his wife and two of his four children were killed, while he was driving the car they were all in. He was taken to hospital unconscious and remained in a confused state for 1 week after the accident, being unable to remember any details of that period. The only physical injury he sustained that required treatment was an extensive laceration of the skin on the left side of his head.

Following this he was in and out of hospital on several occasions for treatment of depression; 2 years later he was admitted to hospital as he said he was seriously contemplating suicide. During that admission his mood was found to be markedly labile and any mention of his family would cause abrupt crying, which would disappear just as quickly, when the subject was changed. There was a pervasive disturbance of sleep and his appetite was impaired. Physical examination showed a slow, shuffling gait, with incoordination of fine and gross motor movements. His speech was dysarthric and scanning in type. Psychological test results following his accident are shown in Table 17.1. No dysphasia was found but he had marked articulatory difficulties. His mood responded substantially to treatment with a monoamine oxidase inhibitor and his emotional lability was greatly reduced. He returned to his work as a part-time teacher.

Three months before his current admission he began to deteriorate in his level of activity. He lost his concentration, and so was unable to read. He spent most of his time sitting around at home and feeling miserable. He had also noticed his walking was worse after he was started on antidepressant medication by his family practitioner. He began to cry whenever he spoke about his deceased wife and children.

312

Personal history

There as no family history of neurological or psychiatric illness. His birth and early development were normal and he was academically above average at school, later attending university and obtaining a B.A. degree. He did not enjoy his subsequent work as a sales representative and so started training to be a teacher. He had been a teacher for over 20 years when he had his accident. His work record was stable and he was a hard worker. His interpersonal relationships were normal, though he did not have many friends. He was heterosexual and married at the age of 43 years. It was a happy marriage and they had three children and one adopted child. He was living with his son (13 years) and daughter (16 years). His daughter resented him since the accident and his son, who was rarely at home, avoided him, spending most of his time with his friends.

Mr. L.F. was a person with obsessional traits and inclined to introversion. He was an avid reader of economics. There was no history of antisocial behaviour, alcohol or drug abuse.

Past medical history

He had suffered from peptic ulcers in his 20's and was currently under treatment for hypertension, taking a beta blocker and diuretic, which he discontinued prior to his admission to hospital. There were no other previous psychiatric or neurological illnesses.

Mental state and physical examination

He looked older than his years, said he was unable to care for his children now and that there was no future for him. He showed the same lability of mood that he had shown in the past whenever his family were mentioned, and cried easily. His appetite was poor, his libido nonexistent and his sleep disrupted with a prolonged latency and frequent wakenings. He was orientated in all three spheres, his concentration and 5 minute memory were normal. No psychotic phenomena were present. He was occasionally incontinent of urine.

Physical examination showd him to be right-handed. A rotatory nystagmus was present. He was dysarthic and exhibited scanning speech. There was past-pointing when finger/nose coordination was tested. His gait was broad-based and shuffling, and he was unable to perform tandem walking. The rest of his physical examination, including his fundi, was normal.

Investigations

Routine blood testing was normal except for a low serum folate of 1.3 ng/ml (NR = 3-20). His serum B_{12} and a standard EEG were normal. His CAT head scan showed moderate dilatation of all the ventricles including the fourth ventricle, with no evidence of cortical atrophy. A communicating hydrocephalus of the normal pressure type was confirmed by a RIHSA cisternogram.

His depression remained following insertion of a ventriculo-peritoneal shunt but subsequently improved on treatment with impramine. He was given folic acid replacement, physiotherapy, individual and group psychotherapy, and discharged to his home. Social work support and intervention were arranged.

Discussion

As a result of the car accident (the details of the accident never became clear), Mr. L.F.'s life was disrupted. Factors, such as the loss of his wife and two children, his guilt, the altered family dynamics, and his surviving children's resentment towards him, began to play a role in his life and could not be clearly separated from the effects of the post-traumatic cerebral damage he had sustained. Although there were no obvious signs of external trauma to his head, except a laceration, his post-traumatic amnesia of 1 week indicated that he had probably sustained considerable intracranial damage. This was confirmed by psychological testing 2 months after the accident (see Table 17.1).

Table 17.1 Psychological test results in case 17.11

	MONTHS AFTER HEAD INJURY					
	2	7	17	25	Shunt inserted	28
WAIS IQ						
Full scale	94	110	113	108		110
Verbal (V)	106	119	117	113		121
Performance (P)	79	97	106	101		93
V – P	27	22	11	12		28
Wechsler memory quotient	86	114	101	90		105
WRAT SCORES (IQ EQUIVALENT)						
Reading	104	109	110	100		104
Spelling	120	122	118	120		118
Arithmetic	76	130	112	99		109

This table shows that the performance IQ is more sensitive to closed brain trauma than the verbal IQ. The former is at its lowest level shortly after the accident and improves rapidly over the next 5 months until it gradually reaches a plateau. The arithmetic score on the WRAT is considerably influenced by motivational factors, and its variability after the accident is probably substantially due to his depressive mood swings. The reading and spelling parts of the WRAT are influenced by verbal factors and are less affected by motivation and brain injury. The memory quotient also shows a rapid improvement reflecting the improvement in attention, concentration, and immediate memory, that tends to occur in the first 6 to 12 months after such an accident. Improvement in intellectual functions may continue for years, but the rate of progress on serial psychological testing will help to indicate how much improvement can be expected.

A deterioration in intellect, with progressive gait disturbance, and urinary incontinence, in a patient with a severe head injury, suggests the development of normal pressure hydrocephalus (NPH). The gait disturbance was progressive for most of the 4 years after the injury, suggesting that a gradual increase in ventricular size (which characteristically predominantly affects the pyramidal tracts as they wind round the ventricles on their way to control the motor activity of the lower limbs) may have been occurring. The cerebellar signs of nystagmus, dysarthria, scanning speech and past-pointing, indicate that there was vestibulo-cerebellar damage.

Progressive deterioration in intellect in any patient, after an interval following a head injury, should suggest the development of either NPH, a subdural haematoma (particularly if there is a fluctuating impairment of cognition, and a headache), depression, or a dementing process which has been caused, or revealed, by the head injury. Both depression and NPH were present in this patient, and the combination resulted in a deterioration, or a lack of improvement, in all his psychological test scores, when tested 25 months post-traumatically, just prior to his neurosurgery.

NPH can mimic depression as it can cause a marked mental and physical slowing, but in this patient depression was clearly present as well. His emotional lability was part of a post-traumatic personality change, which included an exacerbation of his premorbid obsessional personality traits. The diagnosis of depression, in such a brain damaged patient, may be masked by the "organic" emotional lability and it is important to note any change in biological functions (sleep, libido and appetite), as well as noting what the patient says, rather than looking for a severe and consistently depressed affect. The use of the dexamethasone suppression test would have been diagnostically useful in this patient. However, his response to MAOI drugs during one period, and imipramine on another, with the loss of his emotional lability and depressive ideation, indicated that he had been depressed.

The diagnosis of NPH was further confirmed by his reaction to ventriculo-peritoneal shunting, with a rapid improvement in most intellectual functions, a cessation of urinary incontinence, and a limited improvement in his gait. The decrease in his performance IQ was probably due, in part, to the effects of surgical intervention in his right cerebral hemisphere, where the shunt was inserted.

For further reading on the neuropsychological aspects of closed head injury, the reader is referred to Levin *et al.* (1982) and Smith (1981).

CASE 17.12
HYSTERIA, POLYSYMPTOMATIC ILLNESS
AND PERIPHERAL NEUROPATHY

Mrs. T.S., who was 31 years old, was admitted for investigation of weakness, weight loss and amenorrhoea, of 4 months duration, with muscle pain in her limbs for 1 month.

Four months before her admission she had developed dysuria and urgency of micturition which was treated with nitrofurantoin by her family practitioner. However, shortly after this she developed pain in her left side. She was admitted to a local hospital for treatment and investigation of these symptoms, on two occasions during the next month, with negative findings on each occasion. She experienced periods of disorientation (not knowing where she was) on more than one occasion during these hospitalisations, and on returning home began to have episodes of sleepwalking, with amnesia for the somnambulism, the next day. Her dreams became vivid and on one occasion, while in hospital, she described the experience of feeling in a dreamlike state and seeing visual hallucinations of a doctor walking about pouring out tablets at random. As well as her pain, she was noted to have lost weight.

In view of the negative physical findings and her mental state, she was referred to the local psychiatric department. When first seen there, she was lying, in a dramatic manner, on three chairs, repeatedly asking for water and complaining bitterly about how ill she was. She was later described as presenting the classical appearance of a "hysteric".

Her history revealed difficulties in her relationship between her, her husband and her domineering mother (all of whom were living together). In addition, it was noted that she would keep her husband awake at night, complaining of her pain, was repeatedly vomiting after eating, and was perpetually expressing multiple vague somatic complaints. She was treated as suffering from a depressive illness with hysterical features. She was started on antidepressant treatment, neuroleptics and barbiturates, as an out-patient. As she failed to respond to this treatment she was admitted and was then noted to have absent lower limb reflexes. In view of her loss of weight and neurological signs she was transferred to the National Hospital for Nervous Diseases for further assessment.

Personal history

There was no family history of neurological or psychiatric illness. Both patients were of English origin. Her father had died 8 years before of heart disease, and her mother and two siblings were fit and well. Her early development was normal, she enjoyed school work, was academically average, but was not a good social "mixer" and disliked sports. She was steadily employed as a short-hand typist, from the age of 15 to 26 years, when she stopped because she would become claustrophobic while travelling to work on the underground. She was now working in a new position as a part-time secretary. Her periods began at the age of 15 and, though regular, were associated with severe pain and fainting, in her teenage years. She married at 21 and said that she did not want any children, but had not been using any form of contraception.

Her husband described her as someone who made friends easily, but tended to suppress her emotions. Psychiatric evaluation indicated that she was inclined to be a dependent person, with histrionic personality traits. There was no history of alcohol, drug abuse, previous psychiatric treatment or antisocial behaviour.

She had been a healthy child and had had no serious illnesses or operations, except for a tonsillectomy and several episodes diagnosed as cystitis, each one apparently responding to treatment with nitrofurantoin. There had been no previous neurological illnesses.

Mental state and physical examination

She was found to be miserable and cried easily, though she denied feelings of depression. She was cooperative and gave her history in a clear manner. This was in marked contrast to the agitated, emotionally labile state, she had previously presented in the out-patient department, when she had been unable to give a clear history. There was no evidence of psychotic symptoms. She was oriented in all three spheres, her attention, concentration, immediate and 5 minute memory, were all intact.

On physical examination, she was found to be thin and wasted. She had a bilateral lower motor neurone facial nerve weakness, with a bovine cough. There was a generalised muscle hypotonia and wasting, and she was unable to sit up without the aid of her hands. Her lower limb reflexes were absent and her plantar responses were flexor. Muscle weakness was more marked distally. There was impaired pin prick sensation and dysaesthesia from the level of her waist and below. Her blood pressure was 130/94 mm.Hg and her pulse rate 120/minute. The rest of her examination was normal and no skin rashes were seen.

Investigations

A full blood count was normal, without anaemia or basophilic stippling of her red cells. A urine sample was normal on microscopy and culture. Chest x-ray, lumbar puncture, thyroid function and serum lead levels, were all normal. On several occasions her urine went a deep mahogany colour on being allowed to stand overnight and each time showed a markedly excessive content of urobilinogen and porphobilinogen. Electromyography of the right arm and left leg showed evidence of chronic partial denervation.

Discussion

In the *early stages* of this illness the histrionic presentation of multiple physical complaints, including amenorrhoea, muscle pain, vomiting, loss of weight, and weakness, for which no physical cause could be found, suggested the following diagnoses:

    A. Hysterical conversion.
    B. Depression with histrionic features.
    C. Anorexia nervosa.
    D. An organic illness.

A. Hysterical conversion

The only evidence for this diagnosis is based on the histrionic nature of her clinical presentation, the failure to find an organic cause, and the evidence of interpersonal difficulties between her, her husband and her mother. Also, she was described as having a tendency to suppress her emotions, a finding frequently associated with the histrionic personality type, and exhibiting sleepwalking, which often has a neurotic basis in adults (Kales *et al.*, 1980b). However, there is a considerable lack of evidence to support this diagnosis. There was no history to suggest previous conversion phenomena. Preceding psychological factors of a severity adequate to precipitate this illness were not present, neither were there typical dissociative symptoms, or the positive "organic signs" of hysterical illness. Primary or secondary gain were not clearly present.

B. Depression with histrionic features

The recent onset of her illness, its association with insomnia, anorexia, loss of weight, and her depressed mood (crying), make depression a possible diagnosis in the early stages. However, there was no evidence for a genetic predisposition to an affective illness, which might have been expected in view of the dramatic presentation, with marked biological features. In fact some degree of clinical depression may have been present in this case, but it seems most likely to have been a secondary phenomenon to the primary organic illness.

C. Anorexia nervosa

The presence of amenorrhoea, vomiting, anorexia and weight loss, in a female, are typical of anorexia nervosa. But the onset of this condition is usually around the time of adolescence. The patients are cheerful, deny that they are physically ill and exhibit overactivity. A depressed mood and multiple somatic complaints are not usually present, and though insomnia does occur, it is not complained of. Anorexia nervosa patients who over-eat and induce themselves to vomit, sometimes show variations from this typical picture, and may have profound disturbances of personality (Garfinkel *et al.*, 1980), but this patient was relatively stable premorbidly and did not exhibit bulimia.

D. An organic illness

The patient's description of being in a dream-like state, disorientated and visually hallucinating, strongly suggests that she was delirious on several occasions. Delirium in a patient of this age is unusual and particularly suggests drug or alcohol abuse, infections, multiple sclerosis, or systemic lupus erythematosis (SLE). A urinary tract infection may have been the cause, but the later development of a peripheral neuropathy suggested that other causes should be considered.

A large number of conditions can cause a peripheral neuropathy, including endocrine and metabolic disorders (e.g. diabetes mellitus, uraemia, porphyria), vitamin deficiency (e.g. vitamin B_{12}), toxins (e.g. lead), drugs, infections, and so on. The diagnosis is made easier if absent lower limb reflexes are combined with extensor plantar responses. This combination is typically seen in the following four conditions:

Sub-acute combined degeneration (B_{12} deficiency).
Syphilitic tabo-paresis (general paralysis of the insane with tabes dorsalis).
Friedreich's ataxia.
Motor neurone disease.

However, in this patient the plantar responses were flexor. The combination of abdominal pain, peripheral neuropathy, and excess urobilinogen and porphobilinogen, in the urine, strongly suggest a primary diagnosis of porphyria. The absence of light sensitive rashes makes the porphyria more likely to be the acute intermittent type (AIP), rather than porphyria variegata.

This patient's AIP may have been precipitated by the nitrofurantoin she received at the start of her illness, but this drug is not known to have this effect in porphyria and she had received it many times in the past with no problems. The AIP may have been precipitated by a urinary tract infection, though there was little evidence to support this diagnosis. Her symptoms may have been exacerbated by the barbiturates she received, though the history does not suggest this. Certainly she showed many of the recognised features of this uncommon condition, pain, vomiting, emotional disturbance and a rapidly developing peripheral neuropathy of the predominantly motor type. The absence of a family history in this autosomal dominantly inherited condition may be due to the partial penetrance of the gene or other reasons.

This patient's urine had been negative when tested for porphyrins during her initial assessment for abdominal pain, and repeated testing is necessary sometimes, preferably obtaining a sample during an acute attack of porphyria, before positive results are obtained. Porphyria can cause histrionic behaviour, which may antedate the more typical features of the disorder. It can also cause delirium and mimic most psychiatric disorders.

In some cases patients can produce false positive urine results when receiving phenothiazine drugs, suffering from an infection or lead poisoning. There was no

319

convincing evidence of infection being present and she had not received neuroleptic drugs. Lead poisoning can produce delirium, neurasthenia, gastrointestinal disturbances and pain, as found in this case, but lead neuropathy is purely motor, typically producing a "wrist-drop", and does not impair sensation. Also, lead tends to produce anaemia and basophilic stippling of red blood cells, which were not present in this case. Serum lead levels were normal.

Amenorrhoea, loss of weight and weakeness can also be seen in a variety of other disorders that should be considered in this case. They include those where there is insufficient food intake (chronic infections, inflammatory disorders, uraemia, Addison's disease, etc.); those where there is excessive utilisation of food (hyperthyroidism, tuberculosis, etc.); and those where there is malabsorption (Hart, 1979).

CASE 17.13
ACUTE ONSET OF LEFT-SIDED NEUROLOGICAL SIGNS

Mr. P.E., a 49-year-old farmer, was admitted for investigation of a headache and a tendency to bump into objects on his left side.

He was physically quite well until 2 months beforehand. At that time he was riding his bicycle and "suddenly felt the road come up to meet him" — so he stopped for a few minutes, but his conscious level was unimpaired. He remounted his bicycle when the feeling had gone. He remained well until 11 days before his admission, when he began bumping into objects, which he did not seem to notice, on his left side, and developed a right-sided headache. In addition his wife noted he was tending to drag his left leg while walking and was having difficulty dressing himself in the mornings, putting his clothes on in the wrong order. On one occasion, after going to bed, she had to put his left leg into bed as he had "forgotten" to do so. When walking up his drive at home, he would tend to walk diagonally to the right now, instead of straight up the path.

Personal history

His mother and father had both had cerebrovascular accidents, when in their old age, his mother dying as a result of hers. His father was still alive. He had one sibling who was mentally and physically healthy. The patient's early development was normal, he was academically average at school and had no difficulty in forming interpersonal relationships. He did not abuse alcohol or drugs, and there was no history of antisocial behaviour. He had had two operations for inguinal hernias. He was sensitive to penicillin. There was no history of neurological or psychiatric illness.

Mental state and physical examination

He was pleasant and cooperated during the interview, but appeared relatively unconcerned about his disability. His mood was otherwise normal. No psychotic phenomena were present. He was fully orientated in all three spheres, but he was easily distracted. It was noted that he tended to ignore his left arm and left leg, but on direct questioning he denied any trouble with them, although later he admitted that he had noticed some clumsiness of his left hand which would "get in the way". He also admitted that it was now "much more convenient to put things in the right pocket", though he had used both the left and right pockets to the same extent, in the past. He felt his left and right hands looked and felt normal and he had noticed no difference between them.

He had difficulty judging the distance between, and the relative positions of, objects placed in his left visual field, but had no such difficulty with objects in his right visual field.

    Q. "Draw a four-pointed star".
    A. (See Figure 17.3).

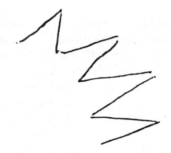

Figure 17.3   Drawing of a star (Case 17.13).

    Q. "Draw a house".
    A. (See Figure 17.4).

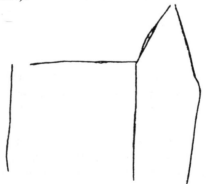

Figure 17.4   Drawing of a house (Case 17.13)

When the examining physician indicated a part of his own body and asked Mr. P.G. to say whether it was on the left or right side, he consistently made errors, despite having his attention drawn to the correct answer after each mistake. He had less difficulty in naming which side parts of his own body were on. He also had difficulty describing familiar routes or remembering the arrangement of rooms in his own house.

His speech was normal and he understood all his instructions. He wrote his name and address correctly, but his writing was noticed to gradually move over to the right half of the paper, as he neglected the left side. He was able to read, but frequently omitted to read words on the left side of the page.

He was unable to identify objects, such as a hair clip, with his left hand, though he could with his right hand. When two objects were presented to him, one to each hand, he would feel the right one first and then put it down and concentrate on identifying the object in his left hand.

He had difficulty constructing patterns with coloured blocks, which could not be explained on the basis of visual inattention or a visual field deficit.

On physical examination he was found to be right-handed. He had a left homonymous hemianopsia, without macula sparing. There was a mild left hemiparesis and an extensor plantar response on the left. Sensory inattention was present on the left side, when he was tested with bilateral simultaneous pin pricks, though he perceived the pin prick on the left side when his attention was drawn to it. Appreciation of vibration, light touch and temperature, were all normal on the left side, when his inattention was overcome, but postural sense and two-point discrimination were impaired on this side. Physical examination was otherwise normal, his pulse rate was 90/minute and regular, his blood pressure = 140/90 mm.Hg.

Investigations

Routine blood tests and chest radiograph were normal. An EEG showed a low voltage disorganised pattern, with slow activity that was maximal in the right parieto-occipital region. Ventriculography demonstrated a large right parietal mass, which was found to be inoperable at operation. A glioma was diagnosed following biopsy.

Discussion

The presentation of this illness indicates the presence of some form of neurological disorder, and the salient points for consideration are the type and site of the lesion in the brain.

This patient shows the clinical features associated with a lesion in the region of the right parietal lobe, notably visual, motor and sensory neglect, and sensory inattention, on the left side of his body, dressing apraxia, constructional apraxia, and anosognosia. Impairment of two-point discrimination and postural sense, on the left side, indicated involvement of the right postcentral gyrus region.

The left hemiplegia and Babinski response supported an involvement of the right precentral gyrus region or its associated subcortical connections. He also exhibited the parietal lobe signs of spatial and left–right disorientation, though they have limited lateralising significance.

Instead of a lower contralateral quadrantanopsic field defect, this patient had a hemianopic field defect, which suggested either a lesion deep in the parietal lobe, involving the optic radiations subserving the upper and lower visual fields, or a lesion in the occipital lobe. The latter was less likely in view of the macula sparing.

Impaired awareness of the contralateral side of the body is one of the striking signs of acute parietal lobe disease, and it is usually associated with the right parietal lobe. It can vary in severity from a mild degree of inattention, elicited by bilateral sensory stimulation, to a lack of concern about a hemiparesis (anosodiaphoria), to the more extreme denial of disability (anosognosia). In some cases there is denial of the existence of the body to the left of the midline (hemidepersonalisation or hemisomatognosia), or the patient may experience a subjective distortion of his perception of part of his body, e.g. a limb feeling excessively heavy or unusually light. These experiences do not usually attain the level of a delusion. However, the patient may produce false explanations to explain why his paralysed limb is not moving, and in some cases paranoid reactions may occur and he may think that someone has substituted another limb for his own.

Experiences of this type, such as anosognosia, are often transient. If they are recurrent, they may have an ictal basis.

If there is a lesion of the left parietal lobe, such experiences are less common and, if they do occur, they tend to involve both sides of the body. Bizarre experiences may occasionally occur in such cases, e.g. the patient may feel that he has died and his body does not belong to him. Such experiences are similar to the nihilistic delusions found in psychotically depressed patients (Cotard's syndrome), and sometimes they may even mimic a depersonalisation experience. Segmental depersonalisation is occasionally seen with parietal lobe disease and involves the patient denying responsibility for the production of his or her, own excreta, e.g. faeces or the products of menstruation.

In most cases when a patient complains of the aforementioned experiences, other organic features will be present, if the aetiology is organic brain disease. However, there may be a striking similarity between the complaints of patients with disorders of body image, whether they appear to be associated with a psychiatric disorder or are a result of organic brain disease. In one documented case unilateral neglect was found to be associated with a small area of atrophy in the contralateral parietal lobe, no other cerebral pathology or psychiatric disorder being found (Critchley, 1953).

For a detailed and elegant description of the different clinical phenomena that can develop with parietal lobe disease, the reader is referred to Critchley (1953).

CASE 17.14
ACUTE PARANOID PSYCHOSIS IN A YOUNG MAN

Mr. D.W., a 26-year-old caucasian, was employed as a manager for a soft drinks firm. He was admitted to the hospital via the emergency department, with a 2 week history of bizarre behaviour.

He had been under financial pressure for several months and in order to earn more money he had begun working excessively, sometimes 16 hours a day, for the previous 2 weeks. Two days prior to his admission his wife, who had been away on holiday, spoke to him over the telephone and found that he was incoherent and talking very rapidly. She hurriedly returned home, and finding him behaving in an agitated and disturbed manner, took him to the hospital.

Personal history

There was no family history of psychiatric or neurological illness. He was the second of two siblings. His early development was unremarkable with no difficulties in his interpersonal relationships with his peers and adults. He was above average academically at school, subsequently obtaining a diploma in market administration at college. He had been working for his current company ever since then and had been highly successful in his work. His psychosexual development was normal, he was of heterosexual orientation and had been happily married for 6 years, with no children. His wife had always encouraged him, sometimes excessively, to get on in his work. He had always been rather jealous of his wife, overpossessive and inclined to be a solitary type of person who, at times, could exhibit histrionic behaviour. In general he was well adjusted and had been so prior to his current breakdown.

Past medical history

There was no history of seizures or any other neurological problems. According to his wife he had had one previous admission to a psychiatric unit 1 year before, for a virtually identical illness. At that time, following extreme pressure at work and worried about his father's illness, he had developed paranoid ideas, agitation and a tendency to be verbally hostile to others, with a lack of insight. He had improved, only receiving treatment with drugs, and was discharged in 2 weeks, on no medication.

Mental state and physical examination

He was found to be agitated and complaining of being unable to sleep. He was episodically mute, in an elective way, cooperative at other times, but inclined to be irritable and negativistic. He was suspicious of the intentions of the medical staff and exhibited a pressure of speech. There was some degree of disorientation for time, when he was acutely agitated, but this settled in 24 to 48 hours and his cognitive functions were then found to be quite intact. No psychotic phenomena were present on examination, but he described a disturbing experience, whilst travelling alone in a car a week before admission, when he had seen "someone sitting in his car with a black hole where his face should have been". This vision did not have the substance of a true perception and had a "dream-like" quality. There had been no auditory hallucinations. His affect was markedly flat but there was no other evidence of an affective disorder.

On physical examination, at the time of admission, he was found to exhibit stereotyped movements of his hands, tapping his fingers together and repetitively interlinking his hands together. His conjunctivae were congested, his pupils dilated, but reacted to light and accommodation. His blood pressure was 150/100 mm.Hg, pulse 64/minute and regular. The rest of the physical examination was within normal limits. He improved substantially several days after admission, though he continued to lack insight, and his abnormal movements ceased.

Investigations

Two urine samples were positive for amphetamines. Normal investigations included serology for syphilis, a fasting glucose, urea and electrolytes, serum calcium, liver function tests, an ESR and full blood count. Other normal results included a fasting glucose. A skull and chest radiograph were normal. The patient took his own discharge before an EEG could be carried out.

Discussion

This man was under considerable pressure from his wife and his financial situation, to succeed at work. In this setting it seems certain, in view of the clinical features and the urine results, that he had taken *stimulant drugs* in order to maintain his prodigious work output. These amphetamines had then led to a characteristic picture of amphetamine psychosis, with over-activity, paranoia, insomnia, "dream-like" experiences, hypervigilance, distractability and over-talkativeness. His flat affect and stereotyped movements of his hands are commonly found with amphetamine abuse. Further indication of drug involvement was provided by his congested conjunctivae, pupillary dilatation and hypertension. This picture can also be caused by other stimulant drugs. Other conditions producing delirium can have a similar short course.

Certain other disorders should be considered. The presence of a "dream-like" state, with visual hallucinations and stereotyped movements, is compatible with a diagnosis of *temporal lobe epilepsy*, but such an attack would be expected to be short-lived (under 5 minutes) and have an acute cessation with subsequent confusion, headache and drowsiness. Occasionally a more prolonged episode involving TLE and a post-ictal psychosis, can occur, but this seems unlikely in view of the absence of any history of epilepsy or any evidence of other factors predisposing to epilepsy. Also, such attacks have more of an intrusive quality and the patient is aware of the alien nature of his experiences, whereas in this case the patient continued to lack insight into his problem and subsequently discharged himself.

Psychiatric disorders which may mimic this picture include *hypomania* and *schizophreniform psychosis*. In either of these there may be pressure of speech, insomnia and overactivity, but the duration of the episode would last more than a few days and auditory hallucinations would be expected to be present, more than visual hallucinations. The "dream-like" quality of this patient's experiences are compatible with acute schizophrenia when the picture is one of oneirophrenia, where impairment of consciousness is present.

A *brief reactive psychosis* would be compatible with this history of a psychotic episode which lasts under 2 weeks, but there is no major precipitating psychosocial stress in this case.

An alternative diagnosis is *factitious disorder with psychological symptoms (Ganser syndrome)*, and though the elective mutism was an unusual feature, his behaviour was generally consistent with his psychotic illness and did not show hysterical conversion features or "talking past the point".

CASE 17.15
STUPOR IN AN ELDERLY WOMAN

Mrs. S.P., a 57-year-old housewife, was brought to the psychiatric emergency department with a history of drowsiness for the past week.

This lady had a history of recurrent depressive episodes since her teens and for several months prior to admission she had become increasingly depressed. She was started on amitriptyline and trifluoperazine by her family practitioner (but it was not clear what doses she was taking). However, 1 week prior to her admission she had become markedly drowsy and so her husband had discontinued her medication and had taken her to a local emergency department, where a diagnosis of retarded depression was made and she was referred to a psychiatric hospital.

Personal history

There was no family history of neurological or psychiatric illness, except for one nephew with a "chronic psychotic illness". The patient was born the first of twins, though her birth and early development were otherwise normal. She left school after grade 11 and subsequently worked as a typist before her marriage at the age of 24 years. She had a close and warm relationship with her six children. Her interpersonal relationships throughout her life had been stable. She was inclined to be somewhat quiet, introverted and obsessional. Her psychosexual development was normal. There was no previous history of drug or alcohol abuse, or antisocial behaviour.

Past medical history

Her previous episodes of depression were usually short-lived, responding to drug treatment, and had never been associated with stupor or other catatonic features. She had been under medical treatment for glaucoma for the past 8 years. For the past 5 years she had been treated for hypertension. There was no history of any neurological disorders.

Mental state and physical examination

She was found to be smiling inappropriately and lethargic, though easily roused. On other occasions she would brighten up and appear to be fully alert for a few minutes. The majority of the time she was mute, slow and somewhat stiff in her movements, and she complained of difficulty in passing her urine.

During a period of psychomotor retardation she was examined and at that time her speech was stereotyped and there was a paucity of thought content. She appeared to be confused and would repeat phrases such as "I don't know which way I am going". There was no evidence of depressive ideation, she denied feelings of depression and, objectively, did not appear depressed. On being asked what day it was she said "thursday", which was incorrect, and continued to perseverate with this response when asked what the month and the year was. She was orientated for person and place. She was easily distracted and was unable to maintain her concentration sufficiently to carry out serial 7's. No psychotic phenomena were elicited.

She had been off all medication for 2 days prior to this examination, except for pilocarpine eye drops for her glaucoma. On examination there was a paucity of spontaneous facial movements. There were moderate snout and pout reflexes, present. A mild bilateral grasp reflex was present and she showed a failure to habituate her blink reflex, on glabella tap. Due to a left-sided cataract, only her right fundus was seen, with some difficulty, and this showed no obvious abnormality. Her pupils were mid-size and responded normally to light. Catalepsy was present and there was some depression of the abdominal reflexes on the right side. Though extrapyramidal rigidity was not present, she exhibited an unsteady gait and required assistance in her walking.

Her temperature was 36.5° C, her pulse 60/minute and regular, and her blood pressure was 145/108 mm.Hg. Her skin was greasy and there was loss of the outer third of her eyebrows.

Investigations

Normal blood tests included a full blood count, fasting glucose, urea and electrolytes, liver function tests, serum calcium and serology for syphilis. Her ESR was 28 mm/Hr. A routine analysis of her urine was normal, and urine screening for drugs was mildly positive for codeine.

An EEG showed a severe disturbance of cerebral activity with abundant diffuse delta and theta activity, most marked over the left anterior region of the head. Bilateral generalised bursts of slow activity were present, suggesting a deep lying cerebral abnormality.

A CAT head screen showed a massive frontal lobe tumour, predominantly on the right side, which subsequently proved to be a malignant glioma, on biopsy. A right frontal lobectomy was unsuccessful and the patient died a couple of weeks later. Postmortem examination confirmed the nature and site of the tumour.

Discussion

The unsteady gait, motor retardation, and primitive reflexes exhibited by this lady, are particularly associated with *frontal lobe lesions*. It is tumours in this region of the brain that are particularly prone to present to the psychiatrist. Slow growing meningiomas are most common, but malignant gliomas produce more marked mental disturbance (Lishman, 1978). Urinary problems are often an early sign of tumours in this region, but the difficulty is one of inhibiting the passage of urine, and not urinary retention. In this case the patient was complaining of difficulty passing urine that was more likely to be the result of the amitryptylline.

Stupor associated with evidence of organic brain disease can be a particular problem in the early stages of *akinetic mutism*, and the *"Locked-In" syndrome*, which can result from a cerebrovascular lesion of the pons or higher regions of the CNS, and this patient was hypertensive. However, these disorders are characterised by almost total immobility, the patients appearing alert primarily by virtue of their eye movements.

This lady's initial incorrect diagnosis was the result of excessive weight being attached to her previous history of recurrent depressive episodes. In fact she showed many features which indicated an organic aetiology for her illness, including perplexity, disorientation, drowsiness with impaired attention, clinically significant primitive reflexes, and an EEG with diffuse slowing, which correlated with her level of arousal, but with features which suggested a focal lesion in the frontal region. Part of the difficulty in the initial stages of a disorder such as this, is that if the patient is mute, it may be difficult to identify the presence of an organic disorder, especially one that is not entirely the result of the drugs that she had been receiving. This is particularly difficult as the urine test indicated that she had been taking codeine, which was not evident from her history. However, codeine poisoning was unlikely in view of her normal respiration, and the absence of hypotension, pin point pupils and muscle hypotonia. *Neuroleptic drugs* of the trifluoperazine type cause extrapyramidal signs, such as the cogwheel rigidity and unsteady gait seen in this case, as their main side effects. This patient also exhibited motor retardation, mutism and catalepsy, which can also be induced by neuroleptics. *Tricyclic antidepressants*, such as amitryptylline, commonly cause delirium, and the marked anticholinergic action of this drug puts the patient at risk of an exacerbation of her glaucoma, urinary retention (which she was complaining of), and the central anticholinergic syndrome (CAS). The latter involves delirium, urinary retention and motor incoordination, all of which were present in this patient. However, agitation, hallucinations, dry skin, flushed face, tachycardia and dilated pupils, unresponsive to light, which also characterise the CAS, were not present.

One other disorder that should be borne in mind is *myxoedema*, as this patient showed drowsiness, motor slowing, bradycardia and a loss of the outer third of her eyebrows. But the other features of this condition, the puffy complexion, coarse dry skin, hypotension, hoarse voice, "delayed-relaxation" of the tendon jerks, and hypothermia, were absent.

CASE 17.16
ACADEMIC AND SOCIAL FAILURE IN A TEENAGER

Mr. C.N., a 17-year-old school boy, was admitted for assessment of the reasons for a deterioration in his school performance.

His parents gave a history of academic difficulties since changing his school 2 years beforehand. This change was occasioned by his previous school closing and his new school made greater academic and social demands on him. One of his current school masters had also taught him at his previous school and said that he had always been slow at his work and poor at sports because of his motor clumsiness, ever since he had known the patient (6 years). He had also tended to be a socially isolated person, with no close friends.

Personal history

His mother had a moderately severe non-fluent dysphasia, following a cerebrovascular accident, one year beforehand. Marked motor clumsiness was reported to be present in most members of the family. His father was physically and mentally well, but had a poor relationship with the patient's mother. There was a poorly documented history of two aunts having mental illness during the Second World War. He had three siblings, one of whom was attending a child guidance clinic for a similar problem; the other two being physically and mentally well.

He was a full-term normal delivery, weighing 3 kgs., talking at 18 months and walking at 2 years. In infancy his emotional response and attachment to his parents were within normal limits. He attended school at the age of 5 years and had always been academically below average. Over the next few years he exhibited considerable difficulty with and little inclination to establish, interpersonal relationships with his peers or elders (including his parents and siblings).

He began to read and write at a similar age to his peers, but his writing failed to progress at the same rate, remaining clumsy and difficult to read. He was nervous and had always tended to bite his nails excessively. He was not sexually active and had no girlfriends, but there was no evidence of sexual deviancy or any other type of antisocial behaviour. There was no history of drug or alcohol abuse. Though he had a few friends he did not feel the need for other people's company and was ill at ease in the presence of others. He was prone to form unusual attachments to the exclusion of all other interests and was currently obsessed with football, exhibiting a remarkable facility for memorising the football results each week, though he did not use this skill for any obvious purpose. He felt, rather unrealistically, that he would be able to play this sport professionally in the future.

Previous medical history

At the age of 7 years he was treated in hospital for a pleuritic chest pain which cleared on antibiotics, but 1 month later irregular muscle twitching occurred involving his head, trunk and arms. It subsequently cleared over the next few weeks. There was no other history of medical or psychiatric illness.

Mental state and physical examination

He was on the ward for 1 month and though he exhibited no markedly abnormal behaviour, he persistently avoided any interpersonal contact.

He was nervous and when a degree of rapport was established, he showed a marked lack of emotional warmth. There was no evidence of depression and there were no psychotic features present. His attention was normal, he was orientated in all three spheres, and 5 minute memory was normal. He did not see himself as having any problems and appeared unconcerned at his lack of social relationships.

On physical examination he was found to be right-handed and 1.83 metres tall. His finger and wrist joints were noted to be hyperextensible, but his skin elasticity appeared normal. His arm span was less than his height and his lower segment length, less than his upper segment. His left upper limb was markedly smaller when compared with his right limb. He was clumsy on finger/thumb coordination and his writing was poorly formed, though syntactically and semantically correct. He had pes cavus bilaterally, but was otherwise physically normal. No abnormality was found on examination of his eyes and this was confirmed by neuro-opthalmalogical assessment.

Investigations

Routine blood testing, including serology for syphilis, was normal. A skull radiograph, EEG and CAT head scan, were also normal. A chest radiograph showed an unexplained elevation of his left hemi-diaphragm. No excess of homocystine was found in his urine.

Psychological testing revealed a WAIS verbal IQ = 114 and a performance IQ = 79. He gave bizarre answers on the picture completion subtest and was impaired in his ability to recognise pictures of common objects photographed from unusual views. He was otherwise able to recognise pictures of common objects and this was regarded as evidence against a primary perceptual impairment. Visual memory was poor, whereas verbal memory was excellent. It was noted that his performance on testing did not conform to any known neurological pattern and he was felt to be exhibiting an incipient thought disorder.

Discussion

In this case the diagnoses that should be considered include the following:

A. Minimal brain dysfunction.
B. Schizoid disorder of adolescence.
C. Schizophrenia.
D. Pervasive developmental disorder.
E. Connective tissue disorders (Marfan's, homocystinuria).

A. Minimal brain dysfunction

It should be emphasised that the diagnosis of MBD is not included in the DSM III and the whole topic is a controversial one. The DSM III does include the diagnostic category of Attention Deficit Disorder, which involves marked inattention and impulsivity, with or without hyperactivity, beginning before the age of 7 years. MBD is used here to imply that this patient was exhibiting a developmental neurological disorder, though not necessarily one resulting from organic brain disease, but maybe a defect of neurological maturation. A genetic component may be indicated by the family history of psychiatric disorder, and such a history has been found in patients with MBD (Morrison and Stewart, 1973).

Mr. C.N.'s case demonstrates some of the features associated with MBD. He has a history of writing disability, poor interpersonal relationships, clumsiness in sports, and shows the soft neurological sign of impairment of fine motor movements. These features taken individually lack clinical significance, but taken together suggest an abnormality of neurological function of a type associated with MBD.

MBD may be associated with social isolation due to rejection by others, because of antisocial behaviour, e.g. impulsiveness and poor frustration tolerance. But this patient rejected social contact, rather than the reverse.

The decreased size of his left upper limb, and a performance IQ that is 35 points less than his verbal IQ, suggest that he has some impairment of function of his right cerebral hemisphere, and that it has been present since early life. His elevated left hemi-diaphragm may be another manifestation of this asymmetry in his physical development, reflecting the trophic function of the CNS in physical development. The absence of other neurological signs could be due to the plasticity of the immature nervous system allowing a degree of compensation for the neurobehavioural effects of an early-onset disorder of neurological function.

B. Schizoid disorder of adolescence

His inability to form adequate peer relationships, his lack of concern over his social isolation, his emotional coldness and his tendency to exhibit eccentric behaviour (such as his obsession with football results), support the presence of a schizoid personality. Personality disorder, as well as a previous history of unequivocal neurological illness, such as encephalitis (Andrulonis *et al.*, 1980), may be associated with MBD.

C. Schizophrenia

A diagnosis of schizophrenia was suggested at one stage in this patient's assessment, but there is no evidence of recent deterioration of social behaviour or intellect. His more recent academic difficulties were, to a degree, an understandable reaction to his entering a school with greater academic and social requirements than his previous school. Schizophrenia occurring in childhood is rare but, like the adult type, typically involves hallucinations, delusions and thought disorder. The former two are absent in this case, but there is some evidence of idiosyncratic thought processes.

Schizoid disorders of adolescence may progress into a schizoid personality disorder of the adult type and, in some cases, schizophrenia develops. Such a development may explain the bizarre responses he gave on psychological testing, but there is little evidence to support this assumption. Schizophrenia developing in a patient with this type of premorbid personality tends to be of the process type, has a poor prognosis, and there is evidence that these patients develop "organic" features on neuropsychological evaluation, and enlarged cerebral ventricles on CAT head scanning, though this remains a somewhat controversial subject.

D. Pervasive Developmental disorder

In cases of this type where a long-standing poor social interaction and bizarre behaviour are found, a past history of a Pervasive Developmental disorder (DSM III), such as infantile autism, must be considered. However, though his writing was clumsy there was no significant abnormality in language development and no abnormal patterns of speech, such as echolalia or pronominal reversal (e.g. using "he" instead of "I"), currently or in the patient's past history.

Impaired social relationships and unusual behaviour are also seen in Childhood Onset Pervasive Developmental disorder which, like Infantile Autism, is profound and incapacitating, often associated with mental subnormality and requiring special educational facilities. However, onset is after 30 months of age, whereas it is before 30 months in autism. In this particular patient the disturbance in social behaviour appeared later than this and, though socially isolated, he had managed to cope at a normal school for over 10 years.

E. *Other organic disorders*

His tallness and hyperextensible joints suggested he may have a connective tissue disorder, such as *homocystinuria* or *Marfan's syndrome*. However, his arm span was less than his height (the reverse being the case in these conditions) and there was no ectopia lentis (dislocated lens) or cardiac abnormalities. Mental deficiency is not seen in Marfan's, but is seen in homocystinuria, however no excess of homocystine was found in his urine. Hyperextensible joints may be an isolated finding of no clinical significance and that is probably the case in this patient, in the absence of other evidence of a connective tissue disorder.

The deformity of his feet raised the possibility that he was suffering from *Friedreich's ataxia*, a recessively inherited, slowly progressive spinocerebellar ataxia, starting in the first two decades of life. Deformities of the vertebral column or feet are usually present, may antedate other features of the condition, and may be the sole manifestation of the gene in formes frustes of the disorder. It is not uncommon for the affected to show cognitive decline, personality disorders, and even psychosis (Lishman, 1978). However, neurological signs, notably cerebellar and posterior column signs, were absent in this patient, which is incompatible with this diagnosis, after such a prolonged history of intellectual and personality difficulties.

The illness in Mr. C.N.'s childhood is unlikely to have significantly contributed to his current problems as he was experiencing difficulties before then. However, *encephalitis* can lead to change in personality and a secondary torsion dystonia (which can cause foot deformities), especially in cases of encephalitis lethargica. Though this illness was not associated with impairment of consciousness, neurological signs or seizures, which would suggest it had been an encephalitis, there is evidence that encephalitis may occasionally occur in an atypical form (Greenough and Davis, 1983).

Similarly other causes of the *torsion dystonias* need brief consideration, but the rapid progression which would be expected in the early onset primary type of torsion dystonia, is not seen here. There is no evidence for perinatal brain damage, Wilson's disease or other basal ganglia disorders (he had a normal cornea and liver function tests, and extrapyramidal signs were absent), to suggest a secondary torsion dystonia.

A diagnosis of Schizoid personality disorder, associated with minimal brain dysfunction, was made, and the family were reassured that no progressive neurological disorder was involved. Appropriate counselling of the patient and family were recommended.

Glossary

This section defines words used in the text. Certain of the definitions are simplified in such a way that those readers who have not been trained in psychiatry can grasp the essence of the word's meaning.

The term *"organic disorder"* is used to refer to those disorders which result from an alteration in the structure or function of the body, in contrast to those caused by psychological factors. The term is most frequently used in the context of an *"organic brain disorder (or syndrome)"* (OBD), which involves a disorder of structure that could reasonably be expected to be visible as an abnormality on the CAT head scan, or a disorder of function that might be revealed by an abnormal EEG. A *"non-organic ("functional" or "psychogenic") disorder (or syndrome)"*, in contrast, is not associated with such abnormalities and involves those conditions that are commonly viewed as being within the psychiatrist's domain, e.g. depression.

The use of the prefix a- and dys- are regarded as being synonymous, where indicated in the glossary, e.g. a(dys-)phasia. This is because of the interchangeable way in which these words are used in clinical practice, though it is semantically incorrect. Finally, though terms such as aphasia are used to describe developmental, as well as acquired disorders, in some texts, they are used here only to refer to the consequences of acquired OBD.

Where reference is made to the dominant cerebral hemisphere this should be taken to refer to the language dominant — usually the left — hemisphere. Conversely, the non-dominant hemisphere is usually on the right side.

ABULIA. A reduction in spontaneous motor activity and thought, resulting in apathy, loss of initiative, etc.

A(DYS-)CALCULIA. An acquired inability to perform calculations, usually resulting from OBD involving the cerebral association cortex.

AFFECT. The experience of emotion, may be subjective or objective (inferred by the behaviour observed).

AGGRESSION: Hostile or destructive behaviour that is directed towards oneself or towards others.

AGNOSIA. An acquired failure to recognise sensory stimuli despite the relevant sensory pathways and conscious level being intact, usually resulting from OBD involving the cerebral association cortex.

A(DYS)GRAPHIA. An acquired impairment of the ability to write, usually resulting from OBD involving the cerebral association cortex.

AKATHISIA. Motor restlessness accompanied by an unpleasant subjective feeling of restlessness.

AKINESIA. A reduction of motor activity.

A(DYS-)LEXIA. An acquired impairment of the ability to read, usually resulting from OBD involving the cerebral association cortex.

A(DYS-)NOMIA. An acquired word finding difficulty, usually resulting from OBD involving the cerebral association cortex.

ANOSOGNOSIA. An acquired indifference to, or a lack of awareness of, a physical disability (usually the result of a lesion of the non-dominant cerebral hemisphere).

ANTICHOLINERGIC. Interferes with conduction in the central and peripheral cholinergic (mainly parasympathetic) nerves.

ANTIDEPRESSANT. Reduces or eliminates depression. When applied to drugs, includes the monoamine oxidase inhibitors (MAOI) and non-MAOI (tricyclic antidepressants, etc.) drugs.

ANTISOCIAL PERSONALITY. A persistent, severe developmental inability to form mature and lasting peer relationships, with an associated tendency to come into conflict with society's laws.

ANXIOLYTIC. Reduces anxiety and its associated symptoms. When used in relation to drugs, refers to the minor tranquillisers (benzodiazepines, etc.) and other drugs with a sedative effect.

A(DYS-)PHASIA. An acquired disorder of the production or comprehension of language, which affects its semantic and syntactic aspects, and usually results from OBD involving the cerebral association cortex of the dominant cerebral hemisphere.

APHEMIA. An acquired impairment of verbal expression resulting from a lesion undercutting Broca's area and affecting the process of articulation.

APRAXIA. An acquired impairment of skilled movements despite the relevant motor pathways being intact, resulting from OBD involving the cerebral association cortex.

A(DYS-)PROSODY. An acquired impairment of the finer aspects of the voice (melody, intonation, emphasis, rhythm), usually resulting from OBD involving the cerebral association cortex.

ASSOCIATION CORTEX. Those areas in the cerebral cortex which serve the higher cortical functions of refining, processing and integrating, nervous impulses received from, and passed to, subcortical structures.

ASTEREOGNOSIS. An acquired inability to identify a familiar object by touch alone, despite intact subcortical pathways and a normal conscious level, usually resulting from OBD involving the cerebral association cortex.

ATTENTION. The ability to selectively and appropriately attend to certain essential aspects of the environment.

AUTOMATISM. The retention of normal posture and muscle tone while performing simple or complex movements, despite an impairment of the conscious level.

BRIEF REACTIVE PSYCHOSIS. A psychotic illness lasting less than 2 weeks and precipitated by some major psychosocial stress.

CATAPLEXY. A sudden loss of muscle tone, which may be focal or generalised, and causes falling if the lower limbs are involved.

CATATONIC. Involving an excess, a deficiency or some other abnormality of motor activity. *See* mutism and stereotypy. May be organic or non-organic in origin.

CEREBRAL PALSY. A movement disorder resulting from organic brain disease occurring during the perinatal period.

CHOREA. An involuntary, sudden, rapid, variable, purposeless movement.

COGNITION. A non-specific term encompassing the higher cortical functions of perceiving, conceiving, remembering, reasoning, imagining and judging.

CONFABULATION. A falsification of memory, occurring in association with memory impairment resulting from OBD.

CONSTRUCTIONAL APRAXIA. An acquired inability to construct patterns by drawing or arranging objects, usually resulting from OBD involving the cerebral association cortex.

CONVERSION PHENOMENON. A physical sign that is produced unconsciously as a result of some psychological conflict or need.

DELIRIUM. An acute, usually reversible, global impairment of cognition, resulting from an organic disorder of brain function.

DELUSION. A false unshakeable belief, that cannot be understood in the context of the patient's social or cultural background. (It is systematised if it is persistent and forms part of a complex system based on one particular theme).

DEMENTIA. A chronic, often irreversible, global impairment of cognition, associated with an abnormality of brain structure.

DEPRESSION. A disturbance of mood involving feelings of misery and sadness. It can be neurotic (*see* neurosis) or psychotic (*see* psychosis). In either type the nature of the symptoms tend to be congruent with the mood.

DEVELOPMENTAL. Congenital or arising during the first decade of life.

DIENCEPHALON. The area of the brain including the thalamus, hypothalamus, subthalamus and epithalamus.

DISSOCIATION. An altered state of consciousness, which serves an unconscious purpose, and often involves the isolation of an idea from its associated emotional tone.

DYSPHORIC. An unpleasant mood state.

DYSTONIA. Involuntary muscle movements that are slow, sustained and contort the affected part of the body.

EPILEPSY. Recurrent, transient alterations of behaviour, resulting from an abnormal and excessive discharge of cerebral neurones.

EPISODIC DYSCONTROL. Intermittent outbursts of aggression that occur out of proportion to any provoking event.

FLIGHT OF IDEAS. The experience of ideas (completed or fragmentary) rapidly entering conscious awareness. Usually accompanies pressure of speech.

FUGUE. Wandering behaviour occurring while the patient is in a dissociated state.

HALLUCINATION. A sensory perception in the absence of an appropriate sensory stimulus (excluding dreams).

HALLUCINOSIS. A hallucination occurring in association with otherwise normal cognition and clear consciousness.

HISTRIONIC PERSONALITY. A persistent, severe developmental disorder of emotional maturation, often resulting in emotional instability and superficiality, dependency and sexual maladjustment.

HYPOMANIA. An elated mood associated with motor overactivity, flight of ideas (which result in pressure of speech) and the positive symptoms of psychosis.

ICTAL. Any behaviour or experience that is the direct result of an epileptic discharge.

ILLUSION. The distortion of a real perception.

INTER-ICTAL. Unrelated to an excessive and abnormal discharge of neural tissue, but occurring in someone who is prone to such (epileptic) discharges, at other times.

LA BELLE INDIFFÉRENCE. An attitude of unconcern in a patient, that is inappropriate in relation to the apparent severity of his illness.

MAJOR TRANQUILLISER. *See* neuroleptic.

MALINGERING. The deliberate production of symptoms or signs in order to mimic physical illness.

MINOR TRANQUILLISER. *See* anxiolytic.

MINIMAL BRAIN DYSFUNCTION. A poorly defined syndrome involving certain behaviours and/or neurological signs, of uncertain origin and significance. Usually taken to refer to hyperactivity and disorders of attention and impulse control.

MONOAMINE OXIDASE INHIBITOR. *See* antidepressant.

MOTOR IMPERSISTENCE. An involuntary inability to continue a particular pattern of motor behaviour, despite understanding instructions to the contrary.

MUTISM. An absence of verbal expression.

MYOCLONUS. A shock-like contraction of part of a muscle, a whole muscle or a group of muscles.

MYOTONIA. Delayed relaxation involving skeletal muscles.

NEGATIVE SYMPTOMS OF PSYCHOSIS. Those symptoms that show relatively little response (compared with the positive symptoms) to neuroleptic treatment—asociality, affective flattening, poverty of speech, impaired attention and abulia.

NEUROLEPTIC. An antipsychotic drug, most effective in treating the positive symptoms of psychosis, producing relatively little sedation (phenothiazines, butyrophenones etc.). Also referred to as major tranquillisers.

NEUROSIS. A non-organic mental disorder, unassociated with the positive symptoms of psychosis and not fully understandable in the context of the patient's personality.

NON-ORGANIC DISORDER. A "functional" or "psychogenic" disorder. Implies an absence of abnormality of physical structure of function.

ORGANIC BRAIN SYNDROME. A group of symptoms and/or signs that are found in association with an acute or chronic impairment of brain function.

ORGANIC DISORDER. Due to an alteration in the structure and/or function of the body.

PARANOID. Persecutory or grandiose.

PERI-ICTAL. Behaviour or experience that occurs before or after an epileptic discharge, but is not ictal.

PERSONALITY. Those aspects of behaviour that are particularly characteristic of a person's mode of interacting with his surroundings.

POSITIVE SYMPTOMS OF PSYCHOSIS. Those symptoms that tend to respond to neuroleptic treatment—hallucinations, delusions, and disorder of the form of thinking.

POST-ICTAL. Behaviour or experience that occurs immediately following an epileptic discharge, but is not ictal.

PRESSURE OF SPEECH. Rapid production of speech that is difficult to interrupt. In its extreme form there is a disorder of the form of thinking. Usually accompanies flight of ideas.

PSEUDODEMENTIA. Any disorder not involving a global impairment of cognition, but mimicking a dementia. Can be organic or non-organic.

PSYCHOGENIC DISORDER. *See* non-organic disorder.

PSYCHOPATHIC PERSONALITY. *See* antisocial personality.

PSYCHOSIS. Any disorder involving the positive symptoms of psychosis. (*See* positive symptoms of psychosis.)

SCHIZO-AFFECTIVE. Involving features compatible with both a schizophrenic and an affective disorder.

SCHIZOID PERSONALITY. A persistent, severe developmental failure to respond emotionally to others. This results in an emotionally cold and aloof personality.

SCHIZOPHRENIA. A non-organic psychosis with a failure to return to the premorbid level of functioning for a period greater than 6 months. The clinical symptoms are not dominated by, or understandable as the result of any mood disorder present.

SCHIZOPHRENIFORM DISORDER. A schizophrenic illness of a duration greater than 2 weeks, but less than 6 months.

SCHIZOTYPAL PERSONALITY. A persistent, severe developmental abnormality involving idiosyncratic thinking and behaviour, and the experience of perceptual abnormalities. Though there may be some similarity with schizophrenia, psychosis is not present.

SPEECH DISORDER. An acquired impairment of verbal expression, due to OBD affecting the neuromuscular mechanisms concerned, e.g. dysarthria.

STEREOTYPY. Purposeless behaviour, that is carried out repetitively.

TARDIVE DYSKINESIA. A movement disorder, usually occurring as a delayed result of neuroleptic use. Typically involves rhythmic, involuntary, stereotyped movements of the mouth, jaws and tongue.

THOUGHT DISORDER. A non-specific term referring to an abnormality of the form, content, stream or possession of ideas.

TIC. Abrupt, repetitive, involuntary activity, involving a group of functionally related muscles.

TRICYCLIC ANTIDEPRESSANT. *See* antidepressant.

VORBEIREDEN. A verbal response that, though incorrect, indicates the question is understood and the correct response is known.

References

Abenson, M. H. (1970). "EEGs in chronic schizophrenia", *Br. J. Psychiat.*, **116**, 421–425.

Abrams, R., and Taylor, M. A. (1976). "Catatonia. A prospective clinical study", *Arch. Gen. Psychiat.*, **33**, 579–581.

Abrams, R., Taylor, M. A., and Stolvrow, K. A. C. (1979). "Catatonia and mania: Patterns of cerebral dysfunction", *Biol. Psychiat.*, **19**, 111–117.

Ackner, B. (1954a). "Depersonalisation: I. Aetiology and phenomenology", *J. Ment. Sci.*, **100**, 838–853.

Ackner, B. (1954b). "Depersonalisation: II. Clinical syndromes", *J. Ment. Sci.*, **100**, 854–872.

Alarcon, R. D., Dickinson, W. A., and Dohn, H. H. (1982). "Flashback phenomena. Clinical and diagnostic dilemmas", *J. Nerv. Ment. Dis.*, **170**, 217–223.

Alberman, E. (1978). "Perinatal mortality rates", *Br. J. Hosp. Med.*, **20**, 439–443.

Albert, M. L. (1978). "Subcortical Dementia", in *Alzheimer's Disease: Senile Dementia and Related Disorders* (Eds. R. Katzman, R. D. Terry and K. L. Bick), pp.173–180, Raven Press, New York.

Albert, M. L., Feldman, R. G., and Willis, A. C. (1974). "The 'subcortical dementia' of progressive supranuclear palsy", *J. Neurol. Neuros. Psychiat.*, **37**, 121–130.

Alexander, M. P. (1982). "Episodic behaviours due to neurologic disorders other than epilepsy", in *Pseudoseizures* (Eds. T. L. Riley and A. Roy), pp.83–110, Williams and Wilkins, Baltimore.

Alexander, M. P., Stuss, D.T., and Benson, D.F. (1979). "Capgras Syndrome: a reduplicative phenomenon", *Neurology*, **29**, 334–339.

Ali, A. R., Smales, O. R. C., and Aslam, M. (1978). "Surma and lead poisoning", *Br. Med. J.*, **2**, 915–916.

Allison, R. S. (1966). "Perseveration as a sign of diffuse and focal brain damage", *Br. Med. J.*, **2**, 1027–1032.

Amado, H., and Lustman, P. J. (1982). "Attention deficit disorders persisting in adulthood: a review", *Compr. Psychiat.*, **23**, 300–314.

Anderson, E. W., and Mallinson, W. P. (1941). "Psychogenic episodes in the course of major psychoses", *J. Ment. Sci.*, **84**, 383–396.

Anderson, E. W., Trethowan, W. H., and Kenna, J. C. (1959). "An experimental investigation of simulation and pseudo-dementia", *Acta Psychiat. Neurol. Scand.*, **Suppl. 132**, 1–42.

Andreasen, N. C. (1982). "Should the term "Thought Disorder" be revised", *Compr. Psychiat.*, **23**, 291–299.

Andreasen, N. C., Dennert, J. W., Olsen, S. A., and Damasio, A. R. (1982a). "Hemispheric asymmetries and schizophrenia", *Am. J. Psychiat.*, **139**, 427–430.

Andreasen, N. C., and Olsen, S. (1982). "Negative v positive schizophrenia", *Arch. Gen. Psychiat.*, **39**, 789–794.

Andreasen, N. C., Olsen, S. A., Dennert, J. W., and Smith, M. R. (1982b). "Ventricular enlargement in schizophrenia: relationship to positive and negative symptoms", *Arch. Gen. Psychiat.*, **139**, 297–302.

Andrulonis, P. A., Glueck, B. C., Stroebel, C. F., Vogel, N. G., Shapiro, A. L., and Aldridge, D. M. (1980). "Organic brain dysfunction and the Borderline Syndrome", in *Psychiatric Clinics of North America*, **Vol. 4**, 47–66, W. B. Saunders, Toronto.

Annegers, J. F., Hanser, W. A., Elveback, L. R., and Kurland, L. T. (1979). "The risk of epilepsy following febrile convulsions", *Neurology*, **29**, 297–303.

Annett, M. (1973). "Laterality of childhood hemiplegia and the growth of speech and intelligence", *Cortex*, **9**, 4–33.

Antoni, N. (1946). "Dreamy states, epileptic aura, depersonalisation and psychaesthenic fits", *Acta Psychiat. Neurol. Scand.*, **21**, 1–20.

Arieti, S. (1974). *Interpretation of Schizophrenia*, Basic Books, New York.

Atanasiu, P., and Gamet, A. (1978). "Rabies", in *Handbook of Clinical Neurology*, **Vol. 34**, (Eds. P. J. Vinken and G. W. Bruyn), pp.235–274, American Elsevier, New York.

Bagshaw, M. H., Mackworth, N. H., and Pribram, K. H. (1972). "The effect of resections of the inferotemporal cortex or the amygdala on visual orienting and habituation", *Neuropsychologia*, **10**, 153–162.

Bakan, P. (1977). "Left handedness and birth order revisited", *Neuropsychologia*, **15**, 837–839.

Baldwin, M. (1970). "Neurologic syndromes and hallucinations", in *Origin and Mechanisms of Hallucinations* (Ed. W. Keup), pp.3–12, Plenum Press, New York.

Baldwin, M., and Hofmann, A. (1969). "Hallucinations", in *Handbook of Clinical Neurology*, **Vol. 4** (Eds. P. J. Vinken and G. W. Bruyn), pp.327–329, American Elsevier, New York.

Ball, M. J. (1982). "Limbic predilection in Alzheimer Dementia: is reactivated herpes virus involved?" *Can. J. Neurol. Sci.*, **9**, 303–306.

Bannister, R. (1973). *Brain's Clinical Neurology*, Oxford University Press, London.

Barkley, R. A. (1977). "A review of stimulant drug research with hyperactive children", *J. Child Psychol. Psychiat.*, **128**, 127–165.

Bauer, H. G. (1959). "Endocrine and metabolic conditions related to pathology in the hypothalamus. A review", *J. Nerv. Ment. Dis.*, **128**, 323–338.

Bax, M. (1980). "Left hand, right hand", *Develop. Med. Child. Neurol.*, **22**, 567–568.

Bean, W. B. (1967). *Rare Diseases and Lesions. Their Contributions to Clinical Medicine*, Charles C. Thomas, Illinois.

Bear, D. M. (1979a). "Interictal behaviour in temporal lobe epilepsy: possible anatomic and physiologic bases", in *Epilepsy: Neurotransmitters, Behaviour and Pregnancy* (Ed. J. A. Wada), Canadian League Against Epilepsy/Western Institute on Epilepsy.

Bear, D. M. (1979b). "Temporal lobe epilepsy: a syndrome of sensory-limbic hyperconnection", *Cortex*, **15**, 357–384.

Bear, D., and Fedio, P. (1977). "Quantitative analysis of interictal behaviour in temporal lobe epilepsy". *Arch. Neurol.*, **34**, 454–467.

Bear, D., Levin, K., Blumer, D., Chetham, D., and Ryder, J. (1982). "Interictal behaviour in hospitalised temporal lobe epileptics: relationship to idiopathic psychiatric syndromes", *J. Neurol. Neuros. Psychiat.*, **45**, 481–488.

Bearn, A. G. (1972). "Wilson's Disease", in *The Metabolic Basis of Inherited Disease* (Eds. J. B. Stanbury, J. B. Wyngaarden and D. S. Fred), McGraw-Hill, New York.

Bebbington, P. (1979). "Sexual disorders", in *Essentials of Postgraduate Psychiatry* (Eds. P. Hill, R. Murray and A. Thorley), pp.247–275, Academic Press, London.

Beeson, P. B., and McDermott, W. (1971). *Cecil-Loeb Textbook of Medicine*, W. B. Saunders, London.

Bell, R., and Hall, R. C. W. (1977). "The mental status examination", *Am. Fam. Phys.*, **16**, 145–152.

Benson, D. F. (1979). *Aphasia, Alexia, Agraphia*, Churchill Livingstone, London.

Benson, D. F., Cummings, J. L., and Tsai, S. Y. (1982). "Angular gyrus syndrome simulating Alzheimer's disease", *Arch. Neurol.*, **39**, 616–625.

Benson, D. F., and Geschwind, N. (1975). "Psychiatric conditions associated with focal lesions of the central nervous system", in *American Handbook of Psychiatry*, **Vol. 4** (Ed. M. F. Reiser), pp.208–243, Basic Books, New York.

Benson, D. F., Marsden, C. D., and Meadows, J. C. (1974). "The amnesic syndrome of posterior cerebral artery occlusion", *Acta Neurol. Scand.*, **50**, 133–145.

Benson, D. F., Stuss, D. T., Naeser, M. A., Weir, W. S., Kaplan, E. F., and Levine, H. (1981). "The long-term effects of pre-frontal leucotomy", *Arch. Neurol.*, **38**, 165–169.

Benton, A. L., and Spreen, O. (1961). "Visual memory test: the simulation of mental incompetence", *Arch. Gen. Psychiat.*, **4**, 79–83.

Benton, A. L., Van Allen, M. W., and Fogel, M. L. (1964). "Temporal orientation in cerebral disease", *J. Nerv. Ment. Dis.*, **139**, 110–120.

Bentson, J., Reza, M., Winter, J., and Wilson, G. (1978). "Steroids and apparent cerebral atrophy on computed tomography scans", *J. Comput. Assist. Tomog.*, **2**, 16–23.

Berg, J. M., and Kirman, B. H. (1960). "The mentally defective twin", *Br. Med. J.*, **1**, 1911–1917.

Bergin, J. D. (1957). "Rapidly progressing dementia in disseminated sclerosis", *J. Neurol. Neuros. Psychiat.*, **20**, 285–292.

Bergman, H., Borg, S., Hindmarsh, T., Idestiom, C. M., and Mutzell, S. (1980). "Computed tomography of the brain and neuropsychological assessment of male alcoholic patients", in *Addiction and Brain Damage* (Ed. D. Richter), pp.202–214, University Park Press, Baltimore.

Berlyne, N. (1972). "Confabulation", *Br. J. Psychiat.*, **120**, 31–39.

Berrington, W. P., Liddell, D. W., and Foulds, G. A. (1956). "A re-evaluation of the fugue", *J. Ment. Sci.*, **102**, 280–286.

Berrios, G. E. (1981). "Stupor revisited", *Compr. Psychiat.*, **22**, 466–489.

Berrios, G. E. (1982). "Tactile hallucinations: conceptual and historical aspects", *J. Neurol. Neuros. Psychiat.*, **45**, 285–293.

Betts, T. A., Merskey, H., and Pond, D. A. (1976). "Psychiatry", in *A Textbook of Epilepsy* (Eds. J. Laidlaw and A. Richens), pp.145–184, Churchill Livingstone, New York.

Bickerstaff, E. R. (1961). "Impairment of consciousness in migraine", *Lancet*, **381**, 1057–1059.

Bickerstaff, E. R. (1974). "Migraine and facial pain", *Medicine*, **31**, 1804–1818.

Binder, R. L. (1983). "Neurologically silent brain tumors in psychiatric hospital admissions: three cases and a review", *J. Clin. Psychiat.*, **44**, 94–97.

Bird, T. D., and Hall, J. G. (1977). "Clinical neurogenetics", *Neurology (Minneap.)*, **27**, 1057–1060.

Bishop, D. V. M. (1980). "Handedness, clumsiness and cognitive ability", *Develop. Med. Child Neurol.*, **22**, 569–579.

Black, D. W. (1982). "Pathological laughter: a review of the literature", *J. Nerv. Ment. Dis.*, **170**, 67–71.

Blau, J. N., Wiles, C. M. and Solomon, F. S. (1983). "Unilateral somatic symptoms due to hyperventilation", *Br. Med. J.*, **286**, 1109.

Bleckwenn, W. J. (1931). "The use of sodium amytal in catatonia", *Res. Publ. Assoc. Nerv. Ment. Dis.*, **10**, 224–229.

Bleuler, E. P. (1950). *Dementia Praecox*, International Universities Press, New York.

Bleuler, M. (1974). "The long term course of the schizophrenic psychoses", *Psychol. Med.*, **4**, 244–254.

342

Blumer, D. (1970). "Hypersexual episodes in temporal lobe epilepsy", *Am. J. Psychiat.*, **126**, 1099–1106.

Blumer, D., and Benson, D. F. (1975). "Personality changes with frontal and temporal lobe lesions", in *Psychiatric Aspects of Neurologic Disease* (Eds. D. F. Benson and D. Blumer), pp.151–170, Grune and Stratton, New York.

Blumer, D., and Walker, A. E. (1975). "The neural basis of sexual behaviour", in *Psychiatric Aspects of Neurologic Disease* (Eds. D. F. Benson and D. Blumer), pp.199–217, Grune and Stratton, London.

Boddy, J. (1978). *Brain systems and psychological concepts*, John Wiley and Sons, London.

Boll, T. J. (1981). "The Halstead–Reitan neuropsychological battery", in *Handbook of Clinical Neuropsychology* (Eds. S. B. Filskov and T. J. Boll), pp.577–607, John Wiley and Sons, New York.

Bond, A., and Lader, M. (1979). "Benzodiazepines and aggression", in *Psychopharmacology of Aggression* (Ed. M. Sandler), pp.173–182, Raven Press, New York.

Bondareff, W., Baldy, R., and Levy, R. (1981). "Quantitative computed tomography in senile dementia", *Arch. Gen. Psychiat.*, **38**, 1365–1368.

Botez, J. E., Ethier, R., Léveille, J., and Botez, T. (1977). "A syndrome of early recognition of occult hydrocephalus and cerebral atrophy", *Qtrly. J. Med.*, **46**, 365–380.

Botez, M. I. (1982). "Falls", *Br. J. Hosp. Med.*, **28**, 494–503.

Bradshaw, J. R., Thomson, J. L. G., and Campbell, M. J. (1983). "Computed tomography in the investigation of dementia", *Br. Med. J.*, **286**, 277–280.

Braffos, O., and Eltinger, L. (1963). "Psychotic patients with narcolepsy", *Nord. Psychiato. Tidsskr.*, **17**, 220–226.

Braham, J. (1971). "Jakob–Creutzfeldt disease: treatment by amantadine", *Br. Med. J.*, **4**, 212–213.

Braunwald, E. (1980). "Valvular heart disease", in *Harrison's Principles of Internal Medicine* (Eds. K. J. Isselbacher, R. A. Adams, E. Braunwald, R. G. Petersdorf and J. D. Wilson), pp.1096–1112, McGraw-Hill, London.

Breakey, W. R., Goodell, H., Lorenz, P. C., and McHugh, P. R. (1974). "Hallucinogenic drugs as precipitants of schizophrenia", *Psychol. Med.*, **4**, 255–261.

Brenner, I., and Rheuban, W. J. (1978). "The catatonic dilemma", *Am. J. Psychiat.*, **135**, 1242–1243.

Brewer, C., and Perret, L. (1971). "Brain damage due to alcohol consumption: an air encephalographic, psychometric and electroencephalographic study", *Br. J. Psychiat.*, **6**, 170–182.

Brockington, I. F. (1979). "Psychiatric disorders in pregnancy and in the puerperium", *Prescribers Journal*, **19**, 66–71.

Brodal, A. (1969). *Neurological Anatomy in Relation to Clinical Medicine*, Oxford University Press, London.

Bronowski, J. (1956). *Science and Human Values,* p.7, Perennial Library/Harper Row, New York.

Brooks, D. N., and Baddeley, A. D. (1976). "What can amnesic patients learn?" *Neuropsychologia*, **14**, 111–122.

Brown, G., Chadwick, O., and Shaffer, D. (1981). "A prospective study of children with head injuries in adulthood, III: psychiatric sequelae", *Psychol. Med.*, **11**, 63–78.

Brown, W. A. (1981). "The dexamethasone suppression test: clinical applications", *Psychosom.*, **22**, 951–955.

Bruun, R. D., and Shapiro, A. K. (1972). "Differential diagnosis of Gilles de la Tourette's syndrome", *J. Nerv. Ment. Dis.*, **155**, 328–334.

Buchsbaum, M. S., Ingvar, D. H., Kessler, R., Waters, R. N., Cappelletti, J., van Kammen, D. P., King, A. C., Johnson, J. L., Manning, R. G., Flynn, R. W., Mann,

L. S., Bunney, W. E., and Sokoloff, L. (1982). "Cerebral glucography with positron tomography", *Arch. Gen. Psychiat.*, **39**, 251–259.

Budell, J. W. (1976). "Treatment of congenital syphilis", *J. Am. Ven. Dis. Assoc.*, **3**, 168–171.

Bull, J. (1969). "Massive aneurysm at the base of the brain", *Brain*, **92**, 535–570.

Butters, N., and Barton, M. (1970). "Effect of parietal lobe damage on the performance of reversible operations in space", *Neuropsychologia*, **8**, 205–214.

Butters, N., and Brody, B. A. (1968). "The role of the left parietal lobe in the mediation of intra- and cross-modal associations", *Cortex*, **4**, 328–343.

Caine, E. D. (1981). "Pseudodementia", *Arch. Gen. Psychiat.*, **38**, 1359–1364.

Caine, E. D., Hunt, R. D., Weingartner, H., and Ebert, M. H. (1978). "Huntington's dementia", *Arch. Gen. Psychiat.*, **35**, 377–384.

Campbell, S. B., Endman, M. W., and Bernfeld, G. (1977). "A three-year follow-up of hyperactive preschoolers into elementary school", *J. Child Psychol. Psychiat.*, **18**, 239–249.

Cantwell, D. P. (1975). "Genetics of hyperactivity", *J. Child Psychol. Psychiat.*, **16**, 261–264.

Cantwell, D. P. (1979). "Minimal brain dysfunction in adults: evidence from studies of psychiatric illness in the families of hyperactive children", in *Psychiatric Aspects of Minimal Brain Dysfunction in Adults* (Ed. L. Bellak), pp.37–44, Grune and Stratton, New York.

Caplan, L. R., and Schoene, W. D. (1978). "Clinical features of subcortical arteriosclerotic encephalopathy (Bingswanger's disease)", *Neurology*, **28**, 1206–1215.

Caplan, L. R., Thomas, C., and Banks, G. (1982). "Central nervous system complications of 'T's and Blues' ", *Neurology (NY)*, **32**, 623–628.

Caplan, R. M. (1982). *Principles of Obstetrics*, Williams and Wilkins, Baltimore.

Carette, S., Keystone, E. C., and Urowitz, M. B. (1981). "Systemic lupus erythematosus", *Medicine North America*, **1**, 1528–1532.

Carroll, B. J. (1982). "The dexamethasone suppression test for melancholia", *Br. J. Psychiat.*, **140**, 292–304.

Carroll, B. J., Feinberg, M., Greden, J. F., Tarika, J., Albala, A. A., Haskett, R. F., James, N. M., Kronfol, Z., Lohr, N., Steiner, M., deVigne, J. P., and Young, E. (1981). "A specific laboratory test for the diagnosis of melancholia", *Arch. Gen. Psychiat.*, **38**, 15–22.

Casper, R. C., Eckere, E. D., Halmi, K. A., Goldberg, S. C., and Davis, J. M. (1980). "Bulimia", *Arch. Gen. Psychiat.*, **37**, 1030–1035.

Chadwick, O., Rutter, M., and Brown, G. (1981a). "A prospective study of children with head injuries, II: cognitive sequelae", *Psychol. Med.*, **11**, 49–61.

Chadwick, O., Rutter, M., and Shaffer, D. (1981b). "A prospective study of children with head injuries, IV: specific cognitive deficits", *J. Clin. Neuropsychol.*, **3**, 101–120.

Chamberlain, H. D. (1928). "The inheritance of left handedness", *J. Heredity*, **19**, 557–559.

Chedru, F., and Geschwind, N. (1972a). "Disorders of higher cortical functions in acute confusional states", *Cortex*, **8**, 395–411.

Chedru, F., and Geschwind, N. (1972b). "Writing disturbances in acute confusional states", *Neuropsychologia*, **10**, 343–353.

Clare, A. (1979). "Psychosurgery and electroconvulsive therapy", in *Essentials of Postgraduate Psychiatry* (Eds. P. Hill, R. Murray and A. Thorley), pp.649–681, Grune and Stratton, New York.

Cloninger, C. R., and Guze, S. B. (1975). "Hysteria and parental psychiatric illness", *Psychol. Med.*, **5**, 27–31.

Cobb, J. (1979). "Morbid jealousy", *Br. J. Hosp. Med.*, **21**, 511–519.

Cobb, W. A., and Morgan-Hughes, J. A. (1968). "Non-fatal subacute sclerosing leucoencephalitis", *J. Neurol. Neuros. Psychiat.*, **31**, 115–123.

Cohen, L. H., Thale, T., and Tissenbaum, M. J. (1944). "Acetylcholine treatment of schizophrenia", *Arch. Neurol. Psychiat.*, **51**, 171–178.

Cohen, S. (1981). "Adverse effects of marijuana: selected issues", in *Research Developments in Drug and Alcohol Use* (Eds. R. B. Millman, P. Cushman Jr. and J. H. Lowinson), pp.119–124, *Ann. N.Y. Acad. Sci.*, **Vol. 326**.

Coid, J. (1979). "Mania a potu: a critical review of pathological intoxication". *Psychol. Med.*, **9**, 709–719.

Collins, W. C. J., Lanigan, O., and Callaghan, N. (1983). "Plasma prolactin concentrations following epileptic and pseudoseizures", *J. Neurol. Neuros. Psychiat.*, **46**, 505–508.

Cooper, I. S., Amin, I., Riklan, M., Waltz, J. M., and Poon, T. P. (1976). "Chronic cerebellar stimulation in epilepsy: clinical and anatomical studies", *Arch. Neurol.*, **33**, 559–570.

Corbett, J. A., Harris, R., and Robinson, R. (1975). "Epilepsy", in *Mental Retardation and Developmental Disabilities: an Annual Review,* **Vol. 7** (Ed. J. Wortis), pp.79–111, Brunner/Mazel, New York.

Corsellis, J. A. N. (1969). "The pathology of dementia", *Br. J. Hosp. Med.*, **2**, 695–703.

Corsellis, J. A. N., Goldberg, G. J., and Norton, A. R. (1968). " 'Limbic encephalitis' and its association with carcinoma", *Brain*, **91**, 481–496.

Corston, R. N., and Godwin-Austen, R. N. (1982). "Transient global amnesia in four brothers", *J. Neurol. Neuros. Psychiat.*, **45**, 375–377.

Crammer, J. L. (1959). "Periodic psychoses", *Br. Med. J.*, **1**, 545–550.

Crisp, A. H. (1980). "Sleep, activity, nutrition and mood", *Br. J. Psychiat.*, **137**, 1–7.

Critchley, M. (1953). *The Parietal Lobes*, Edward Arnold, London.

Critchley, M. (1962). "Periodic hypersomnia and megaphagia in adolescent males", *Brain*, **85**, 627–657.

Critchley, M. (1970). *Aphasiology*, Edward Arnold, London.

Critchley, M. (1975). "The training of a neurologist", *Int. J. Neurol.*, **9**, 000–000.

Critchley, M., and Earl, C. J. C. (1932). "Tuberose sclerosis and allied conditions", *Brain*, **55**, 311–346.

Crockett, D., Clark, C., and Klonoff, H. (1981). "Introduction—An overview of neuropsychology", in *Handbook of Clinical Neuropsychology* (Eds. S. B. Filskov and T. J. Boll), pp.1–37, John Wiley and Sons, New York.

Crow, T. J. (1980). "Molecular pathology of schizophrenia: more than one disease process", *Br. Med. J.*, **280**, 66–68.

Crow, T. J., and Stevens, M. (1978). "Age disorientation of chronic schizophrenia: the nature of the cognitive deficit", *Br. J. Psychiat.* **133**, 137–142.

Cummings, J., Benson, D. F., and LoVerme, S. (1980). "Reversible dementia", *J. Am. Med. Ass.*, **243**, 2434–2439.

Cummings, J. L., and Duchen, L. W. (1981). "Klüver–Bucy syndrome in Pick's disease: clinical and pathologic correlations", *Neurology (Minneap.)*, **31**, 1415–1422.

Currie, S., Heathfield, K. W. G., Henson, R. A., and Scott, D. F. (1971). "Clinical course and prognosis of temporal lobe epilepsy. A survey of 666 patients", *Brain*, **94**, 173–190.

Currier, R. D., Jackson, J. F., and Meydrech, E. F. (1982). "Progression rate and age at onset are related in autosomal dominant neurologic diseases", *Neurology (NY)*, **32**, 907–909.

Cutting, J. (1978a). "The relationship between Korsakov's syndrome and 'alcoholic dementia' ", *Br. J. Psychiat.*, **132**, 240–251.

Cutting, J. (1978b). "Specific psychological deficits in alcoholics", *Br. J. Psychiat.*, **133**, 119–122.

Cytryn, L., and Lourie, R. S. (1980). "Mental retardation", in *Comprehensive Textbook of Psychiatry 3* (Eds. H. I. Kaplan, A. M. Freedman and B. J. Sadock), pp.2484–2526, Williams and Wilkins, London.

345

Dahlstrom, W. G., Welsh, G. S., and Dahlstrom, L. E. (1972). *An MMPI Handbook. Volume 1: Clinical Interpretation*, University of Minnesota Press, Minneapolis.

Damasio, A. R., Damasio, H., and Van Hoesen, G. W. (1982). "Prosopagnosia: anatomic basis and behavioural mechanisms", *Neurology (NY)*, **32**, 331–341.

Davies, R. K., and Neil, J. F. (1979). "Cerebral dysrhythmias in schizophrenics: clinical correlates", in *Psychiatric Aspects of Minimal Brain Dysfunction in Adults* (Ed. L. Bellak), pp.139–150, Grune and Stratton, New York.

Davis, K. R., Taveras, J. M., and New, P. F. J. (1975). "Cerebal infarction diagnosis by computerised tomography: analysis and evaluation of findings", *Am. J. Roentgen.*, **124**, 643–660.

Davison, K., and Bagley, C. R. (1969). "Schizophrenia-like psychoses associated with organic disorders of the central nervous system: a review of the literature", in *Current Problems in Neuropsychiatry*, (Ed. R. N. Herrington), pp.113–184, *Br. J. Psychiat.* Special Pub., Headley Bros., Ashford, Kent.

De Jong, R. N. (1970). *The neurological examination*, Harper and Row, New York.

Delgado-Escueta, A. V., Mattson, R. H., King, L., Goldensohn, E. S., Spiegel, H., Madsen, J., Crandall, P., Dreifuss, F., and Porter, R. J. (1981). "The nature of aggression during epileptic seizures", *New Eng. J. Med.*, **305**, 711–716.

Demanet, J. C. (1976). "Usefulness of noradrenaline and tyramine infusion tests in the diagnosis of orthostatic hypotension", *Cardiology*, **Suppl. 61**, 213–224.

De Renzi, E., and Faglioni, P. (1967). "The relationship between visuo-spatial impairment and constructional apraxia", *Cortex*, **3**, 327–342.

Detre, T. P., and Jarecki, H. G. (1971). *Modern Psychiatric Treatment*, pp.203–216, Lippincott, Philadelphia.

DeVaul, R. A., and Hall, R. C. W. (1980). "Hallucinations", in *Psychiatric Presentations of Medical Illness* (Ed. R. C. W. Hall), pp.91–103, Spectrum Pub., New York.

De Villasante, M. T., and Taveras, J. M. (1976). "Computerized tomography in acute head trauma", *Am. J. Roentgenol.*, **126**, 765–778.

Dewan, M. J., Pandurangi, A. K., Boucher, M. L., Levy, B. F., and Major, L. F. (1982). "Abnormal dexamethasone suppression test results in chronic schizophrenic patients", *Am. J. Psychiat.*, **139**, 1501–1503.

Dewhurst, K. (1969). "The neurosyphilitic psychoses today: a survey of 91 cases", *Br. J. Psychiat.*, **115**, 31–38.

Dewhurst, K., and Beard, A. W. (1970). "Sudden religious conversions in temporal lobe epilepsy", *Br. J. Psychiat.*, **117**, 497–507.

Dewhurst, K., Oliver, J., Trick, K. L. K., and McKnight, A. L. (1969). "Neuropsychiatric aspects of Huntington's disease", *Confina Neurologica*, **31**, 258–268.

Dewhurst, K., and Pearson, J. (1955). "Visual hallucinations of the self in organic disease", *J. Neurol. Neuros. Psychiat.*, **18**, 53–57.

Dietch, J. T. (1981). "Diagnosis of organic anxiety disorders", *Psychosom.*, **22**, 661–669.

DiMascio, A., Shader, R. I., and Harmatz, J. (1969). "Psychotropic drugs and induced hostility", *Psychosom.*, **Suppl. 10**, 46–47.

Dobbing, J., and Smart, J. L. (1974). "Vulnerability of developing brain and behaviour", *Br. Med. Bull.*, **30**, 164–168.

Dongier, S. (1959). "Statistical study of clinical and electroencephalographic manifestations of 536 psychotic episodes occurring in 516 epileptics between clinical seizures", *Epilepsia*, **1**, 117–142.

Dooling, E. C., and Richardson, E. P. (1976). "Delayed encephalopathy after strangling", *Arch. Neurol.*, **33**, 196–199.

Doyle, F. H., Gore, J. C., Pennock, J. M., Bydder, G. M., Orr, J. S., Steiner, R. E., Young, I. R., Burl, M., Clow, H., Gilderdale, D. J., Bailes, D. R., and Walters, P. E. (1981). "Imaging of the brain by nuclear magnetic resonance", *Lancet*, **2**, 53–57.

Drever, J. (1964). *A Dictionary of Psychology* (Revised by H. Wallerstein), Penguin Books, London.

346

Drewe, E. A. (1974). "The effect of type and area of brain lesion on Wisconsin Card Sorting test performance", *Cortex*, **10**, 159–170.

DSM III (1980). *Diagnostic and Statistical Manual of Mental Disorders* (Third Edition), American Psychiatric Association, Washington.

Ducas, J., and Robson, H. G. (1981). "Cerebrospinal fluid penicillin levels during therapy for latent syphilis", *J. Am. Med. Assoc.*, **246**, 2583–2584.

Dyken, P. R., and Miller, M. D. (1980). *Facial features of neurological syndromes*, C. V. Mosby, Missouri.

Ellis, C., and Fidler, J. (1982). "Drugs in pregnancy: adverse reactions", *Br. J. Hosp. Med.*, **28**, 575–584.

Ervin, F., Epstein, A. W., and King, H. E. (1955). "Behaviour of epileptic and non-epileptic patients with 'temporal spikes' ", *A.M.A. Arch. Neurol. Psychiat.*, **74**, 488–497.

Evans, N. J. R. (1982). "Cranial computerized tomography in clinical psychiatry: 100 consecutive cases", *Compr. Psychiat.*, **23**, 445–450.

Ewing, D. J., Campbell, I. W., Murray, A., Neilson, J. M. M., and Clarke, B. F. (1978). "Immediate heart-rate response to standing: simple test for autonomic neuropathy in diabetes", *Br. Med. J.*, **1**, 145–147.

Falconer, M. A. (1969). "The surgical treatment of temporal lobe epilepsy", in *Current Problems in Neuropsychiatry. Schizophrenia, Epilepsy, and the Temporal Lobe* (Ed. R. N. Herrington), pp.95–101, Headley Bros., Kent.

Famuyiwa, O. O., Eccleston, D., Donaldson, A. A., and Garside, R. F. (1979). "Tardive dyskinesia and dementia", *Br. J. Psychiat.*, **135**, 500–508.

Feldman, M., and Bender, M. B. (1970). "Visual illusions and hallucinations in parieto-occipital lesions of the brain", in *Origins and Mechanisms of Hallucinations* (Ed. W. Kemp), pp.23–35, Plenum Press, New York.

Fenton, G. W. (1972). "Epilepsy and automatism", *Br. J. Hosp. Med.*, **7**, 57–64.

Fenton, G. W. (1975). "Clinical disorders of sleep", *Br. J. Hosp. Med.*, **14**, 120–145.

Feussner, J. R., Linfors, E. W., Blessing, C. L., and Starmer, C. F. (1981). "Computed toography in alcohol withdrawal seizures", *Ann. Int. Med.*, **94**, 519–522.

Field, H. (1981). "Post-traumatic syndrome" (Ltr to ed.), *J. Roy. Soc. Med.*, **74**, 941–942.

Filskov, S. B., and Boll, T. J. (Eds.) (1981). *Handbook of Clinical Neuropsychology*, John Wiley and Sons, New York.

Filskov, S. B., and Leli, D. A. (1981). "Assessment of the individual in neuropsychological practice", in *Handbook of Clinical Neuropsychology* (Eds. S. B. Filskov and T. J. Boll), pp.545–576, John Wiley and Sons, New York.

Fischman, R. H. (1982). "Multiple sclerosis: a new perspective on epidemiologic patterns", *Neurology (NY)*, **32**, 864–870.

Fisher, C. M. (1979). "Syncope of obscure origin", *Can. J. Neurol. Sci.*, **6**, 7–20.

Fisher, C. M. (1980). "Late-life migraine accompaniments as a cause of unexplained transient ischaemic attacks", *Can. J. Neurol. Sci.*, **7**, 9–18.

Fisher, C. M. (1982a). "Lacunar strokes and infarcts: a review", *Neurology (NY)*, **32**, 871–876.

Fisher, C. M. (1982b). "Transient global amnesia", *Arch. Neurol.*, **39**, 605–608.

Fisher, C. M. (1982c). "Hydrocephalus as a cause of disturbances of gait in the elderly", *Neurology (NY)*, **32**, 1358–1363.

Fisher, C. M., and Adams, R. H. (1964). "Transient global amnesia", *Acta Neurol. Scand.*, **40 (Suppl. 9)**, 7–83.

Fitzgerald, P. A., and Wells, C. E. (1977). "Hallucinations as a conversion reaction", *Dis. Nerv. Sys.*, **38**, 381–383.

Flor-Henry, P. (1969). "Psychosis and temporal lobe epilepsy", *Epilepsia*, **10**, 363–395.

Flor-Henry, P. (1978). "Gender, hemispheric specialization and psychopathology", *Soc. Sci. Med.*, **12B**, 155–162.

Foster, J. B., Leiguarda, R., and Tilley, P. J. B. (1976). "Brain damage in National Hunt jockeys", *Lancet*, **1**, 981–983.

Franzen, G., and Ingvar, D. H. (1975). "Abnormal distribution of cerebral activity in chronic schizophrenia", *J. Psychiat. Res.*, **12**, 199–214.

Frederiks, J. A. M. (1969). "The agnosias", in *Handbook of Clinical Neurology*, **Vol. 4** (Eds. P. J. Vinken and G. W. Bruyn), pp.13–47, North Holland, New York.

Freemon, F. R. (1976). "Evaluation of patients with progressive intellectual deterioration", *Arch. Neurol.*, **33**, 658–659.

Frieske, D. A., and Wilson, W. P. (1966). "Formal qualities of hallucinations: a comparative study of the visual hallucinations in patients with schizophrenic, organic and affective psychoses", in *Psychopathology of Schizophrenia* (Eds. P. H. Hoch and J. Zubin), pp.49–62, Grune and Stratton, New York.

Friis, M. L., Broeng-Nielsen, B., Sindrup, E. H., Lund, M., Fogh-Anderson, P., and Hauge, M. (1981). "Facial clefts among epileptic patients", *Arch. Neurol.*, **38**, 227–229.

Friis, M. L., and Lund, M. (1974). "Stress convulsions", *Arch. Neurol.*, **31**, 155–159.

Frischholz, E. J. (1982). "Hypnotic responsivity and severe psychopathology". Paper presented at the 135th Annual Meeting of the Am. Psychiat. Ass., Toronto, May, 1982.

Gabbard, G. O., Twemlow, S. W., and Jones, F. C. (1982). "Differential Diagnosis of Altered Mind/Body Perception", *Psychiatry*, **45**, 361–369.

Gaind, R. N., and Jacoby, R. (1978). "Benzodiazepines causing aggression", in *Current Themes in Psychiatry I* (Eds. R. N. Gaind and B. L. Hudson), pp.371–379, Macmillan, London.

Gajdusek, D. C., Gibbs, C. J., and Alpers, M. (1966). "Experimental transmission of a Kuru-like syndrome to chimpanzees", *Nature*, **209**, 794–796.

Garfinkel, P. E., Moldofsky, H., and Garner, D. M. (1980). "The Heterogeneity of Anorexia Nervosa", *Arch. Gen. Psychiat.*, **37**, 1036–1040.

Gastaut, H. (1969). "Clinical and electroencephalographical classification of epileptic seizures", *Epilepsia*, **Suppl. 10**, 1–28.

Gastaut, H., Broughton, R., Roger, J., and Tassinari, C. A. (1974). "Generalised non-convulsive seizures without local onset", in *Handbook of Clinical Neurology*, **Vol. 15** (Eds. P. J. Vinken and G. W. Bruyn), pp.130–144, American Elsevier, New York.

Gates, E. M., Kernhonan, J. W., and Craig, W. M. (1950). "Metastatic brain abscess", *Medicine*, **29**, 71–98.

Gawel, M. J. (1983). "Migraine and cluster headaches", *Medicine North America*, **1**, 3007–3010.

Gawler, J., Du Boulay, G., Bull, J. W. D., and Marshall, J. (1976). "A comparison of computer assisted tomography (EMI scanner) with conventional neuroradiologic methods in the investigation of patients clinically suspected of intracranial tumor", *J. Can. Ass. Radiol.*, **27**, 157–169.

Gelenberg, A. J. (1976). "The catatonic syndrome", *Lancet*, **1**, 1339–1341.

Gelenberg, A. J., and Mandel, M. R. (1977). "Catatonic reactions to high-potency neuroleptic drugs", *Arch. Gen. Psychiat.*, **34**, 947–950.

Gelineau, J. (1980). "De la narcolepsie", *Gazette des Hôpitaux (Paris)*, **53**, 626–628.

Gerson, S. N., Benson, D. F., and Frazier, S. H. (1977). "Diagnosis: schizophrenia versus posterior aphasia", *Am. J. Psychiat.*, **134**, 966–969.

Geschwind, N. (1965). "Disconnexion syndromes in animals and man", *Brain*, **88**, 237–294, 585–644.

Geschwind, N. (1979). "Specializations of the Human Brain", *Sci. Am.*, **241**, 158–168.

Geschwind, N. (1982). "Disorders of attention: a frontier in neuropsychology", *Phil. Trans. R. Soc. Lond.*, **B298**, 173–185.

Ghoneim, M. H. and Mewaldt, S. P. (1977). "Studies on human memory: the interactions of diazepam, scopolamine and physostigmine", *Psychopharmacol.*, **52**, 1–6.

348

Gibbs, C. J., and Gajdusek, D. C. (1969). "Infection as the etiology of spongiform encephalopathy (Creutzfeldt–Jacob disease)", *Science,* 165, 1023–1025.

Gilbert, G. J. (1964). "Periodic hypersomnia and bulimia: The Kleine–Levin syndrome", *Neurology,* 14, 844–850.

Gilliatt, R. W., and Pratt, R. T. C. (1952). "Disorders of perception and performance in a case of right-sided cerebral thrombosis", *J. Neurol. Neuros. Psychiat.,* 15, 264–271.

Girgis, M. (1971). "The orbital surface of the frontal lobe of the brain and mental disorders", *Acta Psychiat. Scand.,* **Suppl. 222,** 1–58.

Gittleson, N. L., and Richardson, T. D. E. (1973). "Myasthenia gravis and schizophrenia—a rare combination", *Br. J. Psychiat.,* 122, 343–344.

Gjessing, L. R. (1974). "A review of periodic catatonia", *Biol. Psychiat.,* 8, 23–45.

Glen, A. I. M. (1979). "Choice of therapeutic agents in Alzheimer's disease", in *Alzheimer's disease* (Eds. A. I. M. Glenn and L. J. Whalley), pp.140–147, Churchill Livingstone, New York.

Goddard, G. V., McIntyre, D. C. and Leech, C. K. (1969). "A permanent change in brain function resulting from daily electrical stimulation", *Exp. Neurol.,* 25, 295–330.

Golden, C. J. (1979). *Clinical Interpretation of Objective Psychological Tests,* Grune and Stratton, New York.

Golden, C. J., Graber, B., Moses, Jr., J. A. and Zatz, L. M. (1980a). "Differentiation of chronic schizophrenics with and without ventricular enlargement, by the Luria–Nebraska Neuropsychological Battery", *Int. J. Neurosci.,* 11, 131–138.

Golden, C. J., Moses, Jr., J. A., Zelazowski, R., Graber, B., Zatz, L. M., Horvath, T. B., and Berger, P. A. (1980b). "Cerebral ventricular size and neuropsychological impairment in young chronic schizophrenics", *Arch. Gen. Psychiat.,* 37, 619–623.

Goldensohn, E. S. (1979). "Use of the EEG for Evaluation of Focal Intracranial Lesions", in *Current Practice of Clinical Electroencephalography* (Eds. D. W. Klass and D. D. Daly), pp.307–341, Raven Press, New York.

Gomez, M. R., Kuntz, N. L., and Westmoreland, B. F. (1982). "Tuberose sclerosis, early onset of seizures, and mental subnormality: Study of discordant homozygous twins", *Neurology (NY),* 32, 604–611.

Goodwin, D. W., Alderson, P., and Rosenthal, R. (1971). "Clinical significance of hallucinations in psychiatric disorders", *Arch. Gen. Psychiat.,* 24, 76–80.

Gordon, E. B., and Sim, M. (1967). "The EEG in presenile dementia", *J. Neurol. Neuros. Psychiat.,* 30, 285–291.

Graham, J. R. (1977). *The MMPI: A Practical Guide,* Oxford University Press, New York.

Graham, P., and Rutter, M. (1968). "Organic brain dysfunction and child psychiatric disorders", *Br. Med. J.,* 3, 697–700.

Granacher, Jr., R. P. (1981). "Differential diagnosis of tardive dyskinesia: an overview". *Am. J. Psychiat.,* 138, 1288–1297.

Granacher, R. P., and Baldessarini, R. J. (1976). "Physostigmine. Its use in acute anticholinergic syndrome with antidepressant and anti-Parkinson drugs", *Arch. Gen. Psychiat.,* 32, 375–380.

Grant, I., and Mohns, L. (1976). "Chronic cerebral effects of alcohol and drug abuse", *Int. J. Addict.,* 10, 833–920.

Greenbaum, J. V., and Lurie, L. A. (1948). "Encephalitis as a causative factor in behaviour disorders of children", *J. Am. Med. Ass.,* 136, 923–930.

Greenough, A., and Davis, J. A. (1983). "Encephalitis lethargica: mystery of the past or undiagnosed disease of the present" (Ltr to ed.), *Lancet,* 1, 922–923.

Greenwood, R., Bhalla, A., Gordon, A., and Roberts, J. (1983). "Behaviour disturbances during recovery from herpes simplex encephalitis", *J. Neurol. Neuros. Psychiat.,* 46, 809–817.

Grimes, J. D. (1983). "Parkinsonism", in *Medicine North America,* 1, 2936–2945.

Gross, M. D., and Wilson, W. C. (1974). *Minimal Brain Dysfunction: A Clinical Study of Incidence, Diagnosis and Treatment in Over 1,000 Children*, Brunner/Mazel, New York.

Guberman, A. (1982). "Psychogenic pseudoseizures in non-epileptic patients", *Can. J. Psychiat.*, **27**, 401–404.

Gulick, T. A., Spinks, I. P., and King, D. W. (1982). "Pseudoseizures: ictal phenomena", *Neurology (NY)*, **32**, 24–30.

Guthkelch, A. N. (1981). "Post-traumatic syndrome" (Ltr to ed.), *J. Roy. Soc. Med.*, **74**, 940.

Hachinski, V. (1981). "Fits or faints?", *Medicine North America*, **1**, 2915–2917.

Hall, R. C. W., Feinsilver, D. L., and Holt, R. E. (1981a). "Anticholinergic psychosis: differential diagnosis and management", *Psychosom.*, **22**, 581–587.

Hall, R. C. W., Popkin, M. K., Stickney, S. K., and Gardner, E. R. (1979). "Presentation of the 'steroid psychoses' ", *J. Nerv. Ment. Dis.*, **167**, 229–236.

Hall, R. C. W., Stickney, S. K., and Gardner, E. R. (1981b). "Psychiatric symptoms in patients with systemic lupus erythematosis", *Psychosom.*, **22**, 15–24.

Halliday, A. M. (1980). "How useful are evoked potentials in clinical diagnosis", in *Current Clinical Neurophysiology* (Ed. C. E. Henry), pp.555–570, American Elsevier, New York.

Halliday, A. M., and Mason, A. A. (1964). "The effect of hypnotic anaesthesia on cortical responses", *J. Neurol. Neuros. Psychiat.*, **27**, 300–312.

Hamilton, M. (1974). *Fish's Clinical Psychopathology*, Wright, Bristol.

Hanson, J. W. (1979). "Anticonvulsants and the fetus: the fetal hydantoin syndrome and related problems", in *Epilepsy: Neurotransmitters, Behaviour and Pregnancy* (Ed. J. A. Wada), Canadian League Against Epilepsy/Western Institute on Epilepsy.

Hanson, J. W., and Smith, D. W. (1975). "The fetal hydantoin syndrome", *J. Paediatr.*, **87**, 285–290.

Hanson, J. W., Streissguth, A. P., and Smith, D. W. (1978). "The effects of moderate alcohol consumption during pregnancy on fetal growth and morphogenesis", *J. Paediatr.*, **92**, 457–460.

Hardyck, C., and Petrinovitch, L. F. (1977). "Left handedness", *Psychol. Bull.*, **84**, 385–404.

Hare, E. H. (1973). "A short note on pseudohallucinations", *Br. J. Psychiat.*, **122**, 469–476.

Harlow, J. M. (1868). "Recovery from the passage of an iron bar through the head", *Pub. Mass. Med. Soc.*, **2**, 329–346.

Harner, R. N. (1975). "EEG evaluation of the patient with dementia", in *Psychiatric Aspects of Neurological Disease* (Eds. D. F. Benson and D. Blumer), pp.63–82, Grune and Stratton, New York.

Harper, M. and Roth, M. (1962). "Temporal lobe epilepsy and the phobic anxiety-depersonalisation syndrome", *Compr. Psychiat.*, **3**, 129–151, 215–226.

Hart, F. D. (1979). *French's Index of Differential Diagnosis*, John Wright and Sons, Bristol.

Hart, H., Bax, M., and Jenkins, S. (1978). "The value of a developmental history", *Develop. Med. Child Neurol.*, **20**, 442–452.

Hartman, E. (1972). "Sleep and depression", *New Eng. J. Med.*, **286**, 269.

Hawkins, D. F. (1976). "Effects of drugs taken in pregnancy on the foetus", *J. Mat. Child Health*, **1976**, 24–29.

Hawton, K., Fagg, J., and Marsack, P. (1980). "Association between epilepsy and attempted suicide", *J. Neurol. Neuros. Psychiat.*, **43**, 168–170.

Heath, R. G. (1975). "Brain function and behavior. I. Emotion and sensory phenomena in psychotic patients and in experimental animals", *J. Nerv. Ment. Dis.*, **160**, 159–175.

Heath, R. G., Franklin, D. E., and Shraberg, D. (1979). "Gross pathology of the cerebellum in patients diagnosed and treated as functional psychiatric disorders", *J. Nerv. Ment. Dis.*, **167**, 585–592.

Heathfield, K. W. G. (1967). "Huntington's chorea", *Brain*, **90**, 203–232.

Heaton, R. K., and Crowley, T. J. (1981). "Effects of psychiatric disorders and their somatic treatments on neuropsychological test results", in *Handbook of Clinical Neuropsychology*, (Eds. S. B. Filskov and T. J. Boll), pp.481–525, John Wiley and Sons, New York.

Heaton, R. K., Smith, H. H., Lehman, R. A. W., and Vogt, A. T. (1978). "Prospects for faking believable deficits on neuropsychological testing", *J. Consult. Clin. Psychol.*, **46**, 892–900.

Hebb, D. O. (1972). *Textbook of Psychology*, p.250, W. B. Saunders, Philadelphia.

Hecaen, H., and Albert, M. (1975). "Disorders of mental functioning related to frontal lobe pathology", in *Psychiatric Aspects of Neurologic Disease* (Eds. D. F. Benson and D. Blumer), pp.137–149, Grune and Stratton, New York.

Heilman, K. M., Scholes, R., and Watson, R. T. (1975). "Auditory affective agnosia: Disturbed comprehension of affective speech", *J. Neurol. Neuros. Psychiat.*, **38**, 69–72.

Heimburger, R. F., Small, I. F., Milstein, V., and Moore, D. (1978). "Stereotaxic amygdalotomy for epilepsy with aggressive behaviour, convulsive and behavioural disorders", *Appl. Neurophysiol.*, **41**, 43–51.

Heinz, E. R., Martinez, J., and Haenggeli, A. (1977). "Reversibility of cerebral atrophy in anorexia nervosa and Cushing's Syndrome", *J. Comput. Assist. Tomog.*, **1**, 415–418.

Hemsi, L. K., Whitehead, A., and Post, F. (1968). "Cognitive functioning and cerebral arousal in elderly depressives and dements", *J. Psychosom. Res.*, **12**, 145–156.

Henry, J. A., and Woodruff, G. H. A. (1978). "A diagnostic sign in states of apparent unconsciousness", *Lancet*, **2**, 920–921.

Hermann, B. P., and Riel, P. (1981). "Interictal personality and behavioral traits in temporal lobe and generalised epilepsy", *Cortex*, **17**, 125–128.

Heston, L. L., Mastri, R., Anderson, V. W., and White, J. (1981). "Dementia of the Alzheimer Type", *Arch. Gen. Psychiat.*, **38**, 1085–1090.

Heyman, A. (1971). "Syncope and hyperventilation", in *Cecil-Loeb Textbook of Medicine* (Eds. P. B. Beeson and W. McDermott), pp.167–171, W. B. Saunders, Philadelphia.

Hickam, J. B. (1971). "Pulmonary hypertension", in *Cecil-Loeb Textbook of Medicine* (Eds. P. B. Beeson and W. McDermott), pp.937–946, W. B. Saunders, Philadelphia.

Hilgard, E. R., and Hilgard, J. R. (1975). *Hypnosis in the Relief of Pain*, Kaufmann, California.

Hill, A. L. (1978). "Savants: mentally retarded individuals with special skills", in *International Review of Research in Mental Retardation*, **vol. 9**, (Ed. N. R. Ellis), pp.277–298, Academic Press, New York.

Hill, D. (1952). "EEG in episodic psychotic and psychopathic behaviour", *Electroencephalogr. Clin. Neurophysiol.*, **4**, 419–442.

Hill, D., and Watterson, D. H. (1942). "Electroencephalographic studies of psychopathic personalities", *J. Neurol. Psychiat.*, **5**, 47–65.

Hill, P. (1979). "Forensic psychiatry", in *Essentials of Postgraduate Psychiatry* (Eds. P. Hill, R. Murray and A. Thorley), pp.531–566, Academic Press, London.

Himmelhoch, J., Pincus, J., Tucker, G., and Detre, T. (1970). "Sub-acute encephalitis: behavioural and neurological aspects", *Br. J. Psychiat.*, **116**, 531–538.

Hitchcock, E. (1979). "Amygdalotomy for aggression", in *Psychopharmacology of Aggression* (Ed. M. Sandler), pp.205–215, Raven Press, New York.

Hollingsworth, M. (1977). "Drugs and pregnancy", *Clin. Obst. Gynaec.*, **4**, 502–520.

Holt, R. E., Rawat, S., Beresford, T. P., and Hall, R. C. W. (1982). "Computed tomography of the brain and the psychiatric consultation", *Psychosom.*, **28**, 1007–1019.

Horowitz, M. J., and Adams, J. E. (1970). "Hallucinations on brain stimulation: evidence for revision of the Penfield hypothesis", in *Origins and Mechanisms of Hallucinations* (Ed. W. Keup), pp.13–22, Plenum Press, New York.

Hounsfield, G. N. (1973). "Computerised transverse axial scanning (Tomography). Part 1. Description of system", *Br. J. Radiol.*, **46**, 1016–1022.

Howard, R. H., and Brown, A. M. (1970). "Twinning: A marker for biological insults", *Child Develop.*, **41**, 519–530.

Huckman, M. J., Fox, J., and Topel, J. (1975). "The validity of criteria for the evaluation of cerebral atrophy by computerised tomography", *Radiology*, **116**, 85–92.

Huessy, H. R., Cohen, S. M., Blair, C. L., and Rood, P. (1979). "Clinical explorations in adult minimal brain dysfunction", in *Psychiatric Aspects of Minimal Brain Dysfunction in Adults* (Ed. L. Bellak), pp.19–36, Grune and Stratton, New York.

Hughes-Jones, N. C. (1973). *Lecture Notes on Haematology*, p.26, Blackwell, London.

Hunter, R., Blackwood, W., and Bull, J. (1968). "Three cases of frontal meningiomas presenting psychiatrically", *Br. Med. J.*, **3**, 9–16.

Hunter, R., and Jones, M. (1966). "Acute lethargica-type encephalitis", *Lancet*, **2**, 1023–1024.

ICD 9 (1978). *International Classification of Diseases, Injuries and Causes of Death, Ninth Revision, Mental Disorders Section*, World Health Organisation, Geneva.

Illingworth, R. S. (1979). *The Normal Child*, Churchill Livingstone, New York.

Ingvar, D. H., and Franzen, G. (1974). "Distribution of cerebral activity in chronic schizophrenia", *Lancet*, **2**, 1484–1486.

Ingvar, D. H., Sjölund, B., and Ardö, A. (1976). "Correlation between dominant EEG frequency, cerebral oxygen uptake and blood flow", *Electroencephalogr. Clin. Neurophysiol.*, **41**, 268–276.

Institute of Psychiatry (1973). *Notes on Eliciting and Recording Clinical Information*, Oxford University Press, London.

Itil, D., and Wadud, A. (1975). "Treatment of human aggression with Major Tranquilisers, Antidepressants and Newer Psychotropic Drugs", *J. Nerv. Ment. Dis.*, **160**, 83–99.

Itil, T. M. (1982). "The use of electroencephalography in the practice of psychiatry", *Psychosom.*, **23**, 799–813.

Itil, T. M., and Fink, M. (1966). "Anticholinergic drug-induced delirium: Experimental modification, quantitative EEG, and behavioral correlations", *J. Nerv. Ment. Dis.*, **143**, 492–507.

Itil, T. M., Keskinev, A., and Fink, M. (1966). "Therapeutic studies in 'therapy-resistant' schizophrenic patients", *Compr. Psychiat.*, **7**, 488–493.

Jacob, M. S., Carlen, P. L., Marshman, J. A., and Sellers, E. M. (1981). "Phenyclidine ingestion: drug abuse and psychosis", *Int. J. Addict.*, **16**, 749–758.

Jacobs, L., and Gossman, M. D. (1980). "Three primitive reflexes in normal adults", *Neurology*, **30**, 184–188.

Jacoby, R. (1981). "Dementia, depression and the CT scan", *Psychol. Med.*, **11**, 673–676.

Jacoby, R., and Levy, R. (1980a). "CT scanning and the investigation of dementia: a review", *J. Roy. Soc. Med.*, **73**, 366–369.

Jacoby, R., and Levy, R. (1980b). "Computed tomography in the elderly. 3. Affective disorder", *Br. J. Psychiat.*, **136**, 270–275.

Jacoby, R., Levy, R., and Dawson, J. M. (1980a). "Computed tomography in the elderly. 1. The normal population", *Br. J. Psychiat.*, **136**, 249–255.

Jacoby, R., Levy, R., and Dawson, J. M. (1980b). "Computed tomography in the elderly. 2. Senile dementia—diagnosis and functional impairment", *Br. J. Psychiat.*, **136**, 256–269.

Janota, I. (1981). "Dementia, deep white matter damage and hypertension: 'Bingswanger's disease' ", *Psychol. Med.*, **11**, 39–48.

Jarvik, L. J. (1976). "Genetic modes of transmission relevant to psychopathology", in *Psychiatry and Genetics* (Eds. M. A. Sperber and L. F. Jarvik), pp.1–40, Basic Books, New York.

352

Jastrowitz, M. (1888). "Beiträge zur Localisation im Grosshirn and über deren praktische Verwerthung", *Dtsch. Med. Wochenschr.*, **14**, 81.

Jenkyn, L. R., Walsh, D. B., and Culver, C. M. (1977). "Clinical signs in diffuse cerebral dysfunction", *J. Neurol. Neuros. Psychiat.*, **40**, 956–966.

Jernigan, T. L., Zatz, L. M., Moses, J. A., and Berger, P. A. (1982a). "Computed tomography in schizophrenics and normal volunteers 1. Fluid volume", *Arch. Gen. Psychiat.*, **39**, 765–770.

Jernigan, T. L., Zatz, L. M., Moses, J. A., and Cardellino, J. P. (1982b). "Computed tomography in schizophrenics and normal volunteers 2. Cranial asymmetry", *Arch. Gen. Psychiat.*, **39**, 771–773.

Johnson, G. F. S. (1979). "Psychopharmacology of aggression", in *Limbic Epilepsy and the Dyscontrol Syndrome* (Eds. M. Girgis and L. G. Kiloh), pp.207–218, Elsevier/North-Holland, Amsterdam.

Johnson, R. T. (1982). "The contribution of virologic research to clinical neurology", *New Eng. J. Med.*, **307**, 660–662.

Johnson, W., Schwartz, G., and Barbeau, A. (1962). "Studies on dystonia musculorum deformans", *Arch. Neurol.*, **7**, 301–313.

Johnstone, E. C., Crow, T. J., Frith, C. D., Husband, J., and Kreel, L. (1976). "Cerebral ventricular size and cognitive impairment in chronic schizophrenia", *Lancet*, **2**, 924–926.

Jones, A. (1964). "Transient radiation myelopathy with reference to Lhermitte's sign of electrical paraesthesiae", *Br. J. Radiol.*, **37**, 727–744.

Jones, K. L., Smith, D. W., Ulleland, C. N., and Streissguth, A. P. (1973). "Fetal alcohol syndrome", *Dev. Med. Child Neurol.*, **21**, 244–248.

Jones-Gotman, M., and Milner, B. (1977). "Design fluency: The invention of nonsense drawings after focal cortical lesions", *Neuropsychologia*, **15**, 653–673.

Joynt, R. J., Benton, A. L., and Fogel, M. L. (1962). "Behavioural and pathological correlates of motor impersistence", *Neurology*, **12**, 876–881.

Joyston-Bechal, M. P. (1966). "The clinical features and outcome of stupor", *Br. J. Psychiat.*, **112**, 967–981.

Judd, L. L., and Grant, I. (1978). "Intermediate duration organic mental disorder among polydrug abusing patients", in *Psychiatric Clinics of North America*, **Vol. 1**, (Ed. H. C. Hendrie), pp.153–167, W. B. Saunders, Toronto.

Kales, J. D., Kales, A., Soldatos, C. R., Caldwell, A. B., Charney, D. S., and Martin, E. D. (1980a). "Night Terrors", *Arch. Gen. Psychiat.*, **37**, 1413–1417.

Kales, A., Soldatos, C. R., Caldwell, A. B., Kales, J. D., Humphrey, F. J., Charney, D. S., and Schweitzer, P. K. (1980b). "Somnambulism", *Arch. Gen. Psychiat.*, **37**, 1406–1410.

Kales, A., Soldatos, C. R., and Kales, J. D. (1983). "Sleep disorders", *Medicine North America*, **1**, 3299–3314.

Kanchandani, R., and Howe, J. G. (1982). "Lhermitte's sign in multiple sclerosis: a clinical survey and review of the literature", *J. Neurol. Neuros. Psychiat.*, **45**, 308–312.

Katz, L., Neal, M. W., and Simon, A. (1961). "Observations on psychic mechanisms in organic psychoses of the aged", in *Psychopathology of Ageing* (Eds. P. H. Hoch and J. Zubin), pp.160–181, Grune and Stratton, New York.

Kaufman, D. M. (1981). *Clinical Neurology for Psychiatrists*, Grune and Stratton, New York.

Kay, D. W. K., Beamish, P., and Roth, M. (1964). "Old age mental disorders in Newcastle-upon-Tyne: a study of prevalence", *Br. J. Psychiat.*, **110**, 146–158.

Kelly, D. (1976). "Neurosurgical treatment of psychiatric disorders", in *Recent Advances in Clinical Psychiatry* (Ed. K. Glanville-Grossman), pp.227–261, Churchill Livingstone, London.

Kelly, R. (1981). "The post-traumatic syndrome", *J. Roy. Soc. Med.*, **74**, 242–245.

Kelly, R., and Smith, B. N. (1981). "Post-traumatic syndrome: another myth discredited", *J. Roy. Soc. Med.*, **74**, 275–277.

Kennedy, A., and Neville, J. (1957). "Sudden loss of memory", *Br. Med. J.*, **2**, 428–433.

Khurana, R. K., Nelson, E., Azzarelli, B., and Garcia, J. H. (1980). "Shy–Drager syndrome: Diagnosis and treatment of cholinergic dysfunction", *Neurology (NY)*, **30**, 805–809.

Kim, Y. K., and Umbach, W. (1973). "Combined stereotaxic lesions for treatment of behaviour disorders and severe pain", in *Surgical Approaches in Psychiatry* (Eds. L. V. Laitinen and K. E. Livingston), pp.182–188, Medical and Technical Pub. Co., Lancaster.

King, D. W., Gallagher, B. B., Murvin, A. J., Smith, D. B., Marcus, D. J., Hartlage, L. C., and Ward, L. C. (1982). "Pseudoseizures: Diagnostic evaluation", *Neurology (NY)*, **32**, 18–23.

Kinsbourne, M., and Warrington, E. K. (1962). "A study of finger agnosia", *Brain*, **85**, 47–66.

Klass, D. W., and Daly, D. D. (1979). *Current Practice of Clinical Electroencephalography*, Raven Press, New York.

Klerman, G. L. (1978). "Affective disorders", in *The Harvard Guide to Modern Psychiatry* (Ed. A. M. Nicholi), pp.253–282, Belknap, Harvard.

Klüver, H., and Bucy, P. C. (1939). "Preliminary analysis of functions of the temporal lobe in monkeys", *Arch. Neurol. Psychiat.*, **42**, 979–1000.

Koenig, H. (1968). "Dementia associated with the benign form of multiple sclerosis", *Trans. Am. Neurol. Ass.*, **93**, 227–231.

Koller, W. C., Glatt, S., Wilson, R. S., and Fox, J. H. (1982). "Primitive reflexes and cognitive functions in the elderly", *Ann. Neurol.*, **12**, 302–304.

Kontos, H. A., Richardson, D. W., and Norvell, J. E. (1975). "Norepinephrine depletion in idiopathic orthostatic hypotension", *Ann. Int. Med.*, **82**, 336–341.

Kral, V. A. (1962). "Senescent forgetfulness. Benign and malignant", *Can. Med. Ass. J.*, **86**, 257–260.

Kramer, P. D. (1982). "Insomnia: Importance of the differential diagnosis", *Psychosom.*, **23**, 129–134.

Kurland, M. L. (1979). "Organic brain syndrome with propanolol", *New Eng. J. Med.*, **300**, 366.

Lader, M., and Sartorius, N. (1968). "Anxiety in patients with hysterical conversion symptoms", *J. Neurol. Neuros. Psychiat.*, **31**, 490–495.

Lancet (1976). Editorial: "Brain damage in sport", *Lancet*, **1**, 401–402.

Landolt, H. (1958). "Serial electroencephalographic investigations during psychotic episodes in epileptic patients and during schizophrenic attacks", in *Lectures on Epilepsy* (Ed. A. M. Lorentz de Haas), Elsevier, Amsterdam.

Larson, E. B., Mack, L. A., Watts, B., and Cromwell, L. D. (1981). "Computed tomography in patients with psychiatric illnesses: Advantage of a 'Rule-In' approach", *Ann. Int. Med.*, **95**, 360–364.

Larsson, T., Sjögren, T., and Jacobson, T. (1963). "Senile dementia: a clinical, sociomedical and genetic study", *Acta Psychiat. Scand.*, **Suppl. 167**, 1–259.

Lauter, H., and Meyer, J. E. (1968). "Clinical and nosological concepts of senile dementia", in *Senile Dementia: Clinical and Therapeutic Aspects* (Eds. C. H. Müller and L. Ciompi), pp.531–546, Huber, Bern.

Lauterbur, P. C. (1973). "Image formation by induced local interactions: Examples employing nuclear magnetic resonance", *Nature*, **242**, 190–191.

LeQuesne, P. M. (1982). "Metal-induced diseases of the nervous system", *Br. J. Hosp. Med.*, **28**, 534–538.

Levin, H. S., Benton, A. L., and Grossman, R. G. (1982). *Neurobehavioural consequences of closed head injury*, Oxford University Press, New York.

Levin, H. S., and Grossman, R. G. (1978). "Behavioural sequelae of closed head injury: A quantitative study", *Arch. Neurol.*, **35**, 720–727.

Levin, H. S., Grossman, R. G., Rose, J. E., and Teasdale, G. (1979). "Long-term neuropsychological outcome of closed head injury", *J. Neurosurg.*, **50**, 412–422.

Levin, M. (1956). "Varieties of disorientation", *J. Ment. Sci.*, **102**, 619–623.

Levy, R. (1969). "The neurophysiology of dementia", *Br. J. Hosp. Med.*, **2**, 688–690.

Lezak, M. D. (1976). *Neuropsychological Assessment*, Oxford University Press, New York.

Lindqvist, G., and Norlén, G. (1966). "Korsakoff's syndrome after operation on ruptured ansurysm of the anterior communicating artery", *Acta Psychiat. Scand.*, **42**, 24–34.

Lipowski, Z. J. (1967). "Delirium, clouding of consciousness and confusion", *J. Nerv. Ment. Dis.*, **145**, 227–255.

Lipowski, Z. J. (1980). *Delirium*, Charles C. Thomas, Illinois.

Lishman, W. A. (1968). "Brain damage in relation to psychiatric disability after head injury", *Br. J. Psychiat.*, **114**, 373–410.

Lishman, W. A. (1973). "The psychiatric sequelae of head injury: A review", *Psychol. Med.*, **3**, 304–318.

Lishman, W. A. (1978). *Organic Psychiatry*, Blackwell, London.

Lishman, W. A. (1981). "Cerebral disorder in alcoholism", *Brain*, **104**, 1–20.

Lishman, W. A., Ron, M., and Acker, W. (1980). "Computed tomography of the brain and psychometric assessment of alcoholic patients—A British study", in *Addiction and Brain Damage* (Ed. D. Richter), pp.215–227, University Park Press, Baltimore.

Liversedge, L. A. (1973). "The clinical features of herpes simplex encephalitis (acute necrotising encephalitis)", *Postgrad. Med.J.*, **49**, 383–386.

Logue, V., Durward, M., Pratt, R. T. C., Piercy, M., and Nixon, W. L. B. (1968). "The quality of survival after rupture of an anterior cerebral aneurysm". *Br. J. Psychiat.*, **114**, 137–160.

Lorber, J. (1961). "Long-term follow-up of 100 children who recovered from tuberculous meningitis", *Paediatr.*, **28**, 778–791.

Luchins, D. J. (1982). "Computed tomography in schizophrenia", *Arch. Gen. Psychiat.*, **39**, 859–860.

Luchins, D. J., Weinberger, D. R., and Torrey, E. F. (1981). "HLA-A_2 increased in schizophrenic patients with reversed cerebral asymmetry", *Br. J. Psychiat.*, **138**, 240–243.

Luchins, D. J., Weinberger, D. R., and Wyatt, R. J. (1982). "Schizophrenia and cerebral asymmetry detected by computed tomography", *Am. J. Psychiat.*, **139**, 753–757.

Lueders, H., Lesser, R. P., and Klein, G. (1980). "Pattern evoked potentials", in *Current Clinical Neurophysiology* (Ed. C. E. Henry), pp.467–526, American Elsevier, New York.

Lum, L. C. (1981). "Hyperventilation and anxiety state", *J. Roy. Soc. Med.*, **74**, 1–4.

Luria, A. R. (1973). *The Working Brain*, Penguin Books, London.

Luria, A. R., and Homskaya, E. D. (1964). "Disturbances in the regulative role of speech with frontal lobe lesions", in *The Frontal Granular Cortex and Behaviour* (Eds. J. M. Warren and K. Akert), pp.353–371, McGraw-Hill, New York.

Luria, A. R., Pribram, K. H., and Homskaya. (1964). "An experimental analysis of the behavioral disturbance produced by a left frontal arachnoidal endothelioma (meningioma)", *Neuropsychologia*, **2**, 257–280.

Mahendra, B. (1981). Editorial: "Where have all the catatonics gone", *Psychol. Med.*, **11**, 669–671.

Manu, P. (1983). "Computed tomography in the investigation of dementia" (Ltr to ed.), *Br. Med. J.*, **286**, 1056–1057.

Marinacci, A. A. (1963). "Special types of temporal lobe seizures following ingestion of alcohol", *Bull. L.A. Neurol. Soc.*, **28**, 241–250.

Mark, V. H., and Ervin, F. R. (1980). *Violence and the brain*, Harper and Row, New York.

Marks, V., and Rose, F. C. (1965). *Hypoglycaemia*, Blackwell, Oxford.

Marsden, C. D. (1976a). "The problem of adult onset idiopathic torsion dystonia and other isolated dyskinesias in adult life", in *Advances in Neurology*, Vol. 14 (Eds. R. Eldridge and S. Fahn), pp.259–276, Raven Press, New York.

Marsden, C. D. (1976b). "Neurology", in *A Textbook of Epilepsy* (Eds, J. Laidlaw and A. Richens), pp.15–55, Churchill Livingstone, London.

Marsden, C. D., and Harrison, M. J. G. (1972). "Outcome of investigation of patients with presenile dementia", *Br. Med. J.*, **2**, 249–252.

Marsden, C. D., Tarsy, D., and Baldessarini, R. J. (1975). "Spontaneous and drug-induced movement disorders in psychotic patients", in *Psychiatric Aspects of Neurologic Disease* (Eds. D. F. Benson and D. Blumer), pp.219–266, Grune and Stratton, London.

Matarazzo, J. D. (1979). *Wechsler's Measurement and Appraisal of Adult Intelligence*, Oxford University Press, New York.

Matefy, R. E., Hayes, C., and Hirsch, J. (1978). "Psychedelic drug flashbacks: Subjective reports and biographical data", *Addict. Behav.*, **3**, 165–178.

Matsumoto, H., Loya, G., and Takeuchi, T. (1965). "Fetal Minamata disease: a neuropathological study of two cases of intra-uterine intoxication by a methyl mercury compound", *J. Neuropath. Exp. Neurol.*, **24**, 563–574.

Mawdsley, C., and Ferguson, F. R. (1963). "Neurological disease in boxers", *Lancet*, **2**, 795–801.

Mayou, R. (1979). "Psychological reactions to myocardial infarction", *J. Roy. Coll. Phys. Lond.*, **13**, 103–105.

McCormick, C. W. (1983). "Management of transient ischaemic attacks", *Medicine North America*, **1**, 2949–2953.

McDonald, C. (1969). "Clinical heterogeneity in senile dementia", *Br. J. Psychiat.*, **115**, 267–271.

McEvoy, J. and Campbell, T. (1977). "Ganser-like signs in carbon monoxide encephalopathy", *Am. J. Psychiat.*, **134**, 1448.

McFie, J. (1975). *Assessment of Organic Intellectual Impairment*, Academic Press, London.

McGlashan, T. H. (1982). "Aphanisis: The syndrome of pseudo-depression in chronic schizophrenia", *Schizop. Bull.*, **8**, 118–134.

McHugh, P. R. (1964). "Occult hydrocephalus", *Qrtly J. Med.*, **33**, 297–308.

McMahon, S. A., and Greenberg, L. M. (1977). "Serial neurologic examination of hyperactive children", *Paediatr.*, **59**, 584–587.

Meadow, S. R., and Smithells, R. W. (1978). *Lecture Notes on Paediatrics*, Blackwell, London.

Meese, W., Kluge, W., Grumme, T., and Hopfenmüller, W. (1980). "CT evaluation of the CSF spaces of healthy persons", *Neurorad.*, **19**, 131–136.

Mellett, P. (1980). "Current views on the psychophysiology of hypnosis", *Br. J. Hosp. Med.*, **23**, 441–446.

Mena, I., Marin, O., Fuenzalida, S., and Cotzias, G. C. (1967). "Chronic manganese poisoning", *Neurology (Minneap.)*, **17**, 128–136.

Mendelson, W. B., Gillin, J. C., and Wyatt, R. J. (1977). *Human Sleep and Its Disorders*, Plenum Press, New York.

Mercer, B., Wapner, W., and Gardner, H. (1977). "A study of confabulation", *Arch. Neurol.*, **34**, 429–433.

Merritt, H. H. (1979). *A Textbook of Neurology*, Lea and Febiger, Philadelphia.

Merskey, H. (1979). *Analysis of Hysteria*, Bailliere Tindall, London.

Merskey, H., and Buhrich, N. A. (1975). "Hysteria and organic brain disease", *Br. J. Med. Psychol.*, **48**, 359–366.

Merskey, H., and Trimble, M. R. (1979). "Personality, sexual adjustment and brain lesions in patients with conversion symptoms", *Am. J. Psychiat.*, **136**, 179–182.

Mertens, H.-G., and Schimrigk, K. (1974). "Differential diagnosis of intra-cranial space-occupying lesions", in *Handbook of Clinical Neurology*, **Vol. 16** (Eds. P. J. Vinken and G. W. Bruyn), pp.209–253, American Elsevier, New York.

Mesulam, M. M. (1981). "Dissociative states with abnormal temporal lobe EEG", *Arch. Neurol.*, **38**, 176–181.

Mesulam, M. M., Waxman, S. G., Geschwind, N., and Sabin, T. D. (1976). "Acute confusional states with right middle cerebral artery infarctions", *J. Neurol. Neuros. Psychiat.*, **39**, 84–89.

Metrakos, K., and Metrakos, J. D. (1961). "Genetics of convulsive disorders: II. Genetic and encephalographic studies in centrencephalic epilepsy", *Neurology*, **11**, 474.

Miller, E. (1974). "Dementia as accelerated ageing of the nervous system; some psychological and methodological considerations", *Age and Ageing*, **3**, 197–202.

Milner, B. (1964). "Some effects of frontal lobectomy in Man", in *The Frontal Granular Cortex and Behaviour* (Eds. J. M. Warrn and K. Akert), pp.313–334, McGraw-Hill, New York.

Modai, I., Sirota, P., Cygielman, G., and Wijsenbeek, H. (1980). "Conversive hallucinations", *J. Nerv. Ment. Dis.*, **168**, 564–565.

Mohr, J. P., Walters, W. C., and Duncan, G. W. (1975). "Thalamic haemorrhage and aphasia", *Brain Lang.*, **2**, 3–17.

Monroe, R. R. (1979). "Epileptoid mechanism in episodic dyscontrol of aggressive criminals", in *Psychiatric Aspects of Minimal Brain Dysfunction in Adults* (Ed. L. Bellak), pp.113–125, Grune and Stratton, New York.

Moore, D. P. (1977). "Rapid treatment of delirium in critically ill patients", *Am. J. Psychiat.*, **134**, 1431–1432.

Morrison, J. R. (1973). "Catatonia: retarded and excited types", *Arch. Gen. Psychiat.*, **28**, 39–41.

Morrison, J. R., and Stewart, M. (1973). "The psychiatric status of the legal families of adopted hyperactive children", *Arch. Gen. Psychiat.*, **28**, 888–891.

Moss, P. D., and McEvedy, C. P. (1966). "An epidemic of overbreathing among schoolgirls", *Br. Med. J.*, **2**, 1295–1300.

Mullen, P. (1979). "The phenomenology of disordered mental function", in *Essentials of Postgraduate Psychiatry* (Eds. P. Hill, R. Murray and A. Thorley), pp.25–54, Academic Press, London.

Mullen, P. (1980). "Sleep disorders". Lecture presented on Current Themes in Psychiatry Course, Guy's Hospital, London, March 28th, 1980.

Mungas, D. (1982). "Interictal behavior abnormality in temporal lobe epilepsy", *Arch. Gen. Psychiat.*, **39**, 108–111.

Murphy, T. L., Chalmers, T. C., Eckhardt, R. D., and Davidson, C. S. (1948). "Hepatic coma: clinical and laboratory investigations on forty patients", *New Eng. J. Med.*, **239**, 605–612.

Murray, T. J., and Pryse-Phillips, W. (1983). "Sleep disorders", *Medicine North America*, **1**, 3052–3056.

Naeser, M. A., Gebhardt, C., and Levine, H. L. (1980). "Decreased computerised tomography numbers in patients with presenile dementia", *Arch. Neurol.*, **37**, 401–409.

Naguib, M., and Levy, R. (1982a). "Prediction of outcome in senile dementia—A computed tomography study", *Br. J. Psychiat.*, **140**, 263–267.

Naguib, M., and Levy, R. (1982b). "CT Scanning in senile dementia", *Br. J. Psychiat.*, **141**, 618–620.

Naples, M., and Hackett, T. P. (1978). "The amytal interview. History and current uses", *Psychosom.*, **19**, 98–112.

357

Nasrallah, H. A., Jacoby, C. G., McCalley-Whitters, M., and Kuperman, S. (1982). "Cerebral ventricular enlargement in subtypes of chronic schizophrenia", *Arch. Gen. Psychiat.*, **39**, 774–777.

Nelson, K. B., and Ellenberg, J. H. (1976). "Predictors of epilepsy in children who have experienced febrile convulsions", *New Eng. J. Med.*, **295**, 1029–1033.

Neophytides, A. N., DiChiro, G., Barron, S. A., and Chase, T. N. (1979). "Computerised axial tomography in Huntington's disease and persons at-risk for Huntington's disease", in *Advances in Neurology*, **Vol. 23** (Eds. T. N. Chase, N. S. Wexler and A. Barbeau), pp.185–191, Raven Press, New York.

Nicholi, A. M. (Ed.) (1978). *The Harvard Guide to Modern Psychiatry*, Belknap, Harvard.

Nichols, P. L., and Chen, T. C. (1980). *Minimal Brain Dysfunction: A Prospective Study*, Lawrence Erlbaum Associates, New Jersey.

Norris, C. R., Trench, J. M., and Hook, R. (1982). "Delayed carbon monoxide encephalopathy: clinical and research implications", *J. Clin. Psychiat.*, **43**, 294–295.

Nott, P. N., and Fleminger, J. J. (1975). "Presenile dementia: the difficulties of early diagnosis", *Acta Psychiat. Scand.*, **51**, 210–217.

Nyback, H., Wiesel, F.-A., Berggren, B.-M., and Hindmarsh, T. (1982). "Computed tomography of the brain in patients with acute psychosis and in healthy volunteers", *Acta Psychiat. Scand.*, **65**, 403–414

Ojemann, R. G., Fisher, C. M., Adams, R. D., Sweet, W. H., and New, P. F. J. (1969). "Further experience with the syndrome of "normal" pressure hydrocephalus", *J. Neuros.*, **31**, 279–294.

Okasha, A., and Madkovr, O. (1982). "Cortical and central atrophy in chronic schizophrenia", *Acta Psychiat. Scand.*, **65**, 403–414.

Okuro, T., Ito, M., Konishi, Y., Yoshioka, M., and Nakano, Y. (1980). "Cerebral atrophy following ACTH therapy", *J. Comp. Assist. Tomogr.*, **4**, 20–23.

Oliver, J. E. (1970). "Huntington's chorea in Northamptonshire", *Br. J. Psychiat.*, **116**, 241–253.

Oppenheim, H. (1889). "Zur Pathologie der Grosshirngeschwülste", *Arch. Psychiat.*, **21**, 560.

Oswald, I. (1969). "Sleep and its disorders", in *Handbook of Clinical Neurology*, **Vol. 3** (Eds. P. J. Vinken and G. W. Bruyn), pp.80–111, American Elsevier, New York.

Oswald, I. (1981). Editorial: "Assessment of Insomnia", *Br. Med. J.*, **283**, 874–875.

Owens, D. G. C., Johnstone, E. C., and Frith, C. D. (1982). "Spontaneous involuntary disorders of movement", *Arch. Gen. Psychiat.*, **39**, 452–461.

Oyewumi, L. K., and Lapierre, Y. D. (1981). "Efficiency of lithium in treating mood disorder occurring after brain stem injury", *Am. J. Psychiat.*, **138**, 110–113.

Papez, J. W. (1937). "A proposed mechanism of emotion", *Arch. Neurol. Psychiat.*, **38**, 725–743.

Parkes, J. D. (1982). "Narcolepsy", in *Pseudoseizures* (Eds. T. L. Riley and A. Roy), pp.62–82, Williams and Wilkins, Baltimore.

Partridge, L. (1979). "The evolution and genetics of behaviour", in *Brain, Behaviour and Evolution* (Eds. D. A. Oakley and H. C. Plotkin), pp.1–27, Methuen, London.

Pasamanick, B., and Knobloch, H. (1966). "Retrospective studies on the epidemiology of reproductive casualty: old and new", *Merrill-Palmer Qtrly.*, **12**, 7–26.

Paulson, G. W. (1977). "The Neurological Examination in Dementia", in *Dementia* (Ed. C. E. Wells), pp.169–188, F. A. Davis Co., Philadelphia.

Paulson, G. W., and Gottlieb, G. (1968). "Developmental reflexes: The reappearance of foetal and neonatal reflexes in aged patients", *Brain*, **91**, 37–52.

Penfield, W., and Jasper, H. (1954). *Epilepsy and the Functional Anatomy of the Human Brain*, Little, Brown and Co., Boston.

Penfield, W., and Perot, P. (1963). "The brain's record of auditory and visual experience", *Brain*, **86**, 596–696.

Penn, H., Racy, J., Lapham, L., Mandel, M., and Sandt, J. (1972). "Catatonic behaviour, viral encephalopathy, and death", *Arch. Gen. Psychiat.*, **27**, 758–761.

Perel, J. M., and Dayton, P. G. (1977). "Methylphenidate", in *Psychotherapeutic Drugs: Part III—Applications* (Eds. E. Usdin and I. S. Forrest), pp.1287–1316, Marcel Dekker, New York.

Perret, E. (1974). "The left frontal lobe of Man and the suppression of habitual responses in verbal categorical behaviour", *Neuropsychologia*, **12**, 323–330.

Perry, J. C., and Jacobs, D. (1982). "Overview: Clinical applications of the amytal interview in psychiatric emergency settings", *Am. J. Psychiat.*, **139**, 552–559.

Perry, T. L. (1981). "Homocystinuria", in *Handbook of Clinical Neurology*, **Vol. 42** (Eds. P. J. Vinken and G. W. Bruyn), pp.555–557, American Elsevier, New York.

Peterson, D. B., Sumner, J. W., and Jones, G. A. (1950). "Role of hypnosis in differentiation of epileptic from convulsive-like seizures", *Am. J. Psychiat.*, **107**, 428–432.

Pincus, J. H. (1978). "Hyperventilation syndrome", *Br. J. Hosp. Med.*, **19**, 312–313.

Pincus, J. H., and Tucker, G. (1974). *Behavioural Neurology*, Oxford University Press, London.

Pitt, B. (1974). *Psychogeriatrics*, Churchill Livingstone, Edinburgh.

Plum, F., and Posner, J. B. (1980). *Diagnosis of Stupor and Coma,* F. A. Davis, Philadelphia.

Plum, F., Posner, J. B., and Hain, R. F. (1962). "Delayed neurological deterioration after anoxia", *Arch. Int. Med.*, **110**, 18–25.

Poeck, K. (1974). "Pathophysiology of emotional disorders associated with brain damage", in *Handbook of Clinical Neurology*, **Vol. 3** (Eds. P. J. Vinken and G. W. Gruyn), pp.343–367, American Elsevier, New York.

Poskanzer, D. C. (1975). "Hemiatrophies and hemihypertrophies", in *Handbook of Clinical Neurology*, **Vol. 22** (Eds. P. J. Vinken and G. W. Bruyn), pp.545–554, American Elsevier, New York.

Post, F. (1965). *The Clinical Psychiatry of Late Life*, Pergamon Press, Oxford.

Post, F. (1966). "Somatic and psychic factors in the treatment of elderly psychiatric patients", *J. Psychosom. Res.*, **10**, 13–19.

Post, F. (1968). "The development and progress of senile dementia in relationship to the functional psychiatric disorders of later life", in *Senile Dementia Clinical and Therapeutic Aspects* (Eds. C. Muller and L. Ciompi) Huber, Bern.

Post, F. (1975). "Dementia, Depression, and Pseudodementia", in *Psychiatric Aspects of Neurologic Disease* (Eds. D. F. Benson and D. Blumer), pp.99–120, Grune and Stratton, London.

Post, R. M. (1975). "Cocaine psychoses: A continuum model", *Am. J. Psychiat.*, **132**, 225–231.

Post, R. M., and Kopanda, R. T. (1976). "Cocaine, kindling, and psychosis", *Am. J. Psychiat.*, **133**, 627–634.

Post, R. M., Uhde, T. W., Ballenger, J. C., and Bunney, Jr. W. E. (1982). "Carbamazepine, temporal lobe epilepsy, and manic-depressive illness", in *Advances in Biological Psychiatry* Vol. 8 (Eds W. P. Koella and M. R. Trimble), pp.117–156, Karger, Basel.

Pratt, R. T. C. (1951). "An investigation of the psychiatric aspects of disseminated sclerosis", *J. Neurol. Neuros. Psychiat.*, **14**, 326–335.

Pritchard, J. A., and MacDonald, P. C. (1980). *Williams' Obstetrics*, Appleton-Century-Crofts, New York.

Quitkin, F., Rifkin, A., and Klein, D. F. (1976). "Neurologic soft signs in schizophrenia and character disorders", *Arch. Gen. Psychiat.*, **33**, 845–853.

Ramani, S., Quesney, L., Olson, D., and Gumnit, R. (1980). "Diagnosis of hysterical seizures in epileptic patients", *Am. J. Psychiat.*, **137**, 705–709.

Ramsay, R. E. (1979). "Epilepsy in Pregnancy", in *Epilepsy: Neurotransmitters, Behaviour and Pregnancy* (Ed. J. A. Wada), Canadian League Against Epilepsy/ Western Institute on Epilepsy.

Rapoport, J. L., Buchsbaum, M. S., and Weingartner, H. (1980). "Dextroamphetamine: its cognitive and behavioural effects in normal and hyperactive boys and normal men", *Arch. Gen. Psychiat.*, **37**, 933–943.

Rappaport, M. (1982). "Brain evoked potentials as a tool in psychiatric assessment", *J. Clin. Psychiat.*, **43**, 465–467.

Raskind, M., Peskind, E., Rivard, M.-F., Veitch, R., and Barnes, R. (1982). "Dexamethasone suppression test and cortisol circadian rhythm in primary degenerative dementia", *Am. J. Psychiat.*, **139**, 1468–1471.

Reis, D. J. (1961). "The palmomental reflex", *Arch. Neurol.*, **4**, 486–498.

Reitan, R. M. (1964). "Psychological deficits resulting from cerebral lesions in Man", in *The Frontal Granular Cortex and Behaviour* (Eds. J. M. Warren and K. Akert), pp.295–312, McGraw-Hill, New York.

Remillard, G. M., Andermann, F., Rhi-Sausi, A., and Robbins, N. M. (1977). "Facial asymmetry in patients with temporal lobe epilepsy", *Neurology*, **27**, 109–114.

Reveley, A. M., Reveley, M. A., Clifford, C. A., and Murray, R. M. (1982). "Cerebral ventricular size in twins discordant for schizophrenia", *Lancet*, **1**, 540–541.

Reynolds, E. H. (1982). "The pharmacological management of epilepsy associated with psychological disorders", *Br. J. Psychiat.*, **141**, 549–557.

Reynolds, E. H. (1983). Editorial: "Interictal behaviour in temporal lobe epilepsy", *Br. Med. J.*, **286**, 918–919.

Rieder, R. O., Donnelley, E. F., Herdt, J. R., and Waldman, I. N. (1979). "Sulcal prominence in young chronic schizophrenic patients: CT scan findings associated with impairment on neuropsychological tests", *Psychiat. Res.*, **1**, 1–8.

Riley, J. N., and Walker, D. W. (1978). "Morphological alterations in the hippocampus after long term alcohol consumption in mice", *Science*, **201**, 646–648.

Riley, T. L. (1982). "Syncope and hyperventilation", in *Pseudoseizures* (Eds. T. L. Riley and A. Roy), pp.34–61, Williams and Wilkins, Baltimore.

Roberts, J. K. A. (1983). "Brain structure and function in the schizophrenias: A neurobehavioral approach", *Psychiat. J. Univ. Ottawa*, **8**, 51–66.

Roberts, J. K. A., Robertson, M. M., and Trimble, M. R. (1982). "The lateralising significance of hypergraphia in temporal lobe epilepsy", *J. Neurol. Neuros. Psychiat.*, **45**, 131–138.

Roberts, J. K. A., Trimble, M. R., and Robertson, M. M. (1983). "Schizophrenic psychosis and aqueduct stenosis in adults", *J. Neurol. Neuros. Psychiat.*, **46**, 892–898.

Robertson, E. E., LeRoux, A., and Brown, J. H. (1958). "The clinical differentiation of Pick's disease", *J. Ment. Sci.*, **104**, 1000–1024.

Robinson, A. (1982). "XXY male, Klinefelter syndrome", in *Handbook of Clinical Neurology*, **Vol. 43** (Eds. P. Vinken and G. W. Bruyn), pp.557–558, American Elsevier, New York.

Robinson, J. T., Chitham, R. G., Greenwood, R. M., and Taylor, J. W. (1974). "Chromosome aberrations and LSD: A controlled study of 50 psychiatric patients", *Br. J. Psychiat.*, **125**, 238–244.

Robinson, R. G., and Benson, D. F. (1981). "Depression in aphasic patients: frequency, severity and clinico-pathological correlations", *Brain and Language*, **14**, 282–291.

Rochford, J. M., Detre, T., Tucker, G. J., and Harrow, M. (1970). "Neuropsychological impairments in functional psychiatric diseases", *Arch. Gen. Psychiat.*, **22**, 114–119.

Roff, M., Sells, S. B., and Golden, M. M. (1972). *Social Adjustment and Personality Development in Children*, University of Minnesota Press, Minneapolis.

Romano, J., and Engel, G. L. (1944). "Physiologic and psychologic considerations of delirium", *Med. Clin. N. Am.*, **28**, 629–638.

Ron, M. A., Toone, B. K., Garralda, M. E., and Lishman, W. A. (1979). "Diagnostic accuracy in presenile dementia", *Br. J. Psychiat.*, **134**, 161–168.

Rosenberg, R. N. (1981). "Biochemical genetics of neurologic disease", *New Eng. J. Med.*, **305**, 1181–1193.

Ross, E. D. (1981). "The Aprosodias", *Arch. Neurol.*, **38**, 561–569.

Ross, E. D., and Rush, J. (1981). "Diagnosis and neuroanatomical correlates of depression in brain damaged patients", *Arch. Gen. Psychiat.*, **38**, 1344–1354.

Roth, B., and Bruhova, S. (1969). "Dreams in narcolepsy hypersomnia and dissociated sleep disorders", *Exp. Med. Surg.*, **27**, 187–209.

Roth, B., Nevsimalova, S., and Rechtschaffen, A. (1972). "Hypersomnia with sleep drunkenness", *Arch. Gen. Psychiat.*, **26**, 456–462.

Roth, M. (1955). "The natural history of mental disorder in old age", *J. Ment. Sci.*, **101**, 281–301.

Roth, M., and Myers, D. H. (1969). "The diagnosis of dementia", *Br. J. Hosp. Med.*, **2**, 705–717.

Roy, A. (1979). "Hysterical seizures", *Arch. Neurol.*, **36**, 447.

Rumbaugh, C. L., Bergeron, R. T., Fang, H. C., and McCormick, R. (1971a). "Cerebral angiographic changes in the drug abuse patient", *Radiology*, **101**, 335–344.

Rumbaugh, C. L., Bergeron, R. T., Scanlan, R. S., Teal, J. S., Segall, H. G., Fang, H. C. H., and McCormick, R. (1971b). "Cerebral angiographic secondary to amphetamine abuse in the experimental animal", *Radiology*, **101**, 345–351.

Rutter, M. (1978). "Diagnostic validity in child psychiatry", in *Advances in Biological Psychiatry*, **vol. 2**, S. Karger, Basel.

Rutter, M. (1981). "Psychological sequelae of brain damage in children", *Am. J. Psychiat.*, **138**, 1533–1544.

Rutter, M. (1982). "Syndromes attributed to 'Minimal Brain Dysfunction' in childhood", *Am. J. Psychiat.*, **139**, 21–33.

Rutter, M., Graham, P., and Yule, W. (1970). *A Neuropsychiatric Study in Childhood: Clinics in Developmental Medicine 35/36*, Heinemann/SIMP, London.

Sackner, M. A., Landa, J., Forrest, T., and Greeneltch, D. (1975). "Periodic sleep apnoea: Chronic sleep deprivation related to intermittent upper airway obstruction and central nervous system disturbance", *Chest*, **67**, 164–171.

Sanders, W. L., and Dunn, T. L. (1973). "Creutzfeldt–Jacob disease treated with amantadine", *J. Neurol. Neuros. Psychiat.*, **36**, 581–584.

Saunders, M. G., and Westmoreland, B. F. (1979). "The EEG in evaluation of disorders affecting the brain diffusely", in *Current Practice of Clinical Electroencephalography* (Eds. D. W. Klass and D. D. Daly), pp.343–379, Raven Press, New York.

Schaaf, M., and Payne, C. A. (1966). "Dystonic reactions to prochlorperazine in hypoparathyroidism", *New Eng. J. Med.*, **275**, 991–995.

Schenk, L., and Bear, D. (1981). "Multiple personality and related dissociative phenomena in patients with temporal lobe epilepsy". *Am. J. Psychiat.*, **138**, 1311–1316.

Schlesinger, B. (1950). "Mental changes in intracranial tumours, and related problems", *Confinia Neurologica*, **10**, 225–263, 322–355.

Schneck, M. K., Reisberg, B., and Ferris, S. H. (1982). "An overview of current concepts of Alzheimer's disease", *Am. J. Psychiat.*, **139**, 165–173.

Schneider, K. (1957). "Primäre und Sekundäre Symptome bei der Schizophrenie", *Fortschritte der Neurologie, Psychiatrie und Ihrer Grenzgebiete*, **25**, 487–590.

Schott, G. D., McLeod, A. A., and Jewitt, D. E. (1977). "Cardiac arrhythmias that masquerade as epilepsy", *Br. Med. J.*, **1**, 1454–1457.

Selekler, K., Kansu, T., and Zileli, T. (1981). "Computed tomography in Wilson's disease", *Arch. Neurol.*, **38**, 727–728.

Serafetinides, E. A. (1965). "Aggressiveness in temporal lobe epileptics and its relation to cerebral dysfunction and environmental factors", *Epilepsia*, **6**, 33–42.

Shaffer, D. (1973). "Psychiatric aspects of brain injury in childhood: a review", *Dev. Med. Child. Neurol.*, **15**, 211–220.

Shapiro, B. E., Alexander, M. P., Gardner, H., and Mercer, B. (1981). "Mechanisms of confabulation", *Neurology (NY)*, **31**, 1070–1076.

Shepherd, M. (1961). "Morbid jealousy: some clinical and social aspects of a psychiatric symptom", *J. Ment. Sci.*, **107**, 687–753.

Sherwin, I., Peron-Magnan, P., Bancaud, J., Bonis, A., and Talairach, J. (1982). "Prevalence of psychosis in epilepsy as a function of the laterality of the epileptogenic lesion", *Arch. Neurol.*, **39**, 621–625.

Shields, J. (1977). "Polygenic influences", in *Child Psychiatry* (Eds. M. Rutter and L. Hersov), pp.22–46, Blackwell, London.

Shy, G. M., and Drager, G. A. (1960). "A neurologic syndrome associated with orthostatic hypotension", *Arch. Neurol.*, **2**, 511–527.

Siegel, R. K. (1978). "Cocaine hallucinations", *Am. J. Psychiat.*, **135**, 309–314.

Sim, M. (1974). *Guide to Psychiatry*, Churchill Livingstone, London.

Sim, M. (1979). "Early diagnosis of Alzheimer's disease" in *Alzheimer's disease* (Eds. A. I. M. Glen and L. J. Whalley), pp.78–85, Churchill Livingstone, New York.

Simpson, M. (1976). "Self mutilation", *Br. J. Hosp. Med.*, **16**, 430–438.

Sjögren, T., Sjögren, H., and Lindgren, A. G. H. (1952). "Morbus Alzheimer and Morbus Pick. A genetic clinical and patho-anatomical study", *Acta Psychiat. Neurol. Scand.*, **Suppl. 82**, 1–152.

Slater, E., Beard, A. W., and Glithero, E. (1963). "The schizophrenia-like psychoses of epilepsy", *Br. J. Psychiat.*, **109**, 95–150.

Slater, E., and Glithero, E. (1965). "A follow-up of patients diagnosed as suffering from hysteria", *J. Psychosom. Res.*, **9**, 9–13.

Sleep (1979). Sleep Disorders Classification Committee of the Association of Sleep Disorders Centers and the Association for the Psychophysiological Study of Sleep. "The Diagnostic Classification of Sleep and Arousal Disorders", *Sleep*, **2**, 1–137.

Smith, A. (1981). "Principles underlying human brain functions in neuropsychological sequelae of different neuropathological processes", in *Handbook of Clinical Neuropsychology* (Eds. S. B. Filskov and T. J. Boll), pp.175–226, John Wiley and Sons, New York.

Smith, J. S., and Brandon, S. (1973). "Morbidity from acute carbon monoxide poisoning at three-year follow-up". *Br. Med. J.*, **1**, 318–321.

Smith, J. S., Kiloh, L. G., Ratnavale, G. S., and Grant, D. A. (1976). "The investigation of dementia: The results of 100 consecutive admissions". *Med. J. Aust.*, **2**, 403–405.

Smithells, R. W. (1979). "Fetal alcohol syndrome", *Dev. Med. Child Neurol.*, **21**, 244–248.

Solomon, S. (1980). "Clinical neurology and neuropathology", in *Comprehensive Textbook of Psychiatry 3* (Eds. H. I. Kaplan, A. M. Freedman and B. J. Sadock), pp.273–305, Williams and Wilkins, London.

Solomons, G. (1979). "Child abuse and developmental disabilities", *Develop. Med. Child. Neurol.*, **21**, 101–106.

Solomons, G., Holden, R. H., and Denhoff, E. (1963). "The changing picture of cerebral dysfunction in early childhood", *J. Paediatr.*, **63**, 113–120.

Sourander, P., and Sjögren, H. (1970). "The concept of Alzheimer's disease and its clinical implications", in *Alzheimer's Disease* (Eds. G. E. W. Wolstenholme and M. O'Connor), pp.531–546, Churchill, London.

Sparks, R. W., and Holland, A. L. (1976). "Method: melodic intonation therapy for aphasia", *J. Speech Hear. Dis.*, **41**, 287–297.

Spehlmann, R. (1981). *EEG Primer*, American Elsevier, New York.

Spitzer, R. L., Endicott, J., and Gibbon, M. (1979). "Crossing the border into borderline personality and borderline schizophrenia", *Arch. Gen. Psychiat.*, **36**, 17–24.

Springer, S. P., and Deutsch, G. (1981). *Left Brain, Right Brain*, W. H. Freeman, San Francisco.

Sroufe, L. A. (1976). "Drug treatment of children with behaviour problems", in *Review of Child Development Research*, vol. 4 (Ed. F. D. Horowitz, E. M. Hetherington, S. Scarr-Salapatek and G. M. Siegel), pp.347–407, University of Chicago Press, Chicago.

Stengel, E. (1941). "On the aetiology of fugue states", *J. Ment. Sci.*, 87, 572–599.

Stengel, E. (1943). "A study on the symptomatology and differential diagnosis of Alzheimer's disease and Pick's disease", *J. Ment. Sci.*, 89, 1–20.

Stepien, L. S., Cordeau, J. P., and Rasmussen, T. (1960). "The effect of temporal lobe and hippocampal lesions on auditory and visual recent memory in monkeys", *Brain*, 83, 470–489.

Sternleib, I., and Scheinberg, I. H. (1968). "The detection of Wilson's disease and the prevention of the clinical manifestations in apparently health subjects", in *Wilson's Disease* (Ed. D. Bergsma), p.768, National Foundation, New York.

Stevens, J. R. (1975). "Interictal clinical manifestations of complex partial seizures", in *Advances in Neurology, Vol. 11* (Eds. J. K. Penry and D. D. Daly), pp.85–107, Raven Press, New York.

Stevens, J. R. (1982). "The neuropathology of schizophrenia", *Psychol. Med.*, 12, 695–700.

Stevens, J. R., and Herman, B. P. (1981). "Temporal lobe epilepsy, psychopathology, and violence: the state of the evidence", *Neurology (NY)*, 31, 1127–1132.

Stevens, M., Crow, T. J., Bowman, M. J., and Coles, E. C. (1978). "Age disorientation in schizophrenia: a constant prevalence of 25 per cent in a chronic mental hospital population", *Br. J. Psychiat.*, 133, 130–136.

Stewart, M. A., de Blois, C. S., and Cummings, S. (1980). "Psychiatric disorder in the parents of hyperactive boys and those with conduct disorder", *J. Child Psychol. Psychiat.*, 21, 283–292.

Storey, P. B. (1970). "Brain damage and personality change after subarchnoid haemorrhage", *Br. J. Psychiat.*, 117, 129–142.

Stoudemire, A. (1982). "The differential diagnosis of catatonic states", *Psychosom.*, 23, 245–252.

Strauss, A. A., and Lehtinen, V. (1947). *Psychopathology and Education of the Brain-Injured Child*, Vol. 1, Grune and Stratton, New York.

Strich, S. J. (1956). "Diffuse degeneration of the cerebral white matter in severe dementia following head injury", *J. Neurol. Neuros. Psychiat.*, 19, 163–185.

Ström-Olsen, R., and Carlisle, S. (1971). "Bi-frontal stereotactic tractotomy: a follow-up study of its effects on 210 patients", *Br. J. Psychiat.*, 118, 141–154.

Struve, F. A., Becka, D. R., and Klein, D. F. (1972). "The B-mitten EEG pattern in process and reactive schizophrenia and affective states", *Clin. Electroencephalogr.*, 3, 136–144.

Struve, F. A., and Klein, D. F. (1976). "Diagnostic implications of the B-mitten EEG pattern: relationship to primary and secondary affective dysregulation", *Biol. Psychiat.*, 11, 599–611.

Stuss, D. T., Alexander, M. P., Lieberman, A., and Levine, H. (1978). "An extraordinary form of confabulation", *Neurology*, 28, 1166–1172.

Stuss, D. T., and Benson, D. F. (1982). "Frontal lobe lesions and behaviour", in *Localisation in Neuropsychology* (Ed. A. Kertesz), Academic Press, New York (in press).

Surridge, D. (1969). "An investigation into some psychiatric aspects of multiple sclerosis", *Br. J. Psychiat.*, 155, 749–764.

Sutherland, J. M., Edwards, V. E., and Eadie, M. J. (1975). "Essential (hereditary or senile) tremor", *Med. J. Aust.*, 2, 44–47.

Szyper, M., and Mann (1978). "Anorexia nervosa associated with temporal lobe epilepsy", Presented at the American Academy of Neurology, Los Angeles, April, 1978.

Talland, G. A. (1961). "Confabulation in the Wernicke-Korsakoff syndrome", *J. Nerv. Ment. Dis.*, **132**, 361–381.

Tarter, R. G. (1980). "Brain damage in chronic alcoholics: a review of the psychological evidence", in *Addiction and Brain Damage* (Ed. D. Richter), pp.267–297, University Park Press, Baltimore.

Taylor, D. C. (1972). "Mental state and temporal lobe epilepsy—a correlative account of 100 patients treated surgically", *Epilepsia*, **13**, 727–765.

Taylor, D. C., and Ounsted, C. (1971). "Biological mechanisms influencing the outcome of seizures in response to fever", *Epilepsia*, **12**, 33–45.

Taylor, M. A., and Abrams, R. (1977). "Catatonia", *Arch. Gen. Psychiat.*, **34**, 1223–1225.

Ter-Pogossian, M. M., Phelps, M. G., Hoffman, E. J., and Mullani, N. A. (1975). "A positron-emmission transaxial tomograph for nuclear imaging (PETT)", *Radiology*, **114**, 89–98.

Tharp, B. R. (1969). "The electroencephalogram in transient global amnesia", *Electroencephalogr. Clin. Neurophysiol.*, **26**, 96–99.

Thompson, P. J., and Trimble, M. R. (1982). "Anticonvulsant drugs and cognitive functions", *Epilepsia*, **23**, 531–544.

Thorley, A., and Stern, R. (1979). "Neurosis and personality disorder", in *Essentials of Postgraduate Psychiatry* (Eds. P. Hill, R. Murray and A. Thorley), pp.179–246, Grune and Stratton, New York.

Tomlinson, B. E. (1977). "The pathology of dementia", in *Dementia* (Ed. C. E. Wells), pp.113–153, F. A. Davis, Philadelphia.

Toole, J. F. (1964). Editorial: "Reversed vertebral artery flow and cerebral vascular insufficiency", *Am. Int. Med.*, **61**, 159–162.

Toone, B. K., and Roberts, J. K. A. (1979). "Status epilepticus: an uncommon hysterical conversion syndrome", *J. Nerv. Ment. Dis.*, **69**, 548–552.

Torrey, E. F., and Peterson, M. R. (1974). "Schizophrenia and the limbic system", *Lancet*, **2**, 942–946.

Tourigny-Rivard, M.-F., Raskind, M., and Rivard, D. (1981). "The dexamethasone suppression test in an elderly population", *Biol. Psychiat.*, **16**, 1177–1184.

Tramont, E. C. (1979). "Treponema pallidum", in *Principle and Practice of Infectious Diseases* (Eds. G. L. Mandell, R. G. Douglas, Jr. and J. G. Bennett), pp.1823–1835, John Wiley and Sons, New York.

Trimble, M. R. (1978). "Serum prolactin in epilepsy and hysteria", *Br. Med. J.*, **2**, 1682.

Trimble, M. R. (1981a). *Neuropsychiatry*, John Wiley and Sons, London.

Trimble, M. R. (1981b). "Post-traumatic syndrome" (Ltr to ed.), *J. Roy. Soc. Med.*, **74**, 940–941.

Trimble, M. R., and Grant, I. (1982). "Psychiatric aspects of multiple sclerosis", in *Psychiatric Aspects of Neurologic Disease*, **Vol. 2** (Eds. D. F. Benson and D. Blumer), pp.279–300, Grune and Stratton, New York.

Tsai, L., and Tsuang, M. T. (1981). "How can we avoid unnecessary CT scanning for psychiatric patients", *J. Clin. Psychiat.*, **42**, 452–454.

Tucker, C. J., Detre, T., Harrow, M., and Glaser, G. H. (1965). "Behaviour and symptoms of psychiatric patients and the electroencephalograms", *Arch. Gen. Psychiat.*, **12**, 278–286.

Tucker, D. M., Watson, R. T., and Heilman, K. M. (1977). "Discrimination and evocation of affectively intoned speech in patients with right parietal disease", *Neurology*, **27**, 947–950.

Turner, E. A. (1969). "A surgical approach to the treatment of symptoms in temporal lobe epilepsy", in *Current Problems in Neuropsychiatry: Schizophrenia, Epilepsy, the Temporal Lobe* (Ed. R. N. Herrington), pp.102–105, Headley Bros., Kent.

Turner, R., Rubenstein, A. H., and Foster, D. W. (1981). "Hypoglycaemia", *Medicine North America*, **1**, 1349–1352.

Tweedy, J., Reding, M., Garcia, C., Schulman, P., Deutsch, G., and Antin, S. (1982). "Significance of cortical disinhibition signs", *Neurology (NY)*, **32**, 169–173.

Vassilopoulos, D. (1982). "Criminality" in *Handbook of Clinical Neurology* Vol. **43** (Eds. P. J. Vinken and G. W. Bruyn), pp.204–206, American Elsevier, New York.

Victor, M., Adams, R. D., and Collins, G. H. (1971). *The Wernicke–Korsakoff Syndrome*, Blackwell, Oxford.

Victor, M., and Hope, J. M. (1958). "The phenomenon of auditory hallucinations in chronic alcoholism", *J. Nerv. Ment. Dis.*, **126**, 451–481.

Walsh, K. W. (1978). *Neuropsychology*, Churchill Livingstone, London.

Walton, J. N. (1953). "The Korsakoff Syndrome in spontaneous subarachnoid haemorrhage", *J. Ment. Sci.*, **99**, 521–530.

Ward, N. G., Rowlett, D. B., and Burke, P. (1978). "Sodium amylobarbitone in the differential diagnosis of confusion", *Am. J. Psychiat.*, **135**, 75–78.

Warrington, E. K. (1969). "Constructional apraxia", in *Handbook of Clinical Neurology*, Vol. **4** (Eds. P. J. Vinken and G. W. Bruyn), pp.67–83, American Elsevier, New York.

Warrington, E. K., and Gautier-Smith, P. C. (1977). "Clinical assessment of higher cerebral function", *Medicine*, **34**, 2049–2053.

Watson, C. G., and Thomas, R. W. (1968). "MMPI Profiles of brain damaged and schizophrenic patients", *Percep. Motor Skills*, **27**, 567–573.

Watson, R. T., Valerstein, E., and Heilman, K. M. (1981). "Thalamic neglect", *Arch. Neurol.*, **38**, 501–506.

Waxman, D. (1980). "Clinical applications of hypnosis in psychiatry", *Br. J. Hosp. Med.*, **23**, 456–463.

Wechsler, D. (1944). *The measurement of adult intelligence*, Williams and Wilkins Co., Baltimore.

Weinberger, D. R., Bigelow, L. B., Kleinman, J. E., Klein, S. T., Rosenblatt, J. E., and Wyatt, R. J. (1980a). "Cerebral ventricular enlargement in chronic schizophrenia: its association with poor response to treatment", *Arch. Gen. Psychiat.*, **37**, 11–13.

Weinberger, D. R., Cannon-Spoor, E., Potkin, S. G., and Wyatt, R. J. (1980b). "Poor premorbid adjustment and CT scan abnormalities in chronic schizophrenia", *Am. J. Psychiat.*, **137**, 1410–1413.

Weinberger, D. R., Delisi, L. E., Neophytides, A. N., and Wyatt, R. J. (1981). "Familial aspects of CT scan abnormalities in chronic schizophrenic patients", *Psychiat. Res.*, **4**, 65–71.

Weinberger, D. R., DeLisi, L. E., Perman, G. P., Targum, S., and Wyatt, R. J. (1982). "Computed tomography in schizophreniform disorder and other acute psychiatric disorders", *Arch. Gen. Psych.*, **39**, 778–783.

Weinberger, D. R., and Kelley, M. J. (1977). "Catatonia and malignant syndrome: a possible complication of neuroleptic administration", *J. Nerv. Ment. Dis.*, **165**, 263–268.

Weinberger, D. R., Torrey, E. F., Neophytides, A. N., and Wyatt, R. J. (1979a). "Lateral cerebral ventricular enlargement inchronic schizophrenia", *Arch. Gen. Psychiat.*, **36**, 735–739.

Weinberger, D. R., Torrey, E. F., Neophytides, A. N., and Wyatt, R. J. (1979b). "Structural abnormalities in the cerebral cortex of chronic schizophrenic patient", *Arch. Gen. Psychiat.*, **36**, 935–939.

Weinberger, D. R., and Wyatt, R. J. (1978). "Catatonic stupor and neuroleptic drugs", *J. Am. Med. Ass.*, **239**, 1846.

Weiner, R. D. (1980). "The persistence of electroconvulsive therapy-induced changes in the electroencephalogram", *J. Nerv. Ment. Dis.*, **168**, 224–228.

Weinstein, E. A., and Kahn, R. L. (1955). *Denial of illness: Symbolic and Physiological Aspects*, Charles C. Thomas, Springfield.

Weinstein, E. A., Kahn, R. L., and Sugarman, L. A. (1954). "Serial administration of the 'amytal test' for brain disease", *Arch. Neurol. Psychiat.*, **71**, 217–226.

Weinstein, M. R. (1976). *Journal of Drug Information*, **2**, 94.

Wells, C. E. (1977). "Diagnostic evaluation and treatment in dementia", in *Dementia* (Ed. C. E. Wells), pp.247–276, F. A. Davis, Philadelphia.

Wells, C. E. (1979). "Pseudodementia", *Am. J. Psychiat.*, **136**, 895–900.

Wells, C. E., and Duncan, G. W. (1980). *Neurology for Psychiatrists*, F. A. Davis Company, Philadelphia.

Werboff, J., and Gottlieb, J. S. (1963). "Drugs in pregnancy: behavioural teratology", *Obst. Gyn. Survey*, **18**, 420–423.

Wiggins, J. S., Goldberg, L. R., and Applebaum, M. (1971). "MMPI Content Scales: interpretative norms and correlations with other scales", *J. Consult. Clinic. Psychol.*, **37**, 403–410.

Willanger, R., Thygesen, P., Nielsen, R., and Peterson, O. (1968). "Intellectual impairment and cerebral atrophy", *Danish Med. Bull.*, **15**, 65.

Williams, R. L., and Karacan, I. (1978). *Sleep Disorders*, John Wiley and Sons, New York.

Wolf, J. K. (1980). *Practical Clinical Neurology*, pp.298–321, Med. Exam. Publishing Co., New York.

Wolff, H. G., and Curran, D. (1935). "Nature of delirium and allied states", *A.M.A. Arch. Neurol. Psychiat.*, **33**, 1175–1215.

Wood, C. D. (1958). "Behavioral changes following discrete lesions of temporal lobe structures", *Neurology*, **8**, 215–220.

Woodruff, R. (1966). "The diagnostic use of the amylobarbitone interview among patients with psychotic illnesses", *Br. J. Psychiat.*, **112**, 727–732.

Yahr, M. D. (1974). "Encephalitis lethargica (Von Economo's disease, epidemic encephalitis)", in *Handbook of Clinical Neurology*, **Vol. 34** (Eds. P. J. Vinken and G. W. Bruyn), pp.451–457, American Elsevier, New York.

Yase, Y. (1972). "The pathogenesis of amyotrophic lateral sclerosis", *Lancet*, **2**, 292–296.

Young, I. R., Hall, A. S., and Pallis, C. A. (1981). "Nuclear magnetic resonance imaging of the brain in multiple sclerosis", *Lancet*, **2**, 1063–1066.

Zivin, L., and Ajmone-Marsan, C. (1968). "Incidence and prognostic significance of 'epileptiform' activity in the EEG of non-epileptic subjects", *Brain*, **91**, 751–778.

Zimmerman, I. L., and Woo-Sam, J. M. (1973). *Clinical Interpretation of the Wechsler Adult Intelligence Scale*, Grune and Stratton, New York.

Index

Abreaction, 229, 238
  definition of, 39
Abscess, cerebral, 128, 138, 141
Absence (*see* Petit mal epilepsy)
Abstract thinking, disorders of, 37–38, 72, 169
Abulia, definition of, 333
Acalculia, 73, 79, 293, 294
  definition of, 333
Acute organic brain disorder (*see* Delirium)
Adrenocorticotrophic hormone, 299
Affect, definition of, 333
Affective disorder (*see also* Pseudo-dementia) 141–143, 146–147, 166, 167, 168
Affective syndrome, organic, 274
African trypanosomiasis, 246
After-image, definition of, 261
Ageing and
  cognitive changes, 170
  physical changes, 184–185
Aggression, 145–157
  definition of, 145, 334
Agnosia, 53–54, 73, 169, 172, 184
  auditory (*see* Kluver–Bucy syndrome)
  colour, 82
  definition of, 53, 333
  finger, 73, 76
  visual (*see* Kluver–Bucy syndrome)
  visual object, 82
  visuospatial (*see* Apraxia, constructional)
Agoraphobia, definition of, 228
Agraphia, 52, 73, 162, 166, 168, 293
  definition of, 30, 334
Akathisia, 30, 241
  definition of, 334
Akinesia, 30, 233, 241,

definition of, 30, 334
Akinetic mutism, 238–239, 327
Akinetic seizures, 207
Alcohol, adverse effects of, 9, 15, 35, 154–155, 156, 164, 184, 188, 197, 215, 231, 265
Alcoholic dementia, 172, 175, 177
Alcoholic hallucinosis, 266
Alcoholic idiosyncratic intoxication, 154
Alcoholism, chronic, 23, 80, 81, 127, 147, 155, 160, 213, 245, 255, 262, 296
Alexia, 73, 82, 83, 293
  definition of, 35, 334
Altered consciousness, 220–232
Alveolar hypoventilation, 245, 249, 286
Alzheimer's dementia, 5, 6, 9, 35, 52, 137, 172, 177, 178, 179, 184, 189, 190, 194, 304
  compared with ageing, 170
  Multi-Infarct dementia, 174
  Pick's dementia, 170–171
  senile dementia, 170–171
Amantadine, 191, 242
Ambitendency, definition of, 234
Amnesia
  anterograde, 20, 21, 143, 313
  frontal lobe disorders, 70, 72
  hippocampal, 36, 80, 230, 294
  hysterical (*see* Amnesia, psychogenic)
  mamillo-thalamic, 35, 36, 80, 139, 159, 176, 178
  modality specific, 80, 130
  post-traumatic (*see* Amnesia, anterograde)
  psychogenic, 59, 166, 200, 228–229, 230
  retrograde, 166, 229, 230
  transient global, 229–231
Amotivational syndrome, 24

366